Symposium on medical and surgical diseases of the retina and vitreous

TRANSACTIONS OF THE NEW ORLEANS
ACADEMY OF OPHTHALMOLOGY

Previously published

Transactions of the New Orleans Academy of Ophthalmology

available from The C.V. Mosby Company are listed below:

Symposium on Glaucoma, 1975

Symposium on Neuro-ophthalmology, 1976

Symposium on Retinal Diseases, 1977

Symposium on Strabismus, 1978

Symposium on Cataracts, 1979

Symposium on Medical and Surgical
Diseases of the Cornea, 1980

Symposium on Glaucoma, 1981

Symposium on medical and surgical diseases of the retina and vitreous

TRANSACTIONS OF THE NEW ORLEANS ACADEMY OF OPHTHALMOLOGY

ALAN C. BIRD, M.D., F.R.C.S.

D. JACKSON COLEMAN, M.D.

J. DONALD M. GASS, M.D.

MORTON F. GOLDBERG, M.D.

J. WALLACE McMEEL, M.D., P.C.

G. RICHARD O'CONNOR, M.D.

ARNALL PATZ, M.D.

STEPHEN J. RYAN, M.D.

ROBERT C. WATZKE, M.D.

with 296 illustrations and 1 color plate

The C. V. Mosby Company

ST. LOUIS • TORONTO • LONDON   1983

A TRADITION OF PUBLISHING EXCELLENCE

Editor: Eugenia A. Klein
Developmental editor: Kathryn H. Falk
Manuscript editor: Carl Masthay
Book design: Staff
Production: Margaret B. Bridenbaugh, Judy England

The C.V. Mosby Company
11830 Westline Industrial Drive, St. Louis, Missouri 63141

Library of Congress Cataloging in Publication Data

Symposium on Medical and Surgical Diseases of the
   Retina and Vitreous (1982: New Orleans, La.)
   Symposium on Medical and Surgical Diseases of
   the Retina and Vitreous.

   Thirty-first annual symposium of the New Orleans
Academy of Ophthalmology from March 6-10, 1982.
   Includes index.
   1. Retina—Diseases—Congresses. 2. Retina—
Surgery—Congresses. 3. Vitreous body—Diseases—
Congresses. 4. Vitreous body—Surgery—Congresses.
I. Bird, Alan C. II. New Orleans Academy of
Ophthalmology. III. Title. [DNLM: 1. Ophthalmology—
Congresses. 2. Retina—Surgery—Congresses.
3. Retina diseases—Congresses. 4. Vitreous body—
Congresses. 5. Vitreous body—Surgery—Congresses.
W1 TR226S / WW 270 S98803s 1982]
RE551.S92   1982   617.7′3   82-18781
ISBN 0-8016-3672-8

C/CB/B   9   8   7   6   5   4   3   2   1   01/B/022

Contributors

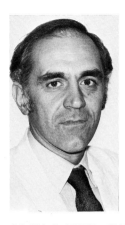

ALAN C. BIRD, M.D., F.R.C.S.

Professor in Clinical Ophthalmology,
Moorfields Eye Hospital,
London, England

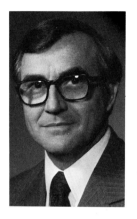

D. JACKSON COLEMAN, M.D.

Professor and Chairman,
Department of Ophthalmology,
The New York Hospital–Cornell Medical Center,
New York, New York

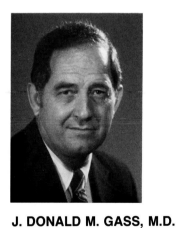

J. DONALD M. GASS, M.D.

Professor,
Department of Ophthalmology,
Bascom Palmer Eye Institute,
University of Miami Medical School,
Miami, Florida

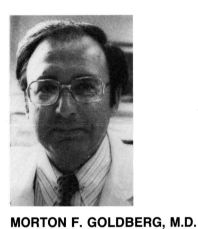

MORTON F. GOLDBERG, M.D.

Professor and Head,
Department of Ophthalmology,
Eye and Ear Infirmary,
University of Illinois,
Chicago, Illinois

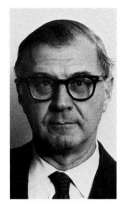

J. WALLACE McMEEL, M.D., P.C.

Surgeon in Ophthalmology,
Massachusetts Eye and Ear Infirmary,
Massachusetts General Hospital, Boston;
Senior Clinical Scientist, Eye Research
Institute of Retina Foundation, Boston;
Assistant Clinical Professor in Ophthalmology,
Harvard Medical School,
Boston, Massachusetts

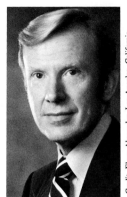

G. RICHARD O'CONNOR, M.D.

Professor of Ophthalmology and Director,
Francis I. Proctor Foundation,
University of California,
San Francisco, California

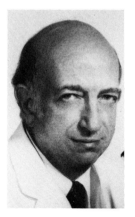

ARNALL PATZ, M.D.

Professor and Chairman,
Department of Ophthalmology,
Wilmer Institute,
The Johns Hopkins University School
    of Medicine and Hospital,
Baltimore, Maryland

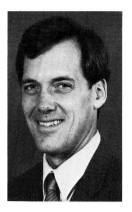

STEPHEN J. RYAN, M.D.

Professor and Chairman,
Department of Ophthalmology,
University of Southern California,
Los Angeles; Medical Director,
Estelle Doheny Eye Foundation,
Los Angeles, California

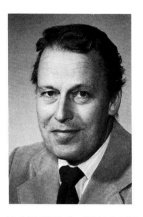

ROBERT C. WATZKE, M.D.

Professor of Ophthalmology,
Department of Ophthalmology,
University Hospitals,
Iowa City, Iowa

We wish to thank
Susan L. Larsen
for her help with the preparation
of this book

Preface

The New Orleans Academy of Ophthalmology convened for its thirty-first annual symposium from March 6 to March 10, 1982. This year's topic of discussion was medical and surgical diseases of the retina and vitreous. Each of our nine guest panelists was chosen for his extensive research and contributions to this exciting field, and each has several representative, original chapters included in this book. To the benefit of all, the Round Table Discussions once again provided the opportunity for our guests to examine and express their viewpoints on various new techniques as well as on current controversial issues. The meeting was as pleasant as it was informative, and we extend our thanks to all who participated. We hope you find the reading enjoyable.

Transactions Committee

Delmar R. Caldwell, M.D., *Chairman*
H. Frank Boswell, M.D.
Robert J. Cangelosi, M.D.
Walter D. Cockerham, M.D.
George S. Ellis, M.D.
Joel P. Pollard, M.D.
Betty Jean Wood, M.D.

Contents

Round table discussions

COLOR PLATE, 336

A Solitary macular lesion in patient with APMPPE (acute posterior multifocal placoid pigment epitheliopathy)

B Multifocal areas of metastatic carcinoma of the lung simulating APMPPE

C Multiple branch vein occlusions in a patient with serpiginous choroiditis

D Multiple gray patches and subretinal fluid in a patient with Harada's disease

E Multifocal outer retinal lesions in a child with diffuse unilateral subacute neuroretinitis

F Hypopigmented choroidal patches in a patient with vitiliginous chorioretinitis (birdshot chorioretinitis)

G Multifocal lesions associated with acute macular neuroretinopathy

H Multifocal choroiditis in sympathetic uveitis.

1

The choroid: its function, evaluation, and surgical management

D. Jackson Coleman
Lloyd M. Wilcox, Jr.*

BACKGROUND

No suborgan tissue in the eye has been the subject of as much scientific speculation as the choroid. Unobtrusively overshadowed by the pigment epithelium and buffered externally by the sclera, the choroid's inaccessible position has not permitted easy diagnostic evaluation or surgical intervention.

In the past decade, there has been much sophisticated study of the structure and function of the choroid. Although little new has been discovered about basic anatomy and physiology, there has been considerable evaluation and conceptualization of the physiologic processes active in this vascular tissue.

The choroid is basically a jacket of erectile tissue composed of capillaries, arteries, veins, and connective tissue (Fig. 1-1) that supports the retina both structurally and physiologically (Tables 1-1 and 1-2). Since blood vessels occupy virtually the entire bulk of the choroid, it is not surprising that this tissue has the highest blood flow in the body on a volume-per-weight basis. The choroid, if considered an organ, has a higher relative blood flow than the kidney does.

Entwining the maze of vascular tubes is a syncytium of nonvascular cells that give the choroid a biochemical and immunologic character. The avascular cells are of negligible bulk to the choroid but contribute to the expansile and contractile borders, which provide the elastic character of this tissue. Part of a collagen-elastic matrix, these resident cells can be divided conveniently into pigmented and nonpigmented types; a branching melanocyte is an example of the former, a mast cell representative of the latter. The pigment of the melanocytes and blood in the perfused vessels give the choroid its characteristic grape purple color (uvea from Latin *uva,* 'grape'). The etymology of choroid ('chorion-like') can be traced to chorion (Greek, 'skin' or 'leather'), or chorionic membrane, another membranous vascular suborgan capable of diffusion. The choroid then is an organized network of tubes emeshed in a superstructure of collagen–elastic tissue with a component of avascular cells as a filler.

---

*M.D., Heed Fellow, Retina-Vitreous Surgery, The New York Hospital, Cornell Medical Center, New York, New York.

1

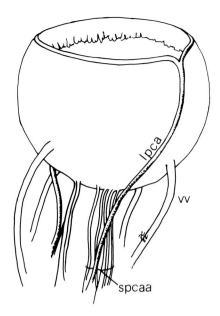

Fig. 1-1. The choroidal jacket surrounding the eye has two long posterior ciliary arteries, *lpca,* supplying the anterior portion, and numerous short posterior ciliary arteries, *spca,* supplying the posterior aspect. *vv,* Vortex vein.

Table 1-1. Macroscopic and physiologic comparison

Choroid	Retina
Fewer arterial bifurcations with each trunk tending to serve a distant terminal choroidal area (lobule)	Many bifurcations and successive subdivisions of arterial tree
Recurrent arteries to anterior choriocapillaris from (1) arterial ring, (2) diverse arterial supply to choriocapillaris, and (3) large-diameter capillaries	End arteries; no anastomoses except at level of capillaries
Anatomic regulation at capillary level because no precapillary sphincter	No precapillary sphincter; almost total perfusion of all capillaries
Physiologic regulation—sympathetic innervation and abundant alpha adrenergic receptors.	Autoregulation; local metabolic factors regulate flow
Stimulation of sympathetic response causes sharp decrease in blood flow	Autoregulation activated with fall in perfusion pressure promoting vasodilatation from local hypoxia and anemia

Table 1-2. Microscopic comparison

	Choriocapillaris (ChCp)	Retinal capillary (RCp)
Lumen	10 to 30 μm, several red blood cells may pass together alongside	5 to 10 μm, often deformation of a single red blood cell to pass through capillary
Anastomoses	Recurrent choroidal arteries to anterior ChCp.; high Po_2 content to venous blood with back flow, that is, retrograde perfusion	End arteries with no anastomoses, except at level of capillaries
Fenestrations	Large fenestrations	No fenestrations; tight junctions
Basement membrane	Continuous but very thin	Endothelium has thick basement membrane
Permeability	Very high, even to high molecular weight proteins; pore size permits proteins to 9×10^5 daltons; calculated pore size about 15 nm[17,47]	Low; impermeable to fluorescein and sodium
Protein content of tissue fluid around capillary	High protein content, net influx of water through retinal pigment epithelium from retina	Low protein content; net outflux of water from retina; dehydrating mechanisms

STRUCTURE
Anatomy of choroid

The choroid lines the inner surface of the sclera and provides a smooth support for the retina. The choroid is divided into three anatomic layers[20,32]—the lamina fusca, the vessel layer, and the choriocapillaris (Fig. 1-2).

Lamina fusca (potential suprachoroidal space)

The lamina fusca is composed of many spongy lamellae of elastic, collagenous, and muscle fibers that anchors the choroid to the sclera and forms a syncytium for the avascular cells. As a collapsed space, it has the potential for accumulating large amounts of fluid. The syncytium is more compact posteriorly in the globe, and the major vessels (ciliary arteries and vortex veins) crossing the lamina fusca tend to keep the space collapsed posterior to the equator.[37] The dilatation of the suprachoroidal space by migrating fluid in an effusion tends to start anteriorly and move circumferentially, very frequently detaching the ciliary body (CB).[15] A choroidal effusion always starts anterior to the equator and moves only slowly posteriorly against collective resistance of the bridging lamellae binding the sclera.[37]

Vessel layer

Large vessel layer (Haller's layer). Internal to the lamina fusca is a vessel layer divided into a large vessel outer layer (Haller's) and a medium-sized vessel inner layer (Sattler's). The larger vessels are predominately veins that drain into the vortex emis-

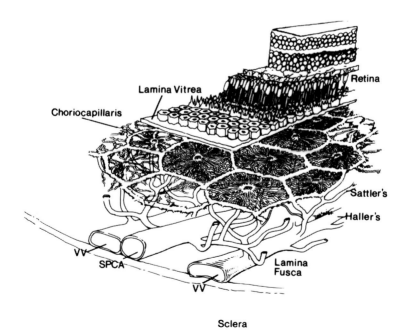

Fig. 1-2. Layers of choroid: lamina fusca, the vessel layer, and the choriocapillaris. Note lobular polygonal pattern of choriocapillaris. *VV,* Vortex vein; *SPCA,* short posterior ciliary artery.

saria, which penetrates the sclera. The arterial supply is derived primarily from the short posterior ciliary arteries (SPCA) posteriorly and the recurrent branches of the long posterior ciliary arteries (LPCA) in the anterior choroid.

Medium-sized vessel layer (Sattler's layer). This layer is the deeper internal layer of arteries and smaller veins. The division between these vessel layers is not distinct, and there is no macroscopic or microscopic marker separating the anatomy of Haller's and Sattler's layers.

Choriocapillaris

Internal to the vessel layer is the choriocapillaris, a single layer of fenestrated capillaries with wide lumens that are arranged in a characteristic lobulated pattern.[28,30,48] The lobular architecture helps explain the perfusion patterns seen with fluorescein angiography and segmental filling characteristic of some choroidopathies.[41,29] Each lobular segment is drained at its periphery by one or more venules, which frequently anastomose. The arterial input to each segment is believed to be relatively independent and there is little possibility for a vascular steal phenomenon. The segments communicate mainly by their draining venular system, though arterioarterial anastomoses have been encountered.[45] With venous obstruction, a damming effect could be capable of supplying adjacent lobules by retrograde flow, with venous blood having a high Po_2.[22] The choriocapillaris is essentially an endothelium-lined tube that is quite porous because of the fenestrations and functional pores in its wall (Fig. 1-3).

Dimension of choroid

The thickness of the choroid is greater at the posterior pole than anterior to the equator. Estimates in the past have largely been made from autopsy material and do not reflect the dynamic aspects of blood flow through the choroid. Necropsy material has suggested choroidal thicknesses in the range of 300 to 350 μm at the posterior pole,[20,44] but these values are made speciously low by shrinkage and dehydration in tissue processing. Recent measurements provided by ultrasound indicate a thickness of 400 to 550 μm. These large values seem to reflect the normally engorged in vivo state.[19] For comparison, the retina is normally 150 to 250 μm thick, and the optic disc has a diameter of 1500 μm.

FUNCTION
General actions

The choroid is believed to have two main physiologic purposes in ocular homeostasis. These putative functions of the choroid involve thermal regulation and metabolic delivery. Additionally, the choroid serves as a reservoir for cells that may participate in the immunologic and inflammatory response for the eye. Lastly, the choroid acts as an elastic, spongy, shock-absorbing coat supporting the sclera and helping to cushion trauma. The general functions are summarized in the following list:

General choroidal functions

1. Thermal
2. Metabolic
3. Immunologic and defensive
4. Structural and supportive

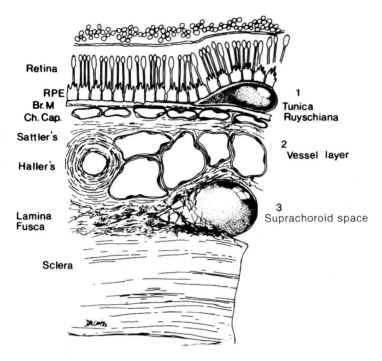

Retina
RPE
Br. M
Ch. Cap.
Sattler's
Haller's
Lamina
Fusca
Sclera

1
Tunica
Ruyschiana

2
Vessel layer

3
Suprachoroid space

Fig. 1-3. Tunica ruyschiana (retinal pigment epithelium, *RPE*), choriocapillaris, *ChCap,* and Bruch's membrane, BrM, taken as a unit. Note the RPE detachment and the suprachoroid detachment.

Thermal regulation

The choroid has long been believed to have a high blood flow. The high-flow state of this tissue has been confirmed over the past decade by very accurate quantitative experiments.[2,49,50,53] This firm knowledge about the high blood flow has led to speculation that the choroid acts as a "heat sink" by controlling temperature rises that might occur when light energy enters the eye, or when there are environmental extremes.[25,24]

Recent experiments, using a thermistor probe placed in the choroid, have tended to support this concept.[38] A rise in temperature was found at the macula with high-intensity light (equivalent of focused light) concomitant with a progressive increase in intraocular pressure. Such a rise in intraocular pressure would be expected to cause a decrease in blood flow, hence a decrease in temperature. In contrast, ambient light (equivalent of unfocused light), or light focused on the peripheral retina, showed a decrease in temperature with an increase in intraocular pressure. These preliminary data suggest, at least at the macula, a thermoregulatory function to the choroid. The thermoregulatory properties may be important in prevention of macular disease. It is possible that light toxicity causes free-radical formation, which leads to increased lipofuscin deposits and senile macular degeneration.[23,51] In this event, a cooling effect on the macula of perhaps only a few degrees may be the critical threshold to prevention of photochemical events that contribute to this process of aging. Free-radical formation, in part induced by light, has been an integral concept in the biology of aging.[46]

Metabolic delivery

The high-flow rate through the choroid is believed to be the driving force behind the inward diffusion of oxygen necessary for metabolism of the vascular outer third of the retina.[2,18,21] Reduced distortion of sensory tissue by blood vessels is an obvious advantage for even photoreceptor distribution.

Inflammatory and immunologic response

A number of cells such as mast cells reside in the choroid, and others, such as plasma cells, visit this plexus from the blood. It is clear that many of the choroidal cellular inhabitants are actively involved in the ocular inflammatory response or immunologic reactions.

Physiologic determinations
Blood flow

Refinement of the labeled microsphere techniques has allowed accurate and reproducible measurements of blood flow in the choroid.[2,3,5,49,50] The experimental technique involves the injection of radioactive spheres that are nearly the size of red blood cells into the central arterial circulation. The microspheres are then distributed to the tissues. The distribution of the spheres is proportional to the blood flow; that is, the more spheres in a tissue, the "hotter" the tissue, hence the greater the flow.[27,36]

On the basis of volume flow per gram of tissue, the choroid is the most vascularized tissue in the body. In a relative comparison (ml/min/gm of tissue) the choroid has three to four times the blood flow of the kidney. Characteristic values for the choroid are 25.4 ± 7.1 versus 6.83 ± 0.45 (ml/min/gm) for the kidney.[50]

Typical blood flow values have been determined in primates and are shown in Fig. 1-4.

Retinal blood flow is considerably less than blood flow to the choroid or blood flow to the iris, ciliary body, and ciliary processes. That the exiguous flow to retina is sufficient to sustain this neural tissue may be explained by the efficient extraction of oxygen (venous Po_2 30 to 40 torrs), the fact that the outer third is supplied by diffusion from the choroid, and all retinal capillaries are continuously perfused.

Choroidal blood flow shows regional variation with the foveal area of choroid (6.49 ± 0.62 ml/min/mm^2) having more than five times the flow of the peripheral choroid (0.76 ± 0.14 mg/min/mm^2).[5]

Control of blood flow

The choroid tends to be regulated by the autonomic nervous system. By contrast, the retina is controlled by local tissue ischemia (hypoxia) in the process of autoregulation.[4,10] There is little or no innervational regulation on the retina vessels per se.[33]

Sympathetic stimulation of the eye innervates alpha adrenergic receptors of choroidal vessels producing a fall in blood flow,[4] or when pharmocologic agents are injected, it can be shown that both alpha and gamma receptors exist.[16]

Vasodilatation of choroidal vessels may occur[43] by stimulation of the seventh cranial nerve or by nerves through the sphenopalatine ganglion. The exact mechanism for the parasympathetic effect on the choroid is unclear.[43] Choroidal vessels may be dilated by a variety of drugs that cause hypotension and a reduction in the perfusion pressure for the choroid. In general, the flow through the choroid should be considered maximal in

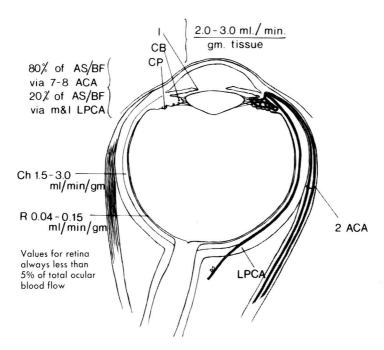

Fig. 1-4. The anterior-segment blood flow, *AS/BF*, from seven or eight anterior ciliary arteries, *ACA*, supply 80% of the blood anterior to the ora serrata. Two long posterior ciliary arteries, *LPCA*, a medial and lateral aspect, *m&l*, supply only 20% of the anterior-segment blood flow. *I*, Iris; *CB*, ciliary body; *CP*, ciliary processes; *Ch*, choroid; *R*, retina; *BF*, blood flow.

normal conditions, with little physiologic reserve for increase above normal. The choroid is a "full-tilt" suborgan, with most alterations in the physiologic state causing a decrease in flow.

Oxygen tensions and the relationships to blood flow

Choroidal extraction or utilization of oxygen is very low, with the venous blood having about a 5% oxygen difference from the arterial side.[11,52]

In primates about 65% to 70% of the retinal oxygen is supplied by choroidal diffusion.[11,53] It is likely that the photoreceptors consume more of this volume than other retinal layers do.[53] The driving force for the oxygen diffusion is probably the high choroidal blood flow with saturated oxygenated blood (high Po_2) acting in a mass-action manner to facilitate diffusion from the outer choroid inward toward the retina.

A compensatory relationship between the choroid and retina seems to exist, such that with mild to moderate increases in intraocular pressure, the retina autoregulates to increase its flow to compensate for pressure-induced reduction in choroidal flow (Fig. 1-5).

Pressure relationship to blood flow

The normal pressure of the central retinal artery entering the eye is probably around 65 mm Hg. This value alone may not seem striking, but one must remember that at the intraocular capillary level, the intravascular pressure must be higher than that of other

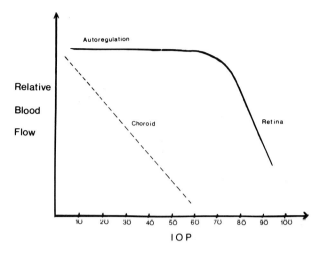

Fig. 1-5. The effect of autoregulation is seen only in the retina. *IOP,* Intraocular pressure. (From Alm, A., and Bill, A.: Acta Physiol. Scand. **84:**306, 1972.)

organs to overcome an abnormally high tissue pressure of 20 mm Hg (that is, intraocular pressure acts as tissue pressure). The central retinal artery pressure then is a major component of the perfusion pressure, but the intraocular pressure also acts as a tissue pressure influencing the venous pressure draining the retina. Additionally, the choroidal blood flow is exquisitely sensitive to changes in intraocular pressure by an inverse relationship.

The choroid is far more sensitive to pressure change than the retina (Fig. 1-5).

With even small-increment increases in intraocular pressure, the blood flow for the choroid declines while the retinal blood flow remains unchanged because of autoregulation.

With a decrease in blood flow, to either choroid or retina, oxygen extraction for both the retina and choroid is increased. A drop in systemic blood pressure reduces the perfusion and is the physiologic equivalent to increasing the intraocular pressure, a concept important in low-tension glaucoma.

Pressure relationship of fluid shifts

The suprachoroidal space (lamina fusca), with a pressure of 1 to 3 mm Hg in the normal physiologic state, is collapsed by an opposing intraocular pressure (acting as a tissue pressure) of 20 mm Hg.[37] For the purpose of this discussion, we are assuming that intravascular pressure or capillary pressure remains normal and does not vary. The intravascular pressure will vary in certain disease states, such as, high episcleral venous pressure.

The suprachoroidal space is analogous to the space between an inner tube and a tire, or the potential layer between the bladder inside a football and its outer pigskin. The choroid must remain ''inflated'' at an ideal pressure against the tire wall of the sclera to keep the space collapsed. The pressure on the choroid is the intraocular pressure, and loss of intraocular pressure always initiates development of the suprachoroidal space.

Tissue fluid of choroid has a high concentration of proteins causing an osmotic

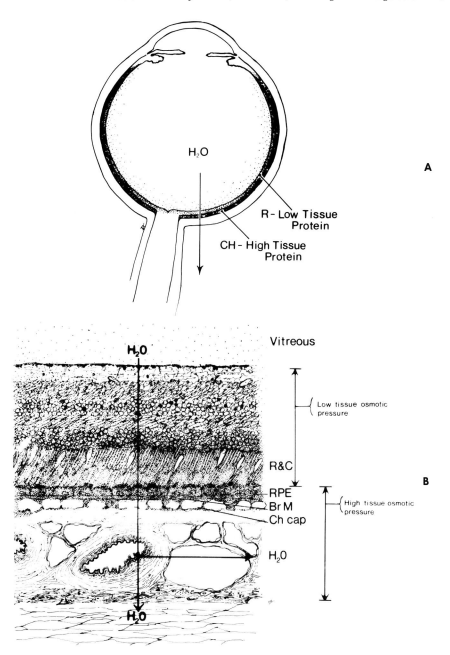

Fig. 1-6. High vitreous water turnover and the mechanism for this egress is influenced by oncotic pressure gradients created by large amounts of protein in the choroid. **A,** Diagram of eye. **B,** Diagram of eye layers.

gradient relative to retina.[8,9] Since the retina has little extracellular space[40] with a low concentration of protein in the tissue fluid, a net flux of water will flow from the retina into the choroid. Additionally, the turnover of vitreal water is high[12,31] and probably exits via the retinal pigment epithelium and choroid (Fig. 1-6). In summary, the water from vitreous and retina is sucked out by the osmotic gradient of the choroid and pumped out by the pigment epithelium.

The relative osmotic pressure of choroid to retina and the pigment epithelial pump account for resorption of fluid from the subretinal space in detachment surgery. Patients with an atrophic choroid are likely to have slow or poor resorption of subretinal fluid. Choroidal detachment retards or prevents absorption of subretinal fluid through that area of the choroid detached. The high turnover of vitreal water and other residing or visiting substances causes the vitreous to be influenced by choroid flow.

SURGICAL CONSIDERATIONS
Surgical anatomy

The choroid can be considered a three-layered suborgan from a surgical perspective. The outer layer is the epichoroid, suprachoroid, or lamina fusca. For the surgeon this layer is the subscleral space that may be incised in order to drain fluid and collapse the space. The second layer is composed of blood vessels (Haller's and Sattler's) that are conceptually separate but are indistinguishable to the surgeon. It is iatrogenic damage to this layer that produces hemorrhage with drainage of subretinal fluid or with excessive cryopexy. The innermost third layer of plaque-like tufts of capillaries, the choriocapillaris (ChCap), is integrally related to Bruch's membrane (BrM) and the retinal pigment epithelium (RPE). The binding of these layers (ChCap, BrM, and RPE) as a anatomic unit was recognized in part in the eighteenth century by the Dutch anatomist Ruysch. The choriocapillaris, Bruch's membrane, and the retinal pigment epithelium is called the tunica ruyschiana.* From a nosologic view, the three layers should be considered a basic unit participating in the pathophysiologic state of macular disease. For the surgeon this inner tripartite layer is a barrier that must be penetrated to release subretinal fluid (Fig. 1-3).

The epichoroid becomes a real space when fluid accumulates beneath the sclera. It is known that the space has been created when a diagnosis of a choroidal detachment is made when one views the characteristic black mound appearance through the pupil. Choroidal detachments, though many are small, are a ubiquitous finding in the initially hypotonous globe. When indicated, the subscleral space can be incised and drained easily, provided that the fluid is localized precisely and entry is exact. Drainage of choroidal effusions is accomplished by localization of the maximum height of choroidal detachment to the closest possible clock hour. At a point 3 to 4 mm posterior to the limbus along the radian, one is likely to locate fluid because the fluid dissects anteriorly, frequently detaching the ciliary body.[14] Additionally with an effusion, there is ciliary body traction from the abnormal pull on the zonules with choroidal displacement. The traction on the ciliary body leads to detachment, hyposecretion, and the incipient stages of cyclitic membrane formation. A solely posterior effusion is a rare event. Since the eye will collapse like a shrunken grape after the release of subscleral fluid, it is suggested that (1) a paracentesis site or pars plana incision be made before drainage so that the eye can be reinflated with saline solution or gas, and (2) a Flieringa ring be used to support the sclera.

---

*After Frederick Ruysch (1638-1731). See Duke-Elder, S.: The anatomy of the visual system, vol. II. In Duke-Elder, S., and Wybar, K.: System of Ophthalmology, St. Louis, 1976, The C.V. Mosby Co., p. 138.

One can create or enlarge the subscleral space or suprachoroidal space by tenting the sclera away from the choroid. One grasps the sclera with forceps perpendicularly to the choroid and pulls externally. With intrascleral suturing, as in retinal or strabismus surgery, this manuever accentuates the suprachoroid, allowing for greater safety by increasing the distance between the choroidal vessels and the needle.

The distended suprachoroid space may also be bridged by stretched lamellae from the vessel layer to sclera and, if the fluid is sufficiently posterior, even major vessels (vortex veins or ciliary arteries) may be encountered traversing the space, trying to hold the choroid to the sclera. By an incision down onto choroid, the epichoroidal space can be appreciated when one gently uses a spatula to push and tease the choroid inward and pulls the sclera gently outward. Such a manuever will tend to rupture some of the bridging fibers. It has been calculated that it takes a 6 gm force to break collectively these bridging fibers.[37] In using a blunt, thin, and malleable spatula to separate the sclera from choroid, one must use great care posterior to the equator so as not to rupture major vessels.

This layer produces the disastrous bleeding complications that may be encountered in retinal detachment surgery. Penetration of a large vessel during drainage of subretinal fluid, or thermal rupture with necrosis from excessive cryopexy, may lead to extensive choroidal hemorrhage. The techniques of producing heavy white cryopexy lesions in areas of thin choroid or of double or triple refreezing in the same area are to be avoided. Hemorrhage sufficient to cause a large choroidal detachment, or a large pool of blood that has ruptured into the subretinal space, is most likely secondary to a rupture of a larger posterior ciliary vessel. By contrast, flecks of blood seen in the subretinal space around the drain site after release of fluid are more likely from tears in the choriocapillaris. In the uncommon case where a choroidal effusion secondary to extensive retinal cryopexy requires drainage, the fluid is often blood tinged, an indication that effusions have a range of pathologic signs from plain transudate to frank blood.

It may be possible to reduce the chances of these hemorrhagic complications if the vessel layer is visualized at a sclerotomy site with magnification and internal transillumination. The large vessels appear bright red and stand in contrast to the dark purple of the pigment. The vessels noted by transillumination may be either arteries or veins since the arteriovenous oxygen difference is small and causes the same bright red appearance.

This unit is integrally involved in macula disease, but the choriocapillaris never loses its attachments to the feeding vessel layer. In contrast to the epichoroid, no space can be created between the vessel layer and the choriocapillaris.

Surgical physiology and pathophysiology of the choroid

Two main conditions may require surgical intervention on the suprachoroid space: (1) choroidal effusion with or without ciliary body detachment and (2) choroidal hemorrhage with or without the expulsive force that produces a rent in the retina. The former condition has been encountered frequently by the glaucoma surgeon, whereas the latter pathologic state is increasingly being referred to the vitreoretinal surgeon. The final common pathologic consequence of both conditions, if persistent and left untreated, can be the formation of a cyclitic membrane leading to phthisis. For an understanding of the pathophysiologic process involved, it is necessary to reemphasize certain aspects of the normal physiologic state.

In choroidal effusion and choroidal hemorrhage, there is development of a potential space that is collapsed under normal conditions. Assuming normal intravascular pressure within the capillary from the arterial to the venous side, this suprachoroidal space remains collapsed primarily because of two physiologic forces: (1) the colloid osmotic force of the choroid and (2) the intraocular pressure that serves as an ersatz tissue force. When these forces are diminished, fluid begins to accumulate in the suprachoroidal space. The question remains unanswered as to whether a pressure change, usually hypotony, precedes or follows the changes in osmotic force and membrane permeability. In choroidal effusion, hypotony is usually recognized as part of the syndrome, but in hemorrhagic choroidal detachment there is almost certainly some disruption of the permeability of capillary membranes in the choroid. The mechanisms to be considered are the pressure alterations, the outward colloid osmotic forces, and the protein and pore size.

Pressure alterations

The rule is that there must be some associated hypotony in choroidal effusion. The suprachoroidal space is at 1 to 3 mm Hg or about 18 mm Hg less than the intraocular pressure; hence the suprachoroidal space remains deflated or compressed. When the intraocular pressure goes to zero or really atmospheric pressure, the elasticity of the choroid and its attachment to the ciliary body pull in such a fashion that a negative pressure is created in the space. The suprachoroid remains a few millimeters of mercury below atmospheric pressure; hence there is a transudation.[7,9,13,37,39] This principle is illustrated in Fig. 1-7.

Colloid osmotic forces outward

The retina has very little extracellular space and only small amounts of extracellular protein relative to choroid.[31] Large amounts of immunoglobulin and albumin are found in the extravascular space relative to the retina and vitreous.[12] Through osmotic pressure, a net flow toward the choroid exists.[7,14,17,39] The choriocapillaris acts as a membrane creating a further protein barrier, thus allowing formation of an osmotic gradient. Thin choroids undoubtedly reabsorb subretinal fluid more slowly, probably because a colloid-poor layer induces relatively lower osmotic pressures.

Protein and pore size

Since pore size in the choriocapillaris has a restricting relationship to the size of the proteins that pass, a change in molecular weight of protein passing through the choriocapillaris would suggest alteration of permeability. It is known that in choroidal effusion the proteins have varying molecular weight where the maximum excluded molecule is between 3.4 to 9.0 $\times$ 10^5 daltons.[17] With a low molecular weight effusion, excluding proteins greater than 3.4 $\times$ 10^5 daltons, the filtration rate is increased. In this process of molecular sieving of the proteins, the bulk flow is inversely proportional to the size molecules passing by diffusional exchange in the capillary. Hence, by looking at the molecular weight of the protein in the effusion fluid one may find a clue to the mechanism of formation.[6,14,17,42] Another pathophysiologic consideration is that the permeability of the capillary remains normal, that is, unchanged, while the intravascular pressure rises, often secondary to elevated episcleral venous pressure.[42] It would seem that

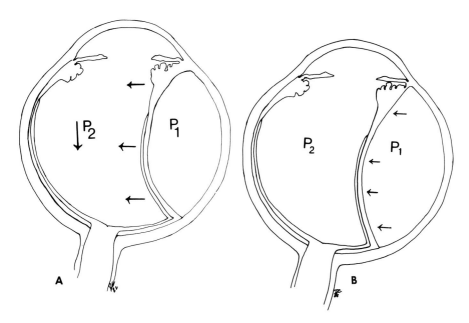

Fig. 1-7. A, Suprachoroidal space pressure, P_1, is normally about 3 mm Hg. Normally the intraocular pressure, P_2, is 20 mm Hg, but with a great decrease in the intraocular pressure such as opening the eye ($P_2 = 0$), a negative pressure is created in the suprachoroidal space ($P_1 = -3$ mm Hg), causing a transudate effusion. **B,** P_1 greatly exceeds the intraocular pressure, P_2. P_2 is caused by excessive intravascular pressures secondary to hemorrhage into the suprachoroidal space.

functional alteration of the capillary does occur in this type of fluid-pressure disturbance.

This undoubtedly occurs in a hemorrhagic effusion of frank choroidal hemorrhage. In expulsive choroidal hemorrhage, vessels break apart under arterial pressure, from disruption of the intima media with arteriosclerotic changes or from necrosis secondary to excessive thermal injury.[1,26,35] The extravasation of blood is under such force as to sunder the bridging lamellae to create the rapidly expanding black mound seen through the pupil. The capillary membrane, with this forceful diapedesis of blood probably ruptures, allowing escape of blood, very high molecular weight protein, and effusion fluid. Since the clot in choroidal hemorrhage is intimately connected to the choroidal lamellae, the decompression procedure should be controlled to prevent further rupture of vessels, lamellae, and dispersion of cells (Fig. 1-7).

> **Clinical example:** With extensive cryopexy during retinal surgery it is possible to have either delayed resorption of subretinal fluid, choroid effusion, or choroidal hemorrhage. Cryopexy most probably alters the choroidal permeability, causes necrosis of small vessels, and may fracture the elastica and intima of large vessels, contributing to any of these three complications.

EVALUATION OF CHOROID

Various physiologic functions of the choroid have been measured in animals with ultrasound, reflective densitometry, and microsphere-injection techniques. In humans, the pigment epithelium reduces the efficacy and accuracy of densitometry, and microspheres are not applicable. Ultrasound thus provides a unique means of measuring human in vivo choroidal thickness. The accuracy of this technique is excellent but limited by occasional interpretative problems in the selection of the anterior boundary of the sclera and the lamina fusca.

Conventional A-scan ultrasonograms provide a reasonable means of discerning choroid in pathologic conditions, but they are not easily interpreted in normal states because of the amplitude similarity of the highly reflective surfaces of choroid and sclera. Similarly, B-scan separation is difficult to interpret in normal eyes but easily discernible in pathologic states (Fig. 1-8). Computerized techniques have allowed us to separate tissue planes with far greater accuracy than with conventional diagnostic displays. Using computerized analysis techniques, we have found that the normal choroid is thicker than previously extrapolated from in vitro measurements. Our data indicate a normal posterior-pole thickness of 400 to 550 μm compared to normal retinal thickness of 200 to 250 μm at the posterior pole.

In abnormal cases, the choroid may be more than 2 mm (2000 μm) thick. Choroidal thickening and detachments are easily recognizable by pattern analysis on both B and A scan since the increased blood or fluid content enhances the choroid-sclera boundary. Diffuse choroidal thickening is commonly seen in hypotony, uveitis, endophthalmitis, and trauma (Fig. 1-9). Localized thickening can also be seen in inflammatory conditions such as scleritis (Fig. 1-10). Choroidal detachments are easily appreciated on B scan

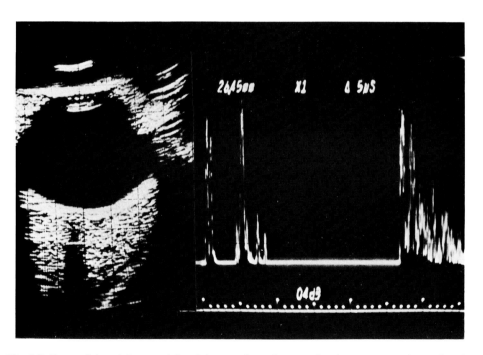

Fig. 1-8. B scan, *left,* and A scan, *right,* of the normal eye demonstrating the appearance of normal ocular and orbital structures on ultrasonic analysis. At normal examining frequencies, such as this 10 MHz scan, the retina, choroid, and scleral layers blend into a high-amplitude complex seen as the concave, limiting boundary of the globe on B scan and seen on the A scan as a high-amplitude complex posteriorly.

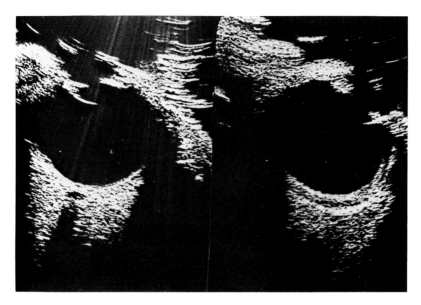

Fig. 1-9. Localized choroidal thickening is seen in this pediatric patient who sustained a blunt injury to the anterior segment. On the axial B scan, *left,* only a subtle distinction of a thicker than normal choroidal layer can be appreciated. In a more inferior plane, there is a distinct separation between the high-amplitude anterior retinal curvature and the posterior scleral layer, allowing a clinical determination of the abnormally thick choroid.

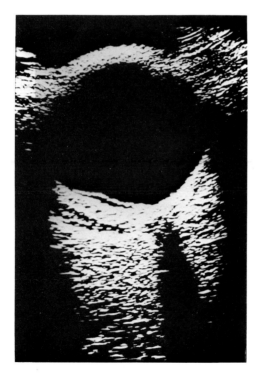

Fig. 1-10. Localized choroidal thickening with associated retinal detachment in a patient with scleritis. Localized separation of the retina extends from the optic nerve head. Inflammatory infiltrate in the episcleral region allows assessment of the increased choroidal thickness in a situation similar to that seen in Fig. 1-9.

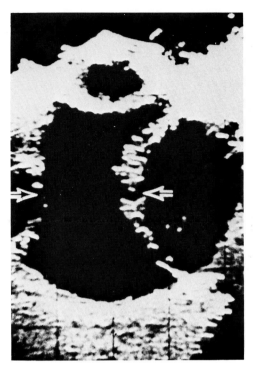

Fig. 1-11. B-scan appearance of choroidal effusion or detachment. In this patient with a flat chamber after an unsuccessful filtering procedure the characteristic "baseball-stitch" configuration of bullous choroidal detachment is seen, *arrows*.

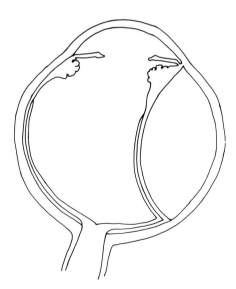

Fig. 1-12. Chorioretinal detachment. The suprachoroidal space can appear prolate on cross section. The expansion can extend anteriorly to the iris root and posteriorly to the vortex veins or rarely to the optic nerve.

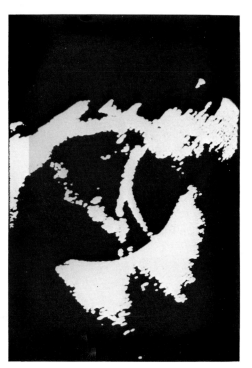

Fig. 1-13. B-scan appearance to total retinal detachment with underlying localized choroidal detachment or effusion. This B scan demonstrates the distinctive points of attachment used in differentiating retinal detachment from choroidal detachment. The retinal detachment inserts at the optic nerve head, whereas the underlying choroidal detachment has more anterior points of attachment, such as the vortex veins. Both the subretinal and subchoroidal fluids are acoustically clear in the scan.

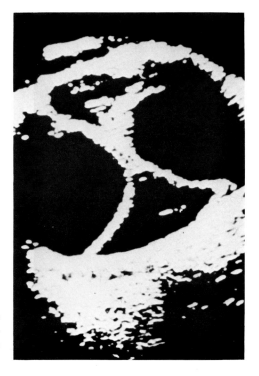

Fig. 1-14. Highly elevated choroidal detachment in the characteristic "kissing choroidal" configuration. Ultrasonography can reliably indicate points of apposition between the choroidal bullae.

and appear as smoothly rounded elevations (Fig. 1-11). Since elevations and detachments of the choroid represent a transmural pressure gradient, these elevations have a characteristic sharply angled intercept with the globe wall. Although the expansion of fluid is pressure directed in a spheroid pattern, the mural constraints of sclera, optic nerve, iris root, and to some extent the vortex veins affect the two-dimensional outline seen on B scan. Consequently, the typical pattern is that of prolate elevation limited by the iris root and optic nerve (Fig. 1-12). In managing patients with choroidal detachment, it is important to determine if there is an associated retinal detachment (Fig. 1-13), or retina-to-retina contact, that is, apposition of retina either to an adjacent bulla or across the eye as in a "kissing-choroidal" elevation (Fig. 1-14). The meridian of maximum elevation should be precisely determined if a sclerotomy is planned.

SURGICAL MANAGEMENT
Objectives and indications

The primary objective in surgery of the choroid is to restore anatomic and physiologic integrity to the ocular tissue. The basic tissue relationships must be reconstituted if the globe has been surgically or traumatically ruptured. Hydrodynamic equilibrium can usually be obtained by use of choroidal drainage and vitreous replacement procedures. Although not all causes of choroidal separation can be satisfactorily managed with these methods alone, an artificial rebalancing of the physiologic state may eventually permit recovery.

Generally effusion is caused by an imbalance of choroidal intravascular pressure to intraocular or tissue pressure. This imbalance can result from (1) an open eye or ciliary epithelial shutdown that lowers the intraocular pressure, or (2) from raised arterial or venous pressures to overwhelm a normal intraocular pressure.

Bellows, Chylack, and Hutchinson[6] reported on a series of 112 eyes and listed eight indications for choroidal surgery. To their list relating mainly to glaucoma, we should add two more indications: (1) combined retinal detachment and choroidal elevation and (2) prolonged retina-to-retina contact with inflammation and incipient adhesions.

Updated concepts in choriovitreoretinal surgery

The use of intraocular gases to expand and maintain the vitreous cavity has added a new dimension to choroidoretinal surgery. The precepts behind choroidal surgery and staged vitreoretinal surgery go beyond the conventional conceptualization of scleral buckling. We have entered an era in ophthalmic surgery where eyes that were definitely lost after expulsive choroidal hemorrhage are now salvageable. We are witnessing a conceptual change in retinal detachment surgery. Earlier techniques relied primarily on an external approach because of the delicacy of the retina. In earlier techniques of buckling, the retina was treated as a passive structure and was placed against the indented choroidoretinal bulge by an externally applied force that was augmented by drainage of subretinal fluid. Our current concepts imply that the retina can be actuated by the active internal forces of gas tamponade. With these newer techniques, the retina can undergo far more manipulation than previously believed. Additionally, because of the need to treat the retina through apposed choroid, at normal or nearly normal thickness, the concept of staged choriovitreoretinal surgery was evolved.

The controlled choroidal drainage must precede detachment surgery by days to weeks. A partial or total vitrectomy is done concomitantly with controlled drainage. These tenets of controlled drainage, gas-fluid exchange, and staged chorioretinal surgery are basic to the new concepts of how to treat these severely damaged eyes.

Controlled choroidal drainage

Ultrasound has greatly augmented our ability to recognize and assess the position of choroidal effusion. Empirically the inferior temporal quadrant has been identified as the safest position for drainage, but this location is not always the point of maximal elevation. The exact quadrant and area of greatest elevation can be accurately determined with ultrasound. If the elevation is increasing with an associated inflammatory component sufficient to warrant surgery, we have found that a controlled drainage will allow

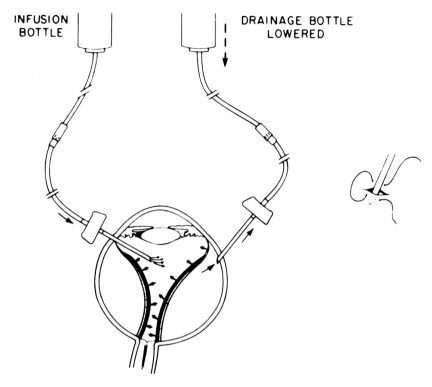

Fig. 1-15. Controlled choroidal drainage utilizes separate infusion lines to the vitreous and suprachoroidal spaces. In this way, a uniform pressure is exerted on the tunica ruyschiana. Slow and limited lowering of the effusion line then permits a corresponding slow drainage of the choroidal fluid, resulting in a more complete evacuation.

more fluid to be evacuated than simple incision into the suprachoroidal space. This technique utilizes two needles, both connected to infusion bottles to act as regulators of positive choroidal force uniformly distributed on the external choroidal surface and the internal retina (Fig. 1-15). The needle passing through the pars plana into the vitreous cavity has a greater infusion pressure than the needle placed through a radial bulge of the choroidal detachment, which is usually pressed back to its normal position as the suprachoroidal space is evacuated.

We generally use 21-gauge butterfly needles because of the short bevel. The bevel is kept parallel to the scleral surface. Lifting of the scleral wound margins and milking of the suprachoroidal space may still be helpful but generally only after the bulk of the fluid has been drained. The drainage procedure is relatively benign, and because of difficulty in achieving total drainage of choroidal fluid, the procedure may need to be repeated before retinal surgery can be performed.

Gas/fluid exchange

Once the choroidal fluid is reasonably evacuated, the retinochoroidal complex may be supported by conventional retinal buckling techniques. Usually, evacuation of the

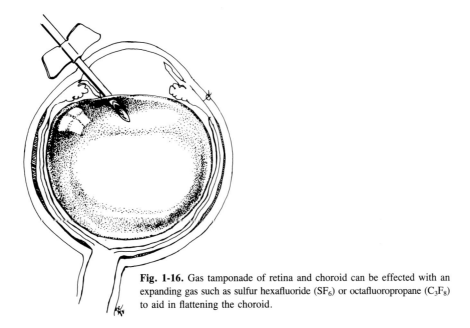

Fig. 1-16. Gas tamponade of retina and choroid can be effected with an expanding gas such as sulfur hexafluoride (SF_6) or octafluoropropane (C_3F_8) to aid in flattening the choroid.

vitreous and replacement with an intraocular gas, such as sulfur hexafluoride (SF_6) or octafluoropropane (C_3F_8), may augment the positive-pressure gradient applied against the choroid and retina and thus preserve the anatomic positioning of retina that has been gained by the drainage (Fig. 1-16). During surgery the gas is injected through the infusion line into the vitreous cavity with subsequent prone positioning of the patient at the end of the operation. The volume must be titrated in terms of the physical properties for expansion of the particular gas.[34,35]

The length of time of maintenance of the tamponade determines the selection of a particular gas.[34,35] The gas-bubble size can be adjusted subsequent to the initial placement both at the end of surgery and postoperatively. After surgery, frequently in an outpatient setting we use a 30-gauge ⅝-inch needle to tap the vitreous, and with alternate evacuation of vitreous fluid and injection of gas, we can obtain a suitable bubble to tamponade the choroid and retina. These controlled drainage-tamponade techniques are the main modalities that constitute active retinal repositioning and mark a distinct evolution from the external (passive) retinal procedures.

Staged chorioretinal surgery

If retinal detachment surgery is required to buckle a definite hole, it is necessary to plan this surgery after the choroid has flattened so that transscleral diathermy or cryopexy can adequately irritate the retinal pigment epithelium and retina. A thick choroid acts as a "heat sink" and thus dissipates the temperature extremes necessary to produce a thermal adhesion. Retinal detachment surgery must be delayed until adequate treatment of the choroid has been performed and the eye shows evidence of choroidal stabilization. This may require one or more weeks. The gas can be reinjected if necessary to maintain the intraocular pressure–choroidal pressure balance. The technique has shown success for dealing with all forms of choroidal detachment including expulsive hemor-

Fig. 1-17. B-scan ultrasonogram of an eye with a recent expulsive choroidal hemorrhage pushing forward to the iris plane.

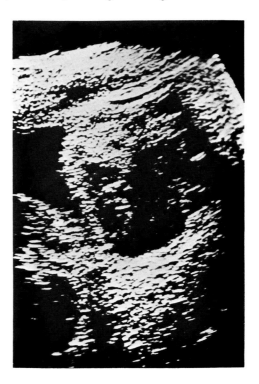

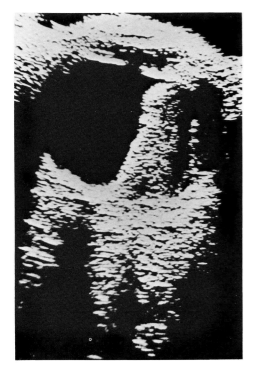

Fig. 1-18. B scan of the same patient shown in Fig. 1-17, 1 month after choroidal drainage. Choroidal elevation remains and a cyclitic membrane is now present.

rhage complicating cataract surgery. A case presentation demonstrates the sequence of operations in such a situation.

CASE REPORT

J.K., an 80-year-old white male with bilateral cataracts underwent planned intracapsular extraction of the left eye on April 15, 1980. After the lens removal, as the sutures were being drawn up, a choroidal expulsive hemorrhage occurred. A sclerotomy was performed and vitreous toileted to permit a tight wound closure. The ciliary body and retina could be seen to fill the pupillary space. The patient was referred to The New York Hospital–Cornell Medical Center on April 17, 1981. Ultrasonography confirmed a massive choroidal hemorrhage with apposition of retina to the posterior iris plane (Fig. 1-17).

A controlled choroidal drainage released the bulk of suprachoroidal fluid, leaving what appeared to be an organized clot that could not be irrigated from the suprachoroidal space. The patient was followed for 1 month during which the choroid showed little further flattening and an anterior cyclitic membrane developed (Fig. 1-18).

On May 20, 1981, an anterior vitrectomy and repeat controlled choroidal drainage were performed. The hemorrhage still could not be completely drained, and so a retinal buckling procedure could not be done, even though visualization of the retina revealed a large retinal tear superiorly. SF_6 gas was instilled, and cryopexy was applied to the tear. Anatomic reattachment of the retina was achieved permitting recovery of 20/200 central vision with full peripheral vision.

SUMMARY

The structure of the choroid has been discussed with special attention to the surgical anatomy. The suprachoroidal space (lamina fusca) created by pathophysiologic conditions is most responsive to surgical entry. The alterations in intraocular pressure, changes in tissue colloid pressures, or ruptures in choroidal vessels may all contribute to choroidal effusion or hemorrhage. Ultrasonography may be used to diagnose these conditions. Choroidal hemorrhage formerly considered almost untreatable should be evaluated for vitreoretinal surgery. Controlled choroidal drainage with vitrectomy, gas-fluid exchange, and a staged secondary retinal detachment procedure is used in extreme cases. Repeat choroidal drainage followed by a staged buckling procedure and internal tamponade by gas may be necessary to achieve a flat choroid and an attached retina.

REFERENCES

1. Aaberg, T.M.: Experimental serous and hemorrhagic uveal edema associated with retinal detachment surgery, Invest. Ophthalmol. **14:**243, 1975.
2. Alm, A., and Bill, A.: Blood flow and oxygen extraction in cat uvea at normal and high intraocular pressures, Acta Physiol. Scand. **80:**19, 1970.
3. Alm, A., and Bill, A.: The oxygen supply to the retina. II. Effects of high intraocular pressure and of increased arterial carbon dioxide tensions on uveal and retinal blood flow in cats, Acta Physiol. Scand. **84:**306, 1972.
4. Alm, A., and Bill, A.: The effect of stimulation of the sympathetic chain on retinal oxygen tension and uveal, retinal and cerebral blood flow in cats, Acta Physiol. Scand. **88:**84, 1973.
5. Alm, A., and Bill, A.: Ocular and optic nerve blood flow at normal and increased intraocular pressures in monkeys, Exp. Eye Res. **15:**15, 1973.
6. Bellows, A.R., Chylack, L.T., and Hutchinson, B.T.: Choroidal effusion during glaucoma surgery in patients with prominent episcleral vessels, Arch. Ophthalmol. **97:**493, 1979.
7. Bellows, A.R., Chylack, L.T., and Hutchinson, B.T.: Choroidal detachment: clinical manifestation, therapy and mechanism of formation, Ophthalmology **88:**1107, 1981.
8. Bill, A.: Capillary permeability to and extravascular dynamics of myoglobin, albumin, and gammaglobulin in the uvea, Acta Physiol. Scand. **73:**204, 1968.
9. Bill A.: A method to determine osmotically effective albumin and gammaglobulin concentrations in tissue fluid, its application to the uvea and a note on the effects of capillary "leaks" on tissue fluid dynamics, Acta Physiol. Scand. **73:**511, 1968.
10. Bill, A.: Blood circulation and fluid dynamics in the eye, Physiol. Rev. **55:**383, 1975.
11. Bill, A.: Ocular circulation. In Moses, R.H., editor: Adler's physiology of the eye, ed. 7, St. Louis, 1981, The C.V. Mosby Co.
12. Cagianut, B., and Verrey, F.: Essai de dépistage du métabolisme hydrique dans les milieux transparents de l'œil humain par injection d'eau lourde dans la chambre antérieure, Ann. d'Ocul. **182:**649, 1949.
13. Capper, S.A., and Leopold, H.: Mechanism of serous choroidal detachment: a review in experimental study, Arch. Ophthalmol. **55:**101, 1956.
14. Chandler, P.A., and Maumenee, A.E.: A major cause of hypotony, Trans. Am. Acad. Ophthalmol. Otolaryngol. **65:**563, 1961.
15. Chandler, P.A., and Maumenee, A.E.: A major cause of hypotony, Am. J. Ophthalmol. **52:**609, 1964.
16. Chandra, S.R., and Friedman, E.: Choroidal blood flow. II. The effect of autonomic agents, Arch. Ophthalmol. **87:**67, 1972.

17. Chylack, L.T., Jr., and Bellows, A.R.: Molecular sieving in suprachoroidal fluid formation in man, Invest. Ophthalmol. Vis. Sci. **17:**420, 1978.
18. Cohan, B.E., and Cohan, S.: Flow and oxygen saturation of blood in the anterior ciliary vein of the dog eye, Am. J. Physiol. **205:**60, 1963.
19. Coleman, D.J., and Lizzi, F.L.: In vivo choroidal thickness measurement, Am. J. Ophthalmol. **88:**369-375, 1979.
20. Duke-Elder, S., and Wybar, K.C.: Anatomy of the visual system. In Duke-Elder, S., editor: System of ophthalmology, St. Louis, 1961, The C.V. Mosby Co.
21. Elgin, S.S.: Arteriovenous oxygen difference across the uveal tract of the dog eye, Invest. Ophthalmol. **3:**417, 1964.
22. Ernest, J.T., Stern, W.H., and Archer, D.B.: Submacular choroidal circulation, Am. J. Ophthalmol. **81:**574, 1976.
23. Feeney-Bruns, L., Berman, E.R., and Rothman, H.: Lipofuscin of human retinal pigment epithelium, Am. J. Ophthalmol. **90:**783, 1980.
24. Friedman, E., and Kuwabara, T.: The retinal pigment epithelium. 4. The damaging effects of radiant energy, Arch. Ophthalmol. **80:**265, 1968.
25. Geeraets, W.J., Williams, R.L., Chan, G., et al.: The loss of light energy in retina and choroid, Arch. Ophthalmol. **64:**158, 1960.
26. Gerald, L.J., Spak, K.E., and Hawkins, R.S.: An all expulsive hemorrhage during intraocular surgery, Trans. Am. Acad. Ophthalmol. Otolaryngol. **77:**119, 1973.
27. Heymann, M.A., Payne, B.D., Hoffman, J.I.E., and Rudolph, A.M.: Blood flow measurements with radionuclide-labelled particles, Prog. Cardiovasc. Dis. **29:**55, 1971.
28. Hayreh, S.S.: Submacula choroidal vascular pattern, Albrecht von Graefes Arch. Klin. Exp. Ophthalmol. **192:**181, 1974.
29. Hayreh, S.S.: Segmental distribution of posterior ciliary artery circulation, **59:**641, 1975.
30. Hayreh, S.S.: Segmental nature of the choroidal vasculature, Br. J. Ophthalmol. **59:**631, 1975.
31. Kinsey, V.E., Grant, M., and Cogan, D.G.: Water movement and the eye, Arch. Ophthalmol. **27:**242, 1942.
32. Last, R.J.: Wolff's Anatomy of the eye and orbit, ed. 6, Philadelphia, 1969, W.B. Saunders Co.
33. Laties, A.: Central retinal artery absence of adrenergic innervation to the intraocular branches, Arch. Ophthalmol. **77:**405, 1967.
34. Lincoff, A., and Kreissig, I.: Intravitreal behavior of perfluorocarbons, Dev. Ophthalmol. **2:**17-23, Basel, 1981, S. Karger AG.
35. Lincoff, H., Mardirossian, J., Lincoff, A., et al.: Intravitreal longevity of three perfluorocarbon gases, Arch. Ophthalmol. **98:**1610-1611, 1980.
36. Malik, A.B., Kaplan, J.E., and Saba, T.M.: Reference sample method for cardiac output and regional blood flow determinations in the rat, J. Appl. Physiol. **40:**472, 1976.
37. Moses, R.A.: Detachment of ciliary body: anatomical and physical considerations, Invest. Ophthalmol. **4:**935, 1965.
38. Parver, L.M., Auker, C., and Carpenter, B.O.: Choroidal blood flow as a heat dissipating mechanism in the macula, Am. J. Ophthalmol. **89:**641, 1980.
39. Pederson, J.E., Gaasterland, D.E., and MacLellan, H.M.: Experimental ciliochoroidal detachment: effect on intraocular pressure and aqueous humor flow, Arch. Ophthalmol. **97:**536, 1979.
40. Pieffer, B.A., Hassell, J.R., and Newsome, D.A.: Composition and interaction of components of monkey vitreous, Invest. Ophthalmol. Vis. Sci. **20:**201, 1981.
41. Rosenblum, P.D., Michels, R.G., Stark, W.J., and Taylor, H.R.: Choroidal ischemia after extracapsular cataract extraction by phacoemulsification of retina, **1:**263, 1981.
42. Ruiz, R.S., and Salmonsen, P.C.: Expulsive choroidal effusion: a complication of intraocular surgery, Arch. Ophthalmol. **94:**69, 1976.
43. Ruskell, G.L.: Facial parasympathetic innervation of the choroidal blood vessels in monkeys, Exp. Eye Res. **12:**1966, 1971.
44. Salzmann, M.: Anatomie und Histologie des menschlichen Augapfels, Leipzig, 1912.
45. Shimizu, K., and Ujiie, K.: Structure of ocular vessels, Tokyo, 1978, Igaku-Shoin.
46. Sinex, F.M.: Molecular genetics of aging. In Finch, C.E., and Hayflick, L., editors: The handbook of the biology of aging, New York, 1977, Van Nostrand Reinhold Co.
47. Spitznas, M., and Real, E.: Fracture faces, fenestrations, and junctions of endothelial cells in human choroidal vessels, Invest. Ophthalmol. **14:**98, 1975.

48. Torczynsky, E., and Tso, M.O.: The architecture of the choriocapillaris at the posterior pole, Am. J. Ophthalmol. **81:**428, 1976.

49. Wilcox, L.M., Keough, E.M., and Connolly, R.J.: Regional ischemia and compensatory vascular dynamics following selective tenotomy in primates, Exp. Eye Res. **33:**353, 1981.

50. Wilcox, L.M., Keough E.M., Connolly, R.J., and Hotte, C.E.: The contribution of blood flow by the anterior ciliary arteries to the anterior segment in the primate eye, Exp. Eye Res. **30:**167, 1980.

51. Wing, G.L., Blanchard, G.C., and Weiter, J.J.: Topography and age relationship of lipofuscin concentration in retinal pigment epithelium, Invest. Ophthalmol. Vis. Sci. **17:**600, 1978.

52. Wise, G.N., Dollery, C.T., and Henkind, P.: The retinal circulation, New York, 1971, Harper & Row, Publishers, chapters 6 and 7.

53. Zuckerman, R., and Weiter, J.J.: Oxygen transport in the bullfrog retina, Exp. Eye Res. **30:**117, 1980.

2

Practical biophysics of photocoagulation

J. Wallace McMeel

Photocoagulation techniques exploit the unique characteristics of the eye that permit transparency of certain wavelengths of light through the ocular media with absorption of this energy at structures that are not transparent to light. The ideal photocoagulation source has a maximum of absorption at the site to be treated but a minimum elsewhere. The photocoagulating source can affect the eye tissue either by producing a thermal reaction, as in all continuous-wave systems, or a physical disruption of tissue, as seen in the Q-switched pulse lasers. Because the latter have as yet not yet come into clinical usage of any significant degree, this discussion directs itself primarily to the thermal aspects of photocoagulation.

Most photocoagulation, fortunately, does not require great precision in either placement of burns or delivery of the energy to the tissue. This includes all the scatter type of treatments not in the immediate vicinity of the disc or macula and much of the treatment now being applied to the anterior segment. Over 90% of the photocoagulation now being administered is in this category.

However, optimal photocoagulation of certain structures requires not only a high degree of precision, but also observation of some of the basic physical laws that relate to optics, thermodynamics, and biophysics that pertain to the intraocular tissues.

LASER BEAM CHARACTERISTICS

For optimal understanding of the photocoagulation, a brief definition of terms is important. Total energy is that delivered at a given power setting over a specific period of time. To have clinical pertinence, one must know the power and the duration of time it is delivered. Also, the area to which the beam is being directy is also important. Thus the power density is the power divided by the exposed area. Once a difference in temperature develops, there is a temperature gradient between the warmer area to the adjacent cooler area, with a dissipation of heat from the former to the latter. If the rate of outflow of heat is equal to the rate of the energy delivered, there will not be a temperature rise. Thus there is a lower limit of power density below which no thermal lesion will be produced. On the other hand, there may be such a rapid buildup of energy that an explosive lesion is produced. Between these two limits, the variations in power density will produce variations in the photocoagulation lesion. The energy can be varied by a change of either the power or the time. Changing the power causes a more noticeable change in the lesion than a change in the duration of time does. Thus a slight change in power may change the severity of the lesion significantly, whereas a slight change in time should change the lesion only slightly.

Heat dissipation is relatively greater with a small spot size than with a large one. Therefore a small spot has a greater opportunity for heat to dissipate than a larger spot with the same power density in the same duration of time. Therefore, in a short burn where there is less time for heat dissipation, only small lesions can be safely produced. In larger lesions, the central area reaches a boiling point and an explosion can be produced. In burns of a longer duration, there is a greater opportunity of dissipation of heat, and it is safer to produce burns of a larger spot size.

The laser beam is prefocused. As the same amount of power is present in all portions of the beam, the power density depends on the cross-section area of the beam. It is greatest at the focal point and becomes less as the diameter of the beam enlarges anteriorly and posteriorly to the focal point. Therefore, when a spot size is increased, the power density decreases if there is no change in the power rating. To maintain an equivalent power density with a change in the size of the spot, one must increase the power on the laser when the spot size is increased. Conversely, to maintain an equivalent power density when the spot size is decreased, the power setting must also be decreased.

BIOPHYSICS OF BEAM ABSORPTION

Optical properties of light as it relates to the ocular tissues are also important considerations in the photocoagulation process. Light may be either scattered or absorbed. Scattering occurs when the light beam strikes particles having refractive indices that differ from that of the interstitial medium. Particles the size of a wavelength of light or longer, produce important scattering, as in a turbid vitreous or cataract. However, this degree of scattering is unrelated to the wavelength of the light. When the particles are smaller than the wavelength of light, scattering, though much less important, becomes related to the wavelength. Because scattering is proportional to the inverse of the fifth power of the wavelength, shorter wavelengths scatter to a greater degree than the longer wavelengths do. Even normal lens and vitreous have this type of scattering of light.

Absorption is the other property of light. The color of a pigment is attributable to its variable absorption coefficient at different wavelengths. Within the eye the three main light-absorptive pigments are xanthophyll, hemoglobin, and melanin. Each has specific characteristics, regarding not only its absorption spectrum, but also the location of each.

Yellow pigment, xanthophyll, is present in two tissues, the lens and the inner retinal layer at the fovea. Although the spectral absorption of each is slightly different, their main absorption band lies between 430 and 490 nm. Unfortunately, the stronger spectral band of the argon laser (488 nm) lies within these limits. The lens xanthophyll becomes progressively greater with age. The presence of macular xanthophyll in the superficial layer of the fovea has great importance in the selection of wavelengths for photocoagulation in the macula.

The oxygenated and reduced forms of hemoglobin have similar but not identical absorption spectra. The maximum coefficients of absorption coincide with two wavelengths of the spectral bands produced by the krypton laser, green (530.9 nm) and yellow (568.1 nm). Each of these bands represents approximately 10% of the power output of the krypton, and so a 12-watt laser is necessary to produce a clinically useful burn. Both the blue (488 nm) and green (514.5 nm) wavelengths of the argon laser are well absorbed by both oxygenated hemoglobin and reduced hemoglobin though somewhat less than krypton green and yellow. There is a sharp decrease in absorption of light from wavelengths longer than 590 nm, and so the red wavelength of krypton (647.1 nm) is minimally absorbed.

Melanin, the ubiquitous brown pigment that determines the coloration of nonalbinos, is abundant in the retina pigment epithelium and the choroid. It does not have specific absorption peaks in the visible spectrum as the other two pigments do. However, its absorption becomes slightly less at the longer wavelengths. Even so, it is the prime pigment that absorbs the red wavelength of the krypton laser because both xanthophyll and hemoglobin have low coefficients of absorption in this portion of the spectrum.

Optimal conditions for photocoagulation of ocular tissue are a maximal absorption within that tissue, so that a temperature rise is produced with minimal energy, and a low and uniform absorption and scattering of light in the tissues lying anteriorly, so that damage to these tissues is minimal. These latter tissues constitute the ocular media. The longer wavelengths are transmitted better, primarily because of a lesser scattering of light. The energy density may be lessened because scattering may enlarge the spot size slightly. Blue light is absorbed by yellow pigment. This is prevalent in nuclear sclerosis. Localized opacities, particularly in the lens, may produce a sharp reduction in energy delivery to the area of retina lying behind them. One must beware of increasing power while treating through these because, once beyond the light-absorbing influence of the opacity, dangerously high-power densities may be inadvertently placed on the retina.

The absorptive tissues themselves constitute the three layers throughout the fundus that extend anteriorly to the ora serrata, plus two sets of structures with special geographic location. The diffusely pigmented tissues are the neurosensory retina, the retina pigment epithelium, and the choroid. The structures with a specific topographic location in the eye are the macula and the retinal vessels.

The neurosensory retina has minimal thermal absorption to all but blue light. Because less scattering of the longer wavelengths of light, there is greater transmission of these wavelengths. Retinal capillaries (5 to 10 μm in diameter) probably absorb less than 5% of light, even for wavelengths for which hemoglobin has its greatest absorption coefficient.

Retina pigment epithelium absorbs the light and converts it to heat. The light-absorbing pigment is melanin. It absorbs all photocoagulating wavelenghts, but the shorter wavelengths are absorbed somewhat more than the longer. However, it is the first layer that absorbs the red wavelength of krypton (647 nm). Because of this absorption, it is a useful wavelength for coagulation at this level because of the minimal scattering and absorption in the ocular media. The choroid has two pigments, melanin and hemoglobin. Thermal trauma produced at this level is less than one might expect with the large amount of energy absorbed because of the heat-dissipating effects of the copious choroidal circulation.

The macula poses a very specific problem because of the concentration of macular xanthophyll at the fovea in the inner layers of the retina. This layer of xanthophyll extends less than a millimeter from the fovea. Macular xanthophyll absorbs wavelengths of 500 nm or less. Thus the blue wavelength (488 nm) of the argon blue laser is significantly more destructive than the green, yellow, and red wavelengths are. These latter pass through the xanthophyll and reach the deeper layers without causing tissue destruction in the superficial layers of the fovea. Because there is an increased melanin pigmentation in the retinal pigment epithelium at the macula, a lower threshold for coagulation using the other wavelengths is required.

Larger retinal vessels constitute linear focal areas of specific wavelength absorption because they contain oxyhemoglobin and hemoglobin. These pigments have a maximal coefficient of absorption very close to the wavelengths of krypton green (531 nm) and krypton yellow (568 nm). Theoretically these wavelengths should be optimal for occluding retinal vessels.

DELIVERY SYSTEM

In addition to the physical and biophysical parameters just noted, certain aspects of the delivery system are important in achieving optimal photocoagulation. These factors relate to precise focusing of the laser beam at the plane where the burns are being made and to the maintenance of exact placement of the beam on the structure being photocoagulated.

Focusing

The optics should ensure that the tissue being coagulated is receiving the spot size and power density that the ophthalmologist has selected on his panel. To achieve this, one must be aware of the following. Two optical systems are superimposed, that of the laser and that of the slitlamp biomicroscope. In the optical system of the slitlamp, an object at the focal plane of the slitlamp forms a sharp image at a plane viewed by the oculars. The observer than sees a sharp image if the oculars are properly focused on this image plane. An observer with a loss of accommodation must either be wearing glasses with correction for distance or have the ocular corrected for distance refractive correction. A reticle (cross hairs) in the ocular, when brought into sharp focus, ensures that the observer has a sharp focus of this image plane. The laser beam is prefocused by the optics of the photocoagulator delivery system to coincide with the plane of the focus of the slitlamp. The laser beam, focused by the photocoagulator optical system, has a cone of light on either side of its focal plane. Thus the spot size is altered by defocusing of the laser beam so that the portion of the cone of light coinciding with the selected diameter is in the plane of focus of the slitlamp. The only time the spot-size readings on the focusing mechanism of the photocoagulator are valid is when the structure to be photocoagulated is at the working distance of the slitlamp. The only time the prefocused slitlamp is at its working distance is when the unaccommodated operator has in sharp focus both the structures to be photocoagulated and the reticle.

The practical utilization of the above facts permits one to have the photocoagulation beam of the size intended by the operator. Although the importance of this is not generally recognized, alterations in the focus of the oculars by only two or three diopters can shift the energy density sufficiently to create hemorrhages instead of useful burns.

To adjust the focus of the photocoagulator properly, one must have the reticle in focus. This can be done by the fogging technique, in which the oculars' setting is +4 and then reduced until the cross hairs are in sharp focus. When in focus and with the spot size set at 50 μm, movement either forward or backward will enlarge the spot on the retina, commensurate to the diameter of the light cone at the plane. The spot size can be similarly altered during photocoagulation by a similar shift.

Beam alignment

The advent of fiber optics as a delivery system for the laser beam has relieved the instrument makers of many problems associated with maintaining alignment of the beam. In the system using mirrors, even minimal misalignment causes significant displacement in the beam with sharp loss of power. Periodic checking on the centration of the beam is the only means of ensuring delivery of the power desired. If one is working with a delivery system still using mirrors, checking must be done, unless one uses a system with a sensor at the final portion of the beam to ensure that the power of that site is within 10% of that at the end of the lasing tube.

Precise beam placement

Observation of the site of photocoagulation during application of the burn is particularly important in two circumstances: (1) photocoagulation where precision of application is important and (2) when a burn of a duration longer than 0.2 seconds is desired. The prime situations for which precise localization of the laser beam and longer burns are needed are in photocoagulation of new vessels at the disc and in submacular neovascularization. If the duration of the burn is three to five tenths of a second, it permits a significantly safer and more effective energy delivery to the tissue than burns of 0.1 second do. Thus an observation system having permanent filters protecting the photocoagulator allows one to monitor both the placement and intensity of the burn. Less desirable is a system in which dense filters fall in front of the observer's tubes to protect the eyes but in so doing block the view of the tissue being burned.

Precision and exact placement of the beam on the structure to be photocoagulated is important not only to observe the burn while it is being made, but also to being able to add a small enough spot so that there is a maximum of energy delivery to the small structure being photocaogulated and a minimum being delivered elsewhere. These small spot sizes (100 μm or less) are indicated when one is treating fine neovascularization. This is unlike treatment of the large vessels, for which spot sizes of 200 to 500 μm are more appropriate. The two sites at which this has clinical pertinence are fine vessels at the disc and fine vessels crossing the angle of the anterior chamber. A spot size of 100 μm or less can be produced only by delivery systems using mirrors. The fiberoptic bundle cannot produce as fine a focus as the mirror system because the light rays from each component fiber of the fiberoptic bundle are reflected from the wall of the fiber at a slightly different angle. This does not permit a totally coherent beam. Even when the spot-size selector indicates a spot of 50 μm, there is little likelihood that it is less than 200 μm.

SUMMARY

A résumé of the important factors in precise photocoagulation as they relate to the characteristics of the photocoagulating beam, the biophysics of pigment absorption by the intraocular tissues, and the pertinent information regarding the delivery system has been presented. Although cases requiring photocoagulation can be successfully treated without these factors being optimal, an increase in precision of one's photocoagulation techniques will result if one is aware of the multiple factors involved in photocoagulation.

3

Retinitis pigmentosa*

Alan C. Bird

During the last 15 years there have been major discoveries in the understanding of the metabolic systems that support the retinal receptors, and it is to be hoped that clinical sciences can take advantage of these advances. I propose to examine certain achievements of workers within different disciplines and to illustrate how these may reflect upon clinical science; it is clear that this summary cannot be comprehensive, but at least is may illustrate the potential benefits of such cooperative work.

CLINICIAN

Retinitis pigmentosa is a solitary manifestation of separate genetically determined disorders in which there is progressive loss of vision and the appearance of characteristic fundus abnormalities. It is likely that each disease contained within this family of disorders has a different etiology, a consideration important to the clinican, the researcher, and the therapist. To the clinician it is essential to be able to identify the inheritance of the disorder in order to give educated genetic advice. It is the responsibility of the clinician to subdivide retinitis pigmentosa into purer samples of disease, since without such a subdivision research is unlikely to be fruitful. It is unreasonable to expect a biochemist to define systemic biochemical abnormalities if blood is analyzed from a series of patients in which each subject has a different disorder. If the cause of retinal degeneration in an animal homolog of human retinitis pigmentosa is identified, the question is then raised as to whether the abnormality is relevant to human disease and, if so, which one. Moreover, if a metabolic abnormality is identified in one disease, it will not necessarily be found in others, and similarly if therapy is effective in one form of the disease, it may not be effective for all patients.

A subdivision of retinitis pigmentosa may be made on the basis of morphologic changes in the fundus, on the basis of inheritance of the disorder, and on the qualitative functional changes identified. Such observations may also give some clues as to the pathogenesis of the different forms of retinitis pigmentosa, or at least indicate in which cell system the primary disorders lie, and will also show in what way the defect interferes with cell function.

---

*Taken in part from Bird, A.C.: The Duke-Elder Lecture, 1981: Retinal receptor dystrophies, Trans. Ophthalmol. Soc. U.K. **101**(Part I):39-47, 1981.

Many attempts have been made by clinicians to subdivide retinitis pigmentosa on the basis of variations in the fundus changes produced and on the clinical behavior of the disorder.

Variation in the amount of pigment within the retina has been remarked upon, but it is unlikely that the "retinitis pigmentosa sine pigmento," as first described by Leber,[64] is a distinct disease entity, since patients with a visual loss but no pigmentation have been observed to develop pigment subsequently.[76,77,97] More recently it has been shown that patients without migration of pigment-containing cells have a short history of visual loss and have mild disease,[80] and it was concluded that these patients had mild or early but classic retinitis pigmentosa. This conclusion was further supported by the histologic observations of Eicholtz[29] who saw characteristic changes in the outer retina and showed that pigment-containing cells were in the retina though they had not been detected ophthalmoscopically.

Unilateral retinitis pigmentosa was reported as early as 1865 by Pedralgia, and ophthalmoscopic observations were corroborated by histopathologic examination 25 years later.[25] As the number of cases accumulated in the literature, the authenticity of the degeneration as being truly genetically determined was questioned. In 1952 François and Verriest reviewed the 56 cases reported up to that time[38] and concluded that only 10 cases were morphologically typical of genetically determined disease and were strictly unilateral. Subsequent reports[20,58] show that minor changes can be demonstrated in the apparently unaffected eye by sophisticated examination in some cases. Furthermore, Carr and Siegel[20] believed that the patients described by them and patients of some previous authors had retinal atrophy because of vascular disease rather than a heritable defect. It should be emphasized that no patient with unilateral retinitis pigmentosa had a family history of disease though in one case the parents were consanguineous.[23]

White deposits at the level of the outer retina, pigment epithelium, and Bruch's membrane have been identified in many patients with retinitis pigmentosa, and the term "retinitis punctata albescens" has been used to identify this variant of the disease. As yet no study has been undertaken to test the possibility that deposition indicates a specific pathogenetic mechanism peculiar to these patients though Deutman[24] expressed the view that retinitis punctata albescens did not necessarily represent a specific condition within retinitis pigmentosa. There is no doubt that white dots in the fundus are common in retinal degeneration because of hypovitaminosis A in dietary deficiency[16,33,65] and in abetalipoproteinemia. Therefore it would seem justifiable to reexamine the proposal that retinitis pigmentosa with prominent white deposits represents a specific disorder within the group of conditions.

Retinitis pigmentosa has been described with involvement of only one sector of the fundus.[11,43] The disease usually affects the lower half of the retina with the loss of visual function in the upper field.[34] Rarely the sectors of involvement by disease are in the superior fundus,[84] the nasal fundus,[99] or the temporal fundus.[2] In most cases the reported inheritance is autosomal dominant and the regional distribution of the disease is common to affected members of the family.[34,43,50,66] However such cases also appear in families with relatives who have affection of the whole fundus,[61] and some are heterozygous X-linked retinitis pigmentosa.[12,61] Krill and co-workers[61] and Bird[12] also showed by fluorescein angiography that minor changes were often more widespread than might be appreciated by opthalmoscopy with white light and that sector retinitis pigmentosa may imply an area of maximum disease rather than an area exclusively involved by disease.

Fluorescein angiography has also been used to demonstrate retinal edema, which occurs in many patients with well-documented retinitis pigmentosa.[37,39,52,73,78] It has been shown that edema may occur in any of the genetic subdivisions of retinitis pigmentosa,[93] and it has been concluded that edema of the retina is a nonspecific response to receptor degeneration rather than indicating a disease entity different from that in patients without edema. The pathogenesis of this response is unknown, and no evidence was found for immunologic changes specific to these patients.[94]

Attempts have been made to subdivide X-linked retinitis pigmentosa using the severity of involvement in heterozygous females as the basis of such a subdivision. In only a few of the early reports was retinal degeneration described in heterozygotes,[53,68] but profound visual loss in heterozygotes was first reported by McKenzie[67] in New Zealand. He studied a family in which there was very strong evidence that retinitis pigmentosa had been inherited as an X-linked disease, and yet there were two women who became blind in the ninth decade of life and two who were younger with less severe visual loss. Eight women appeared to have transmitted the gene to their sons without themselves having symptoms of visual loss. McKenzie concluded that the gene was usually recessive but was sufficiently penetrant to cause disease in a proportion of the females carrying it. The inheritance in this family was termed "X-linked intermediate." In 1960 Kobayashi described a family with even more frequent and severe involvement of the females by disease.[57] In this family five heterozygous females had retinitis pigmentosa, 11 had some stigmas of the disease and four were normal. It was therefore suggested that X-linked disease could be separated into three identifiable conditions: X-linked recessive, X-linked intermediate, and X-linked dominant. However, subsequent experience indicates that there is intrafamilial variation in the severity of disease in heterozygotes and that there is no justification for separating X-linked retinitis pigmentosa on the basis of the severity of the disease in women.[8,12] An abnormal fundus reflex in females heterozygous for X-linked retinitis pigmentosa was described as early as 1914 by Diem.[26] Falls and Cotterman[30] reported that this abnormal reflex was the most common expression of the heterozygous state in their study of a family, and others have emphasized the importance of this opthalmoscopic sign.[36,51,60,85,88,100,101] However Schappert-Kimmijser[90] could identify this abnormal reflex in females of only one family out of eight and concluded that although this sign might be helpful if present, the absence of reflex did not indicate a normal genotype. In our experience these abnormal reflexes are seen consistently in some families and not in others, and the presence or absence of this reflex may represent a means of subdividing X-linked retinitis pigmentosa.

Leber's amaurosis, since its original description, has been considered a distinct disorder. In a study by Alström and Olson[3] it appeared to be a monofactorial autosomal recessive affection though Henkes and Verduin[46] believed that several forms of the disease existed and that at least some were indistinguishable from severe autosomal recessive retinitis pigmentosa. Although there is no doubt that Leber's amaurosis presents a unique problem to the clinician, there is little justification for the distinction from autosomal recessive retinitis pigmentosa.

Of all the clinical variants of retinitis pigmentosa described, in sectorial retinitis pigmentosa only is there sufficient evidence to accept this variant of retinitis pigmentosa as a disease distinct from others. For retinitis pigmentosa sine pigmento, retinitis pigmentosa with macular edema, retinitis punctata albescens, and unilateral retinitis pigmentosa the evidence is inconclusive or implies that the morphologic variation does not identify a specific disease entity. Whether or not the presence of a tapetal reflex in heterozygotes of X-linked retinitis pigmentosa represents a means of distinguishing two disorders within this genetic group remains to be tested by further observation.

GENETICIST

Recognition of the inheritance of retinitis pigmentosa allows the disease to be divided into three categories: autosomal dominant, autosomal recessive, and X linked.

The original studies of relative genetic frequency reported from Belgium and Switzerland appear to show that X-linked disease was rare, autosomal recessive disease was common, and autosomal dominant disease was present in 10% to 20% of families studied.[4,98] Experience in London is different in that X-linked disease appears to be much more common,[12,55,56] representing 12% to 20% of the total in different analyses.

A second feature of all studies is that in a large percentage of families the mode of inheritance cannot be identified from the family history. About 50% of probands in most reports were either simplex cases or had an affected sibling only. This situation is clearly unsatisfactory both for the clinician attempting to give genetic advice and for the researcher wishing to categorize the disorder.

Marcelle Jay has recently analyzed the probable genetic status of simplex and duplex cases.[54] She has found that there is an excess of males among the affected members, a feature common to many reported series.[75,76] This implies clearly that a significant percentage of these patients have X-linked disease. In such families, other affected males were not identified by history alone and the heterozygous state of female relatives was not identified by clinical examination or else female relatives were not seen. Segregational analysis also demonstrates that it is unlikely that all patients from simpex and duplex families have autosomal recessive disease. This conclusion is in contrast with assumptions made in the past.[81,88] Segregational analysis further showed that most if not all severe disease could be autosomal recessive or X linked but that in mild disease this was most unlikely. The alternative genetic status in these mild cases without affected relatives outside their own sibship could be autosomal dominant with reduced penetrance or variable expressivity, X-linked heterozygotes without identified relatives, or a new autosomal dominant mutation; finally it is conceivable that some of these patients do not have genetic disease but their abnormality represents a phenocopy.

This system is clearly useful for analyzing affected populations but does not help the clinican greatly when faced by a patient wishing genetic advice. It is nevertheless reasonable to assume that in the presence of severe disease children will not be affected though if the individual is male it is clearly necessary to examine his daughters before their childbearing age since they might be heterozygous for X-linked retinitis pigmentosa. If the disease is mild, there is a possibility of children being affected though the disorder is likely also to be mild, with the exception of female heterozygotes for X-linked retinitis pigmentosa whose sons might be severely handicapped. These guidelines emphasize the need for the clinician to make every attempt to determine the inheritance of the disorder by examining affected relatives. This is particularly important when one is faced with severely affected males and mildly affected females where asymptomatic female relatives should be seen.

PSYCHOPHYSICIST

When is was discovered that rods subserved night vision,[22,91,92] it was assumed that the rods were the cells primarily affected by retinitis pigmentosa, since this would explain the initial symptom of poor night vision so typical of the disorders. The initial field defect in retinitis pigmentosa is usually in the midzone corresponding to the ophthalmoscopic changes in the postequatorial fundus. This part of the fundus has a high rod population,[83] but even in early disease visula loss can be identified under photopic conditions to a white light, indicating that both receptor systems are affected in patients with few symptoms. The observation of poor night vision and midzone functional loss are compatible with two separate disease processes. On the one hand, it is possible that the rod cells are affected initially because of a defect in the metabolic processes peculiar to rods, with secondary attrition of cones. Alternatively, the disease process may affect the peripheral receptors preferentially, with rods and cones being equally vulnerable. Several attempts have been made to analyze the quality of visual loss in order to compare rod and cone function. Mandelbaum,[69] demonstrated that in the paracentral region there was loss of sensitivity of both cones and rods but that the sensitivity interval between the two was reduced. Zeavin and Wald[105] found that there was loss of rod function within 25 degrees of fixation, a loss that was complete in some patients, and that more peripheral loss of function could be detected later. They also identified loss of cone sensitivity, but it was not clear to them whether the loss of rod function was initiated at the same time as loss of cone function or later. The function of foveal cones remained normal until very late disease, a finding that differed from the one reported by Mandelbaum[69] and by Haig and Saltzman.[44] The three patients studied by Zeavin and Wald[105] were derived from one family with dominantly inherited disease, and they found identical functional deficit in each.

More recently it has been confirmed that qualitative visual loss in members of a single family is relatively constant but that there is interfamilial variation.[72] In some families, all members appear to have loss of rod sensitivity in the presence of relatively well preserved cone thresholds, whereas in others there is simultaneous degeneration of both rod and cone thresholds. Such analyses of retinal function appear to provide further evidence that there are multiple forms of autosomal dominant retinitis pigmentosa, and they provide a means of subdividing this genetic group. Massof and Finkelstein[72] have also found different patterns of visual loss in patients from simplex and multiplex families. The information derived from these studies may also provide some guide as to the pathogeneses of these disorders. In some conditions there appears to be a metabolic defect that affects rods rather than cones, whereas in others both cones and rods are affected simultaneously in the midperiphery.

ELECTROPHYSIOLOGIST

Soon after its introduction into clinical practice, the electroretinogram (ERG) amplitudes were found to be reduced in retinitis pigmentosa.[5,13,27,35,86] Riggs[86] believed that receptor-cell dysfunction alone was insufficient to account for the absence of the ERG, and he suggested that peripheral receptor degeneration caused short-circuiting between the retina and the choroid so that potentials generated in the retina could not be recorded by a distant corneal electrode. He quoted previous observations by Bush[17] in support of this hypothesis, that is, that multiple perforation of the retina causes extinction of the ERG without causing massive retinal destruction.

More recently it has been shown that in early and mild disease the photopic ERG potentials are reduced in the presence of a normal scotopic response[42] and that with better recording systems and averaging techniques ERG potentials can be recorded in more advanced disease.[6,45] These observations suggest that the reduction of the ERG in retinitis pigmentosa is attributable to receptor dysfunction alone.

By use of a *Ganzfeld* ('total-field') stimulus and an adapting background illumination, qualitative analyses of the ERG in different forms of retinitis pigmentosa have been undertaken. It has been postulated that diminution of the ERG potential in the presence of normal latency implies reduced population of normal receptors whereas a prolonged implicit time implies widespread receptor dysfunction.[8] It was found that in patients of a single pedigree with dominantly inherited retinitis pigmentosa the rod ERG component was reduced in amplitude and in latency and the cone component was normal,[7] whereas in dominant retinitis pigmentosa with reduced penetrance the cone responses were also abnormal.[10] This finding provided additional evidence to support the concept that these were distinct and that the disease process in each was different. Further studies would be required to identify if further subdivision of dominant retinitis pigmentosa could be made on this basis. In X-linked disease, both cone and rod responses were delayed and reduced.[9]

Comparative studies have also been undertaken on members of families identified as having primary rod loss and with midperipheral affection of both cones and rods as identified by Massof and Finkelstein.[72] The ERG responses reflect precisely the changes in function that might have been expected from the psychophysical results, which thus support the proposed subdivision of dominant inheritance with complete penetrance on functional grounds.

PHOTOCHEMISTS

Our knowledge concerning the nature of the defect within the visual receptors has been greatly enhanced by study of rhodopsin kinetics and visual thresholds. It has been demonstrated that the reduction of light sensitivity on rods can be attributed wholly to reduced rhodopsin content in the rod outer segments.[48,87] At first this appears to be difficult to reconcile with the observation that bleaching 5% of rhodopsin increases the rod threshold above that of cones.[89] The apparent anomaly may be explained by the fact that the outer-segment membrane changes accompanying exposure to light[14] may alter rod function independently of the quantity of available bleachable rhodopsin. It is with these considerations in mind that Ripps and co-workers[87] postulated that in retinitis pigmentosa the outer-segment membrane rhodopsin concentration was normal and that the abnormal quantity of rhodopsin but with otherwise normal function could be best explained by rods having short outer segments; the alternative explanation that there is a reduced population of normal rods was not totally excluded.

Ripps, Brin, and Weale[87] recorded the amount of rhodopsin in a patient with vitamin A deficiency whose rod threshold was above that of the cone threshold. This patient appeared to have only a small reduction in rhodopsin and was similar in that regard to partially bleached retina. Clearly this observation has to be repeated but, if confirmed, gives positive evidence that vitamin A deficiency, at whatever metabolic level, is not responsible for reduced rod function in those patients with retinitis pigmentosa in whom rhodopsin measurements have been made. It would seem justifiable to discontinue search for vitamin A metabolic defects in retinitis pigmentosa at present. However, if a patient with retinitis pigmentosa were found to have a significant reduction in rod function but a relatively good preservation of rhodopsin contents, investigation of the vitamin A metabolism would be justifiable and would carry a high chance of success.

It is encouraging to the clinician that studies of rhodopsin kinetics in two conditions of slow dark adaptation has identified totally different pathogenic mechanisms in each. In fundus albipunctatus it has been clearly shown that the slow dark adaptation can be explained by slow regeneration of rhodopsin,[19] whereas in Oguchi's disease rhodopsin regeneration is normal and slow dark adaptation must relate to some other defect in the reestablishment of rod transduction systems.[18]

HISTOPATHOLOGIST

With few exceptions all the histopathologic reports of retinal dystrophies are based on inadequately preserved material and, with one exception, describe the most advanced stages of these disorders.[28] All demonstrate that the retinal receptors and outer retina generally are most affected by disease, with relative preservation of the inner layers of the retina. Electron microscopic studies are few but reveal that in advanced autosomal dominant disease the only remaining photoreceptors in the retina are cones.[59,95]

Our knowledge of photoreceptor changes associated with the early stages of retinitis pigmentosa is limited to a single specimen obtained from a 23-year-old male suffering from X-linked disease.[96] All the remaining photoreceptor cells in this patient exhibited abnormalities, but there were great differences between the central retina and the periphery. Central foveal cones were reduced in number by about half, with the shortened and severely distorted outer segments containing vesiculated and disrupted membranes. Progressively more advanced disruption was seen as the study was extended from the fovea to the midperiphery. In the parafoveal regions the cones had lost their outer segments though the inner segments remained relatively healthy; peripheral to this region there was progressively more disorganization of the inner segment as the distance from the fovea increased. In the area of major atrophy there were only occasional vestiges of cones identified by their swollen ellipsoid nuclei, but in some cases ellipsoids protruded through the outer limiting membrane. In the most peripheral retina the inner and outer segments of both rods and cones became apparent, being progressively more organized as the study moved to the far periphery. In this region both rods and cones had outer segments at least 25% shorter than those from a comparable location in a normal eye, and although the disc membranes of the rods were well ordered and near normal in appearance, those of the cones were both disorientated and vesiculated. Very similar changes were demonstrated by Marshall in an elderly patient who was heterozygous for X-linked retinitis pigmentosa.[71]

These studies demonstrate two interesting features. It appears that there is progressive loss of the outer segment in cones whereas the inner segment may remain relatively healthy and nuclear cell death may occur long after the outer segment is lost. By contrast, rods that were identified appeared to have relatively normal inner segments though slightly shortened. The degree of shortening was less than what had been postulated as a result of psychophysical testing.[87] There must be some doubt concerning the validity of comparing the histopathologic features in one eye with the results derived from psychophysical testing in another. Nevertheless, if such a correlation were made, the shortening of rod outer segments by 25% to 50% is much less than what would have been predicted as a result of rhodopsin estimations where a shortening of 90% would have been necessary. Histopathologic reports tend to support an alternative explanation that reduction in the number of rods together with shortening of the rod outer segments contribute to loss of function.

BASIC SCIENTISTS

During the past 15 years we have seen a great increase in the knowledge of the micrometabolism of retinal cells and in particular of the interaction of photoreceptor cells and the pigment epithelium. The potential value of basic scientific work to clinical ophthalmology can be illustrated by two examples.

It is now several years since the demonstration that rod outer segments were subject to continuous renewal with progressive addition of new discs at the proximal end of the outer segment and the shedding of packets of discs from the outer-segment distal tip.[103,104] The shed outer-segment discs are phagocytosed by the retinal pigment epithelium[15,104] and the disc membranes are degraded as a result of lysosomal activity within the pigment epithelial cells. The potential relevance of this phagocytic role as the pigment epithelium to disease was demonstrated in the Royal College of Surgeons (RCS) rat. In this animal a genetic defect results in the failure of the pigment epithelium to engulf shed outer-segment material so that debris accumulates between the pigment epithelium and photoreceptors, with subsequent degeneration of the photoreceptors.[15,47,63] Several possible metabolic faults could account for this failure. It was possible that outer-segment shedding was abnormal, that the pigment epithelium was incapable of phagocytosing outer-membrane discs, or that the membrane recognition system between the two was at fault. In a very elegant experiment LaVail and Mullen[62] created a rat that had a mosaic of pigmented cells from a normal rat and nonpigmented cells from an RCS rat. The pattern of degeneration in these animals strongly implied that the metabolic fault lay in the pigment epithelial cell rather than in the receptor.

During the last decade cell biochemists have concentrated their efforts on elucidating the mechanisms of cell transduction after the exposure to light. Particularly impressive is the information generated by studies of cyclic nucleotides. In general, these chemical systems appear to act as intracellular messengers and are important in the regulation of cellular function. It has been shown that cyclic guanosine monophosphate (GMP) is highly concentrated in rod outer segments[79] and that the level of cyclic GMP alters with light exposure of the retina.[102] The synthesis of cyclic GMP from guanosine triphosphate (GTP) is catalyzed by the enzyme guanylate cyclase, which has high activity in the rod outer segment.[31,41,106] Cyclic GMP is hydrolyzed to 5'-GMP by phosphodiesterase, which is also concentrated in the rod outer segment and is bound to the outer-segment cell membrane.[21,40,70,74] It is believed that the bleaching of rhodopsin by light enhances phosphodiesterase activity and this promotes hydrolysis of cyclic GMP in rod outer segments. The activation of this enzyme by bleached rhodopsin is rapid and quite compatible with the predicted time frame of rod transduction. With low levels of illumination, bleaching of one molecule of rhodopsin results in hydrolysis of 1000 to 2000 molecules of cyclic GMP within 100 to 300 milliseconds. There is therefore good evidence that this system may provide a means of amplification of the primary physicochemical event and represent an integral part of cell transduction.

An abnormality in cyclic GMP metabolism has been detected in inherited retinal diseases of mice and dogs. In mice homozygous for the RD (retinal degeneration) gene and Irish setters with photoreceptor degeneration there appears to be an abnormal accumulation of cyclic GMP because of abnormally low phosphodiesterase activity, and it has been postulated that this metabolic abnormality is important to the pathogenesis of the disorder.[1,31]

In a recent study by Hollyfield et al.[49] it has been demonstrated that experimental manipulation of cyclic GMP may have a specific effect of retinal photoreceptors. Abnormally high levels of receptor cyclic GMP were induced in organ culture by use of phosphodiesterase inhibitors or by addition of cyclic GMP to the medium. In the non-differentiated retina high levels of cyclic nucleotide prevented receptor cell differentiation, whereas in the differentiated normal retina the nucleotide initiated specific photoreceptor degeneration resembling that seen in human retinitis pigmentosa.

Farber et al.[32] have now shown that in the cone-dominant retinas there is specific concentration of adenosine 35-monophosphate (AMP) is the outer segments, which varies with light. It is clear that the studies undertaken for cyclic GMP metabolism in rods could equally well be undertaken for cyclic AMP in cones, and it is likely that these studies will provide equally important results with respect to one receptor cell function.

CONCLUSION

It is encouraging for the clinician interested in retinal disorders that workers in a variety of special fields have produced a great deal of new information concerning the inheritance of the disorders within retinitis pigmentosa, the functional properties of the diseased retina, and the metabolic characteristics of normal and diseased retinae. It is particularly encouraging that homologs of human disease exist and that there have been major achievements in a search for the pathogenesis of disorders in those animals. It is evident that little of the new knowledge can be applied directly to human disease at present and certainly none has produced any particular clues as to possible treatment of disorders within retinitis pigmentosa. Nevertheless, it is clear that the discoveries made by scientists from each discipline are relevant to work in the related fields and that the potential application to clinical ophthalmology is evident.

REFERENCES

1. Aguirre, G., Farber, D.B., Lolley, R.N., Fletcher, T., and Chader, G.J.: Rod-cone dysplasia in Irish setters: a defect in cyclic GMP metabolism in visual cells, Science **201:**1133-1134, 1978.
2. Alezzandrini, A.: Retinitis pigmentosa in symmetric quadrants, Am. J. Ophthalmol. **60:**1160, 1965.
3. Alström, C.H., and Olson, O.: Heredo-retinopathia congenitalis monohybrida recessiva autosomalis, Hereditas **43:**1-178, 1957.
4. Amman, F., Klein, D., and Franceschetti, A.: Genetic and epidemiological investigations on pigmentary degeneration of the retina and allied disorders in Switzerland, J. Neurol. Sci. **2:**183-196, 1965.
5. Armington, J.C.: Electrical responses of the light adapted eye, J. Optic Soc. Am. **43:**450-456, 1953.
6. Armington, J.C., Gouras, P., Tepas, D.I., and Gunkel, R.: Detection of the electroretinogram in retinitis pigmentosa, Exp. Eye Res. **1:**74-80, 1961.

7. Berson, E.L., Gouras, P., and Gunkel, R.D.: Progressive cone degeneration dominantly inherited, Arch. Ophthalmol. **80:**77, 1968.

8. Berson, E.L., Gouras, P., and Hoff, M.: Temporal aspects of the electroretinogram, Arch. Ophthalmol. **81:**207-214, 1969.

9. Berson, E.L., Gouras, P., and Gunkel, R.D., and Myrianthopoulos, N.C.: Rod and cone responses in sex-linked retinitis pigmentosa, Arch. Ophthalmol. **81:**215-225, 1969.

10. Berson, E.L., Gouras, P., Gunkel, R.D., and Myrianthopoulos, N.C.: Dominant retinitis pigmentosa with reduced penetrance, Arch. Ophthalmol. **81:**226-235, 1969.

11. Bietti, G.B.: Über familiäres Vorkommen von 'Retinitis punctata albescens' (verbunden mit 'Dystrophia marginalis cristallinea corneae'): Glitzern des Glaskörpers und anderen degenerativen Augenveränderungen, Klin. Monatsbl. Augenheilkd. **99:**737-756, 1937.

12. Bird, A.C.: X-linked retinitis pigmentosa, Br. J. Ophthalmol. **59:**177-199, 1975.

13. Björk, A., and Karps, G.: The electroretinogram in retinitis pigmentosa, Acta Ophthalmol. **29:**361-371, 1951.

14. Blasie, J.K.: The location of photopigment molecules in the cross-section of frog retinal receptor disk membranes, Biophys. J. **12:**191-204, 1972.

15. Bok, D., and Hall, M.O.: The role of the pigment epithelium in the etiology of inherited retinal dystrophy in the rat, J. Cell Biol. **49:**664-682, 1971.

16. Bors, F., and Fells, P.: Reversal of the complications of self-induced vitamin A deficiency, Br. J. Ophthalmol. **55:**210, 1971.

17. Bush, N.R.: The electrical responses of the eye before and after perforation of the retina, doctoral thesis, Brown University, 1951; cited by Riggs (see reference 86).

18. Carr, R.E., and Ripps, H.: Rhodopsin kinetics and rod adaptation in Oguchi's disease, Invest. Ophthalmol. **6:**426, 1967.

19. Carr, R.E., Ripps, H., and Siegel, I.M.: Visual pigment kinetics and adaptation in fundus albipunctatus, Docum. Ophthalmol. **4:**193, 1974, The Hague.

20. Carr, R.E., and Siegel, I.M.: Retinal function in patients treated with indomethacin, Am. J. Ophthalmol. **75:**302-306, 1973.

21. Chader, G., Johnson, M., Fletcher, R., and Bensinger, R.: Cyclic nucleotide phosphodiesterase of the bovine retina: activity, subcellular distribution and kinetic parameters, J. Neurochem. **22:**93-99, 1974.

22. Charpentier, A.: De la vision avec diverses parties de la rétine, Arch. Physiol. Norm. et Pathol. ser. 2 (Paris) **4:**894-945, 1877.

23. Cordier, J., Reny, A., and Seigneur, J.P.: Rétinite pigmentaire unilatérale, Bull. Soc. Ophtalmol. Fr. **66:**224-227, 1966.

24. Deutman, A.F.: Rod-cone dystrophy. In Krill, A.E., editor: Hereditary retinal and choroidal diseases, New York, 1977, Harper & Row, Publishers.

25. Deutschmann, R.: Einseitige typische Retinitis pigmentosa mit pathologisch anatomischem Befund, Beitr. Augenheilkd. **1**(3):69-80, 1891.

26. Diem, M.: Retinitis punctata albescens et pigmentosa, Klin. Monatsbl. Augenheilkd. **53:**371, 1914.

27. Dodt, E., and Wadensten, L.: The use of flicker electroretinography in the human eye, Acta Ophthalmol. **32:**165-180, 1954.

28. Duke-Elder, S., and Dobree, J.H.: Diseases of the retina. In Duke-Elder, S., editor: System of ophthalmology, vol. 10, London, 1967, Henry Kimpton (St. Louis, The C.V. Mosby Co.).

29. Eicholtz, W.: Histologie der Retinopathia pigmentosa cum et sine pigmento, Klin. Monatsbl. Augenheilkd. **164:**467-475, 1974.

30. Falls, H.F., and Cotterman, C.W.: Choroido-retinal degeneration: a sex-linked form in which heterozygous women exhibit a tapetal-like retinal reflex, Arch Ophthalmol. **40:**685-703, 1948.

31. Faber, D.B., and Lolley, R.N.: Enzymic basis for cyclic GMP accumulation in degenerative photoreceptor cells of mouse retina, J. Cyclic Nucleotide Res. **2**(3):139-148, 1976.

32. Farber, D.B., Souza, D.W., Chase, D.G., and Lolley, R.N.: Cyclic nucleotides of cone-dominant retina: reduction of cyclic AMP levels by light and by cone degeneration, Invest. Ophthalmol. Vis. Sci. **20**(1):24-31, 1981.

33. Fells P., and Bors, F.: Ocular complications of self-induced vitamin A deficiency, Trans. Ophthalmol. Soc. UK **89:**221, 1969.

34. Fledelius, H., and Simonsen, S.E.: A family with bilateral symmetrical sectorial pigmentary retinal lesion, Acta Ophthalmol. **48:**14-22, 1970.

35. François, J.: L'électro-rétinographie dans les dégénérescences tapéto-rétiniennes périphériques et centrales, Ann. Ocul. **185:**843-856, 1952.

36. François, J.: Chorioretinal degeneration of retinitis pigmentosa of intermediate sex-linked hereditary, Docum. Ophthalmol. **16:**111-127, 1962.

37. François, J., De Laey, J.J., and Verbraeken, H.: L'œdème cystoïde de la macula, Bull. Soc. Belg. Ophtalmol. **161:**708, 1971.

38. François J., and Verriest, G.: Rétinopathie pigmentaire unilatérale, Ophthalmologica **124:**65-88, 1952.

39. ffytche, T.J.: Cystoid maculopathy in retinitis pigmentosa, Trans. Ophthalmol. Soc. UK **92:**265, 1972.

40. Goridis, C., Virmaux, N., Cailla, H.L., and DeLaage, M.A.: Rapid, light-induced changes of retinal cyclia GMP levels, **49**(2):167, 1974.

41. Goridis, C., Virmaux, N., Weller, M., et al.: Role of cyclic nucleotides in photoreceptor function. In Bonting, S.L., editor: Transmitters in the visual process, Oxford, 1976, Pergamon Press, Ltd.

42. Gouras, P., and Carr, R.E.: Electrophysiological studies in early retinitis pigmentosa, Arch. Ophthalmol. **72:**104-110, 1964.

43. Haase, W., and Hellner, K.A.: Über familiäre bilaterale sektorenförmige Retinopathia pigmentosa, Klin. Monatsbl. Augenheilkd. **147:**365, 1965.

44. Haig, C., and Saltzman, S.L.: Correlation of visual acuity and absolute luminance threshold in retinitis pigmentosa, Arch. Ophthalmol. **53:**109, 1955.

45. Henkes, H.E., van der Tweel, L., and van der Gon, J.J.: Selective amplication of the electroretinogram, Ophthalmologica (Basel) **132:**140, 1956.

46. Henkes, H.E., and Verduin, P.C.: Dysgenesis of abiotrophy? A differentiation with the help of the electroretinogram (ERG) and electro-oculogram (EOG) in Leber's congenital amaurosis, Ophthalmologica (Basel) **145:**144-160, 1963.

47. Herron, W.L., Riegel, B.W., Myers, D.E., et al.: Retinal dystrophy in the rat: a pigment epithelial disease, Invest. Ophthalmol. **8:**595-604, 1969.

48. Higham, V.N., and Weale, R.A.: Rhodopsin density and visual threshold in retinitis pigmentosa, Am. J. Ophthalmol. **75:**822-832, 1973.

49. Hollyfield, J.G., Rayborn, M.E., Farber, D.B., and Lolley, R.N.: Selective photoreceptor degeneration. In Hollyfield, J.G., and Vidrio, E.A., editors: Structure of the eye, Amsterdam, 1982, Elsevier-North Holland.

50. Hommer, K.: Das ERG bei sektorenförmiger Retinitis pigmentosa (Retinopathia pigmentosa), Graefes Arch. Ophthalmol. **161:**16-26, 1959.

51. Hussels, I.E.: Une famille atteinte de rétinopathie pigmentaire liée au sexe, de maladie de Parkinson et d'autres troubles neuro-psychiatriques, thesis no. 3064, Geneva, 1967, Médecine et Hygiène.

52. Hyvärinen, L, Maumenee, A.E., Kelly, J., and Cantollino, S.: Fluorescein angiographic findings in retinitis pigmentosa, Am. J. Ophthalmol. **71:**17-26, 1971.

53. Janssen, O.: Inaugural dissertation, Munster, 1938; quoted by François, 1962 (see reference 36).

54. Jay, M.: Personal communication, 1981.

55. Jay, B., and Bird, A.C.: X-linked retinitis pigmentosa, Trans. Am. Ophthalmol. Otolaryngol. **77:**641-651, 1973.

56. Jay, B., Bird, A.C., and Jay, M.: The incidence of the different genetic forms of retinitis pigmentosa, Doc. Ophthalmol. **17:**313-318, 1978, The Hague.

57. Kobayashi, F.: Genetic study on retinitis pigmentosa, Jpn. J. Ophthalmol. **4:**82, 1960.

58. Kolb, H., and Galloway, N.R.: Three cases of unilateral pigmentary degeneration, Br. J. Ophthalmol. **48:**471-479, 1964.

59. Kolb, H., and Gouras, P.: Electron microscopic observations of human retinitis pigmentosa, dominantly inherited, Invest. Ophthalmol. **13:**487-498, 1974.

60. Krill, A.E.: X-chromosomal–linked diseases affecting the eye: status of the heterozygote, Trans. Am. Ophthalmol. **67:**535, 1969.

61. Krill, A.E., Archer, D.B., and Martin, D.: Sector retinitis pigmentosa, Am. J. Ophthalmol. **69:**977, 1970.

62. LaVail, M.M., and Mullen, R.J.: Experimental chimeras, Adv. Exp. Med. Biol. **77:**153-173, 1977.

63. LaVail, M.M., Sidman, R.L., and O'Neil, D.: Photoreceptor–pigment epithelial cell relationships in rats with inherited retinal degeneration: radioautographic and electron microscope evidence for a dual source of extra-lamellar material, J. Cell Biol. **53:**185-209, 1972.

64. Leber, T.: Ueber anomale Formen der Retinitis pigmentosa, Graefes Arch. Ophthalmol. **17**(1):314-341, 1871.

65. Levy, N.S., and Toskes, P.P.: Fundus albipunctatus and vitamin A deficiency, Am. J. Ophthalmol. **78**:926, 1974.

66. Lisch, K.: Isolierte Entwicklungsstörungen, Med. Monatsschr. **14**:720-725, 1960.

67. McKenzie, D.S.: The inheritance of retinitis pigmentosa in one family, Trans. Ophthalmol. Soc. N.Z. **5**:79-82, 1951.

68. McQuarrie, M.D.: Two pedigrees of hereditary blindess in man, J. Genet. **30**:147-153, 1935.

69. Mandelbaum, J.: Dark adaptation: some physiologic and clinical considerations, Arch. Ophthalmol. **26**:203-239, 1941.

70. Manthorpe, M., and McConnell, D.G.: Cyclic nucleotide phosphodiesterases associated with bovine retinal outer segment fragments, Biochem. Biophys. Acta **403**(2):438-445, 1975.

71. Marshall, J.: Personal communication, 1981.

72. Massof, R.W., and Finkelstein, D.: Rod sensitivity relative to cone sensitivity in retinitis pigmentosa, Invest. Ophthalmol. Vis. Sci. **18**:263-272, 1979.

73. Metge, P., Chovet, M., Ebagosti, A., and Tassy, A.: Œdème maculaire cystoïde dans la rétinopathie pigmentaire, Bull. Soc. Ophthalmol. Fr. **74**:119-122, 1974.

74. Miki, N.: [Role of cyclic GMP in visual process: activation of cyclic GMP phosphodiesterase by light and ATP (author's translation)], Protein Nucleic Acid Enzyme (Tokyo) **21**(8):605-611, Aug. 1976.

75. Nettleship, E.: On retinitis pigmentosa and allied diseases, Roy. Lond. Ophthalmol. Hosp. Rep. **17**:1-56, 1907.

76. Nettleship, E.: On retinitis pigmentosa and allied diseases, Roy. Lond. Ophthalmol. Hosp. Rep. **17**:333-426, 1908.

77. Nettleship, E.: A note on the progress of some cases of retinitis pigmentosa sine pigmento and of retinitis pigmentosa punctata albescens, Roy. Lond. Ophthalmol. Hosp. Rep. **19**:123-129, 1914.

78. Notting, J.G.A., and Deutman, A.F.: In de Laey, J.J., editor: International Symposium on Fluoroangiography, Doc. Ophthalmol. **9**:439, 1976.

79. Orr, H.T., Lowry, O.H., Cohen, A.I., et al.: Distribution of 3′,5′-cyclic AMP and 3′,5′-cyclic GMP in rabbit retina in vivo: selective effects of dark and light adaptation and ischemia, Proc. Natl. Acad. Sci. U.S.A. **73**(12):4442-4445, 1976.

80. Pearlman, J.T., Flood, T.P., and Seiff, J.R.: Retinitis pigmentosa without pigment, Am. J. Ophthalmol. **81**:417, 1976.

81. Pearlman, J.T., Saxton, J., Hoffman, G., and Carson, S.: Unilateral retinitis pigmentosa sine pigmento, Br. J. Ophthalmol. **60**:354, 1976.

82. Pedraglia: Klinische Beobachtungen: Retinitis pigmentosa, Klin. Monatsbl. Augenheilkd **3**:114, 1865.

83. Polyak, S.L.: The retina, Chicago, 1941, University of Chicago Press.

84. Ragnetti, E.: Su una forma atipica di retinosi pigmentosa, Boll. Oculist. **41**:617-625, 1962.

85. Ricci, A., Ammann, F., and Franceschetti, A.: Reflet tapétoïde réversible (phénomène de Mizuo inverse) chez des conductrices de rétinopathie pigmentaire récessive liée au sexe, Bull. Soc. Fr. Ophtalmol. **76**:31-35, 1963.

86. Riggs, L.A.: Electroretinography in cases of nightblindness, Am. J. Ophthalmol. **38**:70-78, 1954.

87. Ripps, H., Brin, K.P., and Weale, R.A.: Rhodopsin and visual threshold in retinitis pigmentosa, Invest. Ophthalmol. **17**:735, 1978.

88. Roberts, J.A.F.: An introduction to medical genetics, London, 1959, Oxford University Press.

89. Rushton, W.A.H.: Dark adaptation and the regeneration of rhodopsin, J. Physiol. **156**:166-178, 1961.

90. Schappert-Kimmijser, J.: Les dégénérescences tapéto-rétiniennes du type X chromosomal aux Pays-Bas, Bull. Soc. Fr. Ophthalmol. **76**:122-129, 1963.

91. Schultze, M.: Zur Anatomie und Physiologie der Retina, Arch. Mikr. Anat. **2**:175-286, 1866.

92. Schultze, M.: Über Stäbchen und Zäpfchen der Retina, Arch. Mikr. Anat. **3**:215-267, 1867.

93. Spalton, D.J., Bird, A.C., and Cleary, P.E.: Retinitis pigmentosa and retinal oedema, Br. J. Ophthalmol. **62**:174, 1978.

94. Spalton, D.J., Rahi, A.H.S., and Bird, A.C.: Immunological studies in retinitis pigmentosa associated with retinal vascular leakage, Br. J. Ophthalmol. **62**:183, 1978.

95. Szamier, R.B., and Berson, E.L.: Retinal ultrastructure in advanced retinitis pigmentosa, Invest. Ophalmol. Vis. Sci. **16**(10):947-962, 1977.

96. Szamier, R.B., Berson, E.L., Klein, R., and Meyers, S.: Sex-linked retinitis pigmentosa: ultrastructure of photoreceptor and pigment epithelium, Invest. Ophthalmol. Vis. Sci. **18**(2):145-160, 1979.
97. Usher, C.H.: On the inheritance of retinitis pigmentosa, with notes of cases, Roy. Lond. Ophthalmol. Hosp. Rep. **19**:130-236, 1914.
98. Voipio, H., Grippenburg, V., Raitta, C., and Horsman, H.A.: Retinitis pigmentosa: a preliminary report, Hereditas **52**:247, 1964.
99. Vukovich, V.: Das ERG bei retinitis pigmentosa mit bitemporalem Gesichtsfeldausfall, Graefes Arch. Ophthalmol. **161**:27-31, 1959.
100. Warburg, M., and Simonsen, S.E.: Sex-linked recessive retinitis pigmentosa: a preliminary study of the carriers, Acta Ophthalmol. **46**:494, 1968.
101. Weiner, R.L., and Falls, H.F.: Intermediate sex-linked retinitis pigmentosa, Arch. Ophthalmol. **53**:530-535, 1955.
102. Woodruff, M.L., and Bownds, M.D.: Amplitude, kinetics, and reversibility of a light induced decrease in guanosine 3'5'-cyclic monophosphate in frog photoreceptor membranes, J. Gen. Physiol. **73**(5):629-653, 1979.
103. Young, R.W.: The renewal of photoreceptor cell outer segments, J. Cell Biol. **33**:61-72, 1967.
104. Young, R.W., and Bok, A.: Participation of the retinal pigment epithelium in the rod outer segment renewal process, J. Cell Biol. **42**:392-403, 1969.
105. Zeavin, B.H., and Wald, G.: Rod and cone vision in retinitis pigmentosa, Am. J. Ophthalmol. **42**:253-269, 1956.
106. Zimmerman, W.F., Daemen, F.J., and Bonting, S.L.: Distribution of enzyme activities in subcellular fractions of bovine retina, J. Biol. Chem. **251**:4700-4705, 1976.

4

Subretinal neovascularization

Stephen J. Ryan

Disciform macular degeneration, a term first used by Oeller[37] in 1903, is a clinico-pathologic condition resulting from a variety of diseases affecting the macula. It should be emphasized that the disciform response is not an etiologic diagnosis, but rather a characteristic response of the macula to a condition or disease that affects the retinal pigment epithelium–Bruch's membrane–choriocapillaris complex.[45] Verhoeff and Grossman[55] in 1937 described the histopathologic disciform process and Gass,[19] in his landmark monograph in 1967, described the broad spectrum of the clinical and pathologic manifestations that characterize this entity. Recently, an investigation was conducted to test the various hypotheses regarding the pathogenesis of disciform macular degeneration; these studies were performed on rhesus monkeys *(Macaca mulatta)* in which we had reproducibly induced subretinal neovascularization by argon laser photocoagulation.[43,44]

Although the disciform process was first described over 100 years ago,[38] the basic pathogenesis of this entity has not been clearly established. Originally, it was believed that the etiology and pathology were primarily retinal. Although it was later documented that this hypothesis, which incriminated retinal circulation, was incorrect,[55] Junius and Kuhnt[28] did provide the first major description of the morphologic evolution of the response. In his landmark monograph, Gass[19] correlated the clinical and histopathologic findings as the basis for the pathogenesis of this entity. More recently, Blair and Aaberg,[5] Teeters and Bird,[53,54] Sarks,[47] and Green and Key[25] confirmed and expanded on Gass's findings that the most common cause of the disciform response is senile macular degeneration. However, there are at least 20 other conditions that can result in an identical disciform response: these include angioid streaks,* blunt trauma,† laser therapy,[14,16] myopia,[21] presumed ocular histoplasmosis syndrome,‡ and various idiopathic processes.[8] This last group of conditions affects primarily young adults and results in discrete macular lesions rather than the more typical diffuse retinal pigment epithelial changes of the disciform response associated with senile macular degeneration.

This was funded in part by grant EY01545, National Institutes of Health.
*See references 4, 7, 10-12, 15, 20-22, 24, 26, 49, 51.
†See references 9, 18, 23, 27, 36, 39, 52.
‡See references 13, 19, 30, 35, 40, 42, 46, 56.

Again, it must be emphasized that the disciform process is a response to some other condition and is not an etiologic diagnosis. Maumenee[32-34] stressed that the disciform process is the common macular response to many clinical entities. Correlation of the histologic appearance with the clinical findings in the predisciform state seems to be most promising in providing additional information for understanding the pathogenesis of the disciform process.* In addition, the availability of a reproducible animal model of the neovascularization that characterizes the macular disciform process[2,3,43,44,46] should allow for more rapid proliferation of information on the basic pathogenesis, evolution, and natural history of the disciform response.

MATERIALS AND METHODS

Adult rhesus monkeys *(Macaca mulatta)* were utilized in these studies because of their distinct retinal and choroidal circulation and because they have a macula similar to that in man. In addition, because this primate has been extensively studied in the course of numerous other scientific investigations, details of ocular morphology, physiology, and ultrastructure are well documented.

Base-line fundus photographs and fluorescein angiograms were obtained on each animal before any manipulative procedures; these were repeated on several occasions during follow-up study. Monkeys were sedated with 50 to 100 mg of ketamine or 30 mg phencyclidine, administered intramuscularly; this was followed by an injection of 37 to 70 mg of pentobarbital intravenously. Pupils were dilated with topical 10% phenylephrine HCl and 1% tropicamide. The animals were divided into 10 treatment groups: laser breaks, branch vein occlusion, laser occlusion of both temporal branch veins, laser breaks with ensuing branch vein occlusion, venous occlusion followed by laser breaks, laser breaks and macular vein occlusions at the same session, laser breaks and branch vein occlusion at the same session, laser breaks only (grid method), laser (grid method) with inferotemporal branch vein occlusion at the same session, and application of laser grid.

A length of approximately 2000 µm of the retinal branch vein was occluded by a two-step process; the vein was put into spasm by use of the Coherent Radiation System 900 argon laser delivered through a Zeiss slitlamp with a Goldmann contact lens. Approximately 500 µm, 0.5 second, 200 to 300 milliwatt (mW) spots were delivered to the retinal branch vein; this was followed immediately by 200 µm, 0.5 second, 200 to 500 mW spots. Approximately 150 spots were required to achieve complete occlusion. Eyes were then enucleated and preserved in cold 2% glutaraldehyde–2% paraformaldehyde overnight. Selected lesions were then chosen for histopathologic and ultrastructural correlation.

Sections of selected lesions were exposed to 3-diaminobenzidine and H_2O_2 as substrates for the peroxidase enzyme. Alternate sections were postfixed in osmium tetroxide and embedded in Epon-Araldite for sectioning for electron microscopy. In addition, 1 µm thick sections were stained with toluidine blue for light microscopic correlation. Thin sections were also stained with uranyl acetate and lead citrate for examination with a Zeiss 10 electron microscope.

---

*See references 17, 25, 29, 47, 48, 50, 57.

RESULTS

Table 4-1 shows the number of animals treated and the number that developed subretinal neovascularization in each of the 10 groups.

I. Laser breaks. Two maculas revealed individual cluster breaks in and around them; these produced a whitening of the retina at the laser burn site that was directly proportional to the energy of the laser application. Although choroidal and retinal hemorrhages occurred, these did not correlate well with laser intensity. None of these spots progressed to subretinal neovascularization as determined by fundus photography or fluorescein angiography. Light and electron microscopy of these lesions at 1 and 16 weeks after injury revealed no disruption of Bruch's membrane after laser intensity of less than 500 mW with spots of 50 and 100 μm. There was, however, considerable disruption of the retina and choroid adjacent to Bruch's membrane with herniation of the retina into the choroid and destruction and scarring of the outer retina, retinal pigment epithelium, and adjacent structures, as previously reported after photocoagulation.[1,6,31]

II. Branch vein occlusions. Four monkeys were subjected to laser occlusion of retinal branch veins—three to the inferotemporal vein and one to the superotemporal vein. Retinal and preretinal hemorrhage, which prevented further laser treatment, was not an uncommon complication.

All four of these eyes, which were studied by indirect ophthalmoscopy, fundus stereophotography, and fluorescein angiography, revealed clinical features consistent with retinal vein occlusion. On fluorescein angiography there was the typical delayed venous return, distended and tortuous veins, and dilated capillary beds; fluorescein was seen to leak from dilated capillaries in the area of occlusion.

These four eyes were followed clinically for 7 months; during this time two of the four occlusions remained distinct, both clinically and angiographically. Although the remaining two continued to show some signs of occlusion, this partially recanalized. None of these four eyes progressed to develop subretinal neovascularization.

Table 4-1. Incidence of subretinal neovascularization (SRN) after laser application

	Category	Eyes treated	Eyes with SRN
Group I	Laser breaks only in Bruch's membrane (scatter approach)	2	0
Group II	Branch vein occlusion only	4	0
Group III	Branch vein occlusion (both temporal branches)	5	0
Group IV	Laser breaks followed 1 week later by branch vein occlusion	2	2
Group V	Branch vein occlusion followed 1 week later by laser breaks	2	2
Group VI	Laser breaks and macular vein occlusions at same session	4	3
Group VII	Laser breaks and branch vein occlusion at same session	2	2
Group VIII	Laser breaks only (grid)	5	4
Group IX	Laser breaks (grid) and inferotemporal branch vein occlusion at same session	11	9
Group X	Application of laser grid	29	26

III. Laser occlusion of both temporal branch veins. Both temporal branch veins were occluded in five eyes, all of which developed clinical and fluorescein angiographically confirmed occlusion. One of these eyes developed a fibrous, relatively avascular scar after retinal hemorrhage and edema. In several of these eyes the vitreous remained hazy for weeks, secondary to vitreous hemorrhage. Three of these eyes were followed for 5 months, and the other two were followed for 4 months; no subretinal neovascularization developed.

IV. Laser breaks with ensuing branch vein occlusion. In these eyes, and all eyes used subsequently, a variable number of laser spots was applied in a "sideways-T" formation; the length was along the horizontal raphe in the papillomacular bundle and the top was distal to the fovea, allowing for comparison of the effects in ischemic versus nonischemic retina at a similar distance from the fovea. Some lesions were discrete, whereas others were placed in aggregates so that lesions actually overlapped, thereby forming a confluent scar.

Two eyes in the study had laser breaks followed by inferotemporal branch vein occlusion within 1 week. One eye developed subretinal neovascularization in four of 10 discrete laser spots; neovascularization was first noted as early as 7 weeks after laser treatment. These tufts of neovascularization were located along the horizontal raphe in an area that proved to be ischemic when studied by fluorescein angiography.

The second eye developed subretinal neovascularization in six of 12 discrete laser breaks, all situated along the line of the horizontal raphe. After more than 9 months of follow-up study, this neovascularization persists.

V. Venous occlusion followed by laser breaks. In two eyes, inferotemporal branch vein occlusion occurred first, which was subsequently followed within 1 week by laser breaks. One of these eyes also underwent occlusion of all macular draining veins secondary to recanalization of the branch vein. The other eye, which developed a large macular serous detachment and extensive preretinal, retinal, and choroidal hemorrhage, developed subretinal neovascularization in four of seven discrete laser breaks. As in group IV eyes, these neovascularization tufts were located along the horizontal raphe. During the course of the 7-month follow-up study, most of the neovascularization involuted, leaving only relatively avascular scars.

VI. Laser breaks and macular vein occlusions at the same session. Four eyes were subjected to laser breaks, which were followed immediately by laser coagulation of all macular draining veins. In three of these four eyes the laser breaks progressed to confluent scars. Over the 4- to 5-month follow-up study, two of the eyes revealed new vessels developing and involuting; the other eye revealed two discrete neovascular tufts, which still persist.

VII. Laser breaks and branch vein occlusion at the same session. Two eyes underwent laser breaks immediately followed by inferotemporal branch vein occlusion. Each of these eyes developed extensive subretinal neovascularization that was subsequently confirmed by light and electron microscopy.

Because it was apparent from these pilot studies that subretinal neovascularization could not be reproducibly caused with any degree of certainty by these procedures, other methods were sought. Thus, a celluloid grid was designed that allows for spacing of discrete lesions at various distances from the fovea. This grid is superimposed on a fundus photograph or fluorescein angiogram of the fovea and projected at the time of laser application. This grid pinpoints positions at uniform distances from the center of the capillary free zone of the fovea; distances on the fundus are measured in multiples or fractions of the foveal capillary free zone, which in the rhesus monkey is 200 microns in diameter.[41] In these studies we also used a higher intensity spot (750-950 milliwatts) than in earlier pilot studies; this may well have been a significant factor in the reproducible induction of subretinal neovascularization.

VIII. Laser breaks only (grid method). Subretinal neovascularization developed in four of five eyes in which laser breaks were placed at fixed distances by means of the celluloid grid. These were followed for over three months.

IX. Laser breaks (grid method) with inferotemporal branch vein occlusion at the same session. The combination of branch vein occlusion and laser breaks placed with use of the Celluloid grid resulted in subretinal neovascularization in nine of 11 eyes. These have been followed for 2 to 5 months.

X. Application of laser grid. After the results noted above were obtained, a number of variables were further investigated and a series of laser grid applications were made. The method of laser photocoagulation was then adjusted to produce disruption or a break in Bruch's membrane. The individual laser spots were 100 μm in diameter, 0.1 second in duration, and at 200 to 700 mW. Representative cases are shown in Fig. 4-1 and 4-2. One month after laser photocoagulation eight spots were placed in the macular region in 29 eyes. Of these, 26 developed at least one area of subretinal neovascularization, which progressed over the 3-month follow-up period. At one of the sites of subretinal neovascularization there is seen a retinal choroidal anastomosis (Fig. 4-1), which was also seen in several other eyes in these experiments. Of 216 laser spots applied to the macular region in these eyes, 90 developed unequivocal subretinal neovascularization; this was documented by fluorescein angiography which showed leakage of dye with accumulation in a serous detachment of the sensory retina.

In an effort to determine whether or not the location of a laser burn had a significant effect on development of subretinal neovascularization, laser burns were also applied to the periphery. Approximately two spots were placed in each quadrant in the vicinity of the equator. Serous separation was seen in several cases, as was hemorrhage. In fact, of 18 eyes receiving peripheral laser application to the periphery, only one developed subretinal neovascularization, and in only one single spot. Thus, of a total of 144 peripheral laser spots, only one developed subretinal neovascularization.

To further define the role of location in relation to subretinal neovascularization, a grid of eight spots was applied nasal to the optic nerve head. Fig. 4-2, *A* and *B,* shows the pattern immediately after laser photocoagulation. Ten weeks later there is presence of a fibrous scar with a few small vessels present at the edge; although there is some fluorescein staining on angiography, the pattern is not typical of subretinal neovascularization. Of a total of 32 laser spots applied nasal to the optic nerve head, only one developed any evidence of subretinal neovascularization.

Of the 90 subretinal neovascularization foci induced, 19 remain active; the other 71 eventually underwent involution. Of those that became involuted, the average time from development to involution was 16 weeks, with a standard deviation of 13.2 weeks and a range of 2 to 55 weeks. Of the same 90 sites of subretinal neovascularization, 27 had at least one episode of spontaneous hemorrhage.

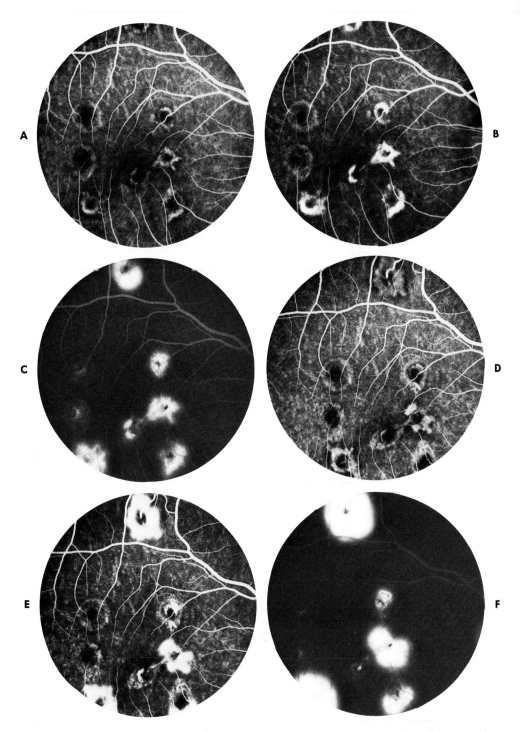

Fig. 4-1. Monkey 495. Laser photocoagulation. **A** to **C,** One month after laser burn. **D** to **F,** Four months after laser burn. **A,** Early venous stage documents beginning subretinal neovascularization at five of the eight sites of laser break. **B,** Middle venous phase demonstrates hyperfluorescence and accumulation of dye at these five sites. **C,** Late venous stage of the angiogram documents leakage of dye at each of these five sites 4 months after laser burn. **D,** Early venous stage. Note that there is retinal choroidal anastomosis at the superiormost site of laser photocoagulation. The beginning of tufts of subretinal neovascularization are apparent in five of the eight sites of laser burn. **E,** Middle venous phase demonstrates leakage of dye becoming more profuse in appearance. **F,** Late venous phase. Note the intense fluorescein stain of the serous fluid beneath the sensory retina. This dye pattern is typical of active subretinal neovascularization. (From Ryan, S.J.: Albrecht von Graefes Arch. Klin. Ophthalmol. **215:**29, 1980.)

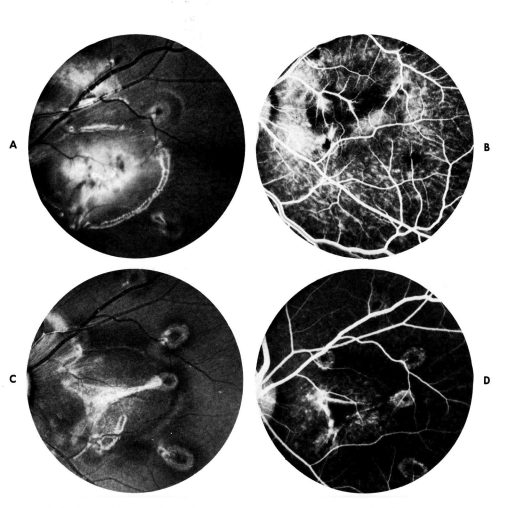

Fig. 4-2. Monkey 499. This monkey underwent application of the laser grid, nasal to the optic nerve head. **A,** Seven weeks after breaks placed by grid, there has been extensive choroidal hemorrhage and leakage of serum from one of the sites closest to the midlevel of the optic nerve head. **B,** The corresponding fluorescein angiogram and arteriovenous phase at this initial stage (7 weeks after grid application) demonstrates blockage related to hemorrhage and ultimately shows diffuse leakage from this site of laser break. **C,** Fundus shows resolution 17 weeks after breaks, predominantly in the form of a fibrous scar. It has assumed a triangular configuration. **D,** Also 17 weeks after breaks, the corresponding fluorescein angiogram in the late venous phase demonstrates that there is staining along the edges of the scar compatible with neovascularization as part of the fibrous scarring process. However, since this is predominantly a fibrotic response rather than active neovascular leak, it is not classified as subretinal neovascularization. (From Ryan, S.J.: Albrecht von Graefes Arch. Klin. Ophthalmol. **215:**29, 1980.)

DISCUSSION

With the ultimate goal of producing subretinal neovascularization in an experimental animal model, argon laser photocoagulation was used to produce breaks in Bruch's membrane. In preliminary studies, such laser-induced breaks did not result in subretinal neovascularization. However, when higher intensities were applied, neovascular tissue did ensue. The Bruch's membrane break by itself is not considered the basis of the neovascularization; rather, it is believed that the inflammatory response, which is elicited by the higher intensity laser photocoagulation, may be the essential feature required for development of subretinal neovascularization. This inflammatory response invariably includes a large population of macrophages; it is believed that these macrophages may release a vasoproliferative factor. In addition, hemorrhage alone may further stimulate the inflammatory response. Local ischemia resulting from the choriocapillaris may also elicit a vasoproliferative response, in association with or without the inflammatory response.

In our studies, the rate of subretinal neovascularization after branch vein occlusion alone was very low (1 of 9 eyes), and the one lesion produced did not, in fact, have the classic appearance of subretinal neovascularization. As later studies showed, the break in Bruch's membrane is far more important than the vein occlusion in the subsequent development of neovascularization. In fact, we no longer employ occlusion of the branch vein in the production of experimental subretinal neovascularization.

Using the grid method for laser application, a reproducible model of subretinal neovascularization was achieved. With this technique, subretinal neovascularization developed in 26 of 29 eyes and in 90 of 216 (42%) spots; the average time for development was 4 weeks.

When laser photocoagulation was applied to the periphery, only one of 144 spots developed subretinal neovascularization; similarly, only one of 32 spots located nasally to the nerve head developed subretinal neovascularization. This would seem to support the clinical observation that the macular region is far more susceptible to subretinal neovascularization than the peripheral retinais.

It should also be noted that the majority of neovascularization sites eventually involuted, on an average within 16 weeks after induction. On the other hand, other of these sites have remained actively neovascular for more than 18 months.

Histopathologic studies have helped us understand the pathogenesis of the disciform response; however, many variables are difficult to study in a clinical situation and detailed pathologic and ultrastructural studies cannot be correlated directly with clinical observations, particularly at early phases of the condition. Although we acknowledge that the etiology of this animal model is not that of human senile macular degeneration, the technique reported here does result in subretinal neovascularization, which is the determinant of the disciform response. Morphologic correlation at various stages of evolution in this animal model will provide a better understanding of the clinical observations and concepts related to disciform macular degeneration; such correlation is clearly an important goal for future research.

REFERENCES

1. Apple, D.J.: Histopathology of xenon arc and argon laser photocoagulation. In L'Esperance, F.A., Jr., editor: Current diagnosis and management of chorioretinal diseases, St. Louis, 1977, The C.V. Mosby Co.
2. Archer, D.B.: Neovascularization of the retina, Trans. Ophthalmol. Soc. U.K. **96:**471, 1976.

3. Archer, D.B., Ernest, J.T., and Newell, F.W.: Classification of branch retinal vein obstruction, Trans. Am. Acad. Ophthalmol. Otolaryngol. **78:**148, 1974.

4. Behr, C.: Ein weiterer Beitrag zur Anatomie und zur Pathogenese der scheibenförmigen Degeneration am hinteren Augenpol, Z. Augenheilkd. **75:**216, 1931.

5. Blair, C.J., and Aaberg, T.M.: Massive subretinal exudation associated with senile macular degeneration, Am. J. Ophthalmol. **71:**639, 1971.

6. Campbell, C.J., Rittler, M.C., and Swope, C.H.: The ocular effects produced by experimental lasers. IV. The argon laser, Am. J. Ophthalmol. **67:**672, 1969.

7. Clay, G.E., and Baird, J.M.: Angioid streaks of the choroid and pseudoxanthoma elasticum, South. Med. J. **31:**127, 1938.

8. Cleasby, G.W.: Idiopathic focal subretinal neovascularization, Am. J. Ophthalmol. **81:**590, 1976.

9. Doyne, R.W.: Choroidal and retinal changes: the result of blows on the eyes, Trans. Ophthalmol. Soc. U.K. **9:**128, 1889.

10. Doyne, R.W., and Stephenson, S.: Retinitis circinata, Trans. Ophthalmol. Soc. U.K. **24:**91, 1904.

11. Elwyn, H.: Heredodegenerations and heredoconstitutional defects of the retina, Arch. Ophthalmol. **53:**619, 1955.

12. Feingold, M.: Senile external exudative macular retinitis with remarks on similar tumor formation in a case of angioid streaks, Trans. Am. Ophthalmol. Soc. **22:**268, 1924.

13. Fine, S.L., and Patz, A.: Comparison of xenon arc and argon laser photocoagulation in ocular histoplasmosis, Int. Ophthalmol. Clin. **15:**259, 1975.

14. Fine, S.L., Patz, A., and Orth, D.: Subretinal neovascularization developing after prophylactic argon laser photocoagulation of atrophic macular scar, Am. J. Ophthalmol. **82:**352, 1976.

15. François, J., and Deweer, J.P.: Dégénérescence maculaire sénile et hérédité, Ann. d'Ocul. **185:**136, 1952.

16. François, J., and de Laey, J.J., and Cambie, E.: Neovascularization after argon laser photocoagulation of macular lesions, Am. J. Ophthalmol. **79:**206, 1975.

17. Frank, R.N., Green, W.R., and Pollack, I.P.: Senile macular degeneration: clinicopathologic correlations of a case in the predisciform stage, Am. J. Ophthalmol. **75:**587, 1973.

18. Fuller, B., and Gitter, K.A.: Traumatic choroidal rupture with late serous detachment of the macula: report of successful argon laser treatment, Arch. Ophthalmol. **89:**354, 1973.

19. Gass, J.D.M.: Pathogenesis of disciform detachment of the neuroepithelium, Am. J. Ophthalmol. **63:**573, 1967.

20. Gass, J.D.M., and Clarkson, J.G.: Angioid streaks and disciform macular detachment in Paget's disease (osteitis deformans), Am. J. Ophthalmol. **75:**576, 1973.

21. Gass, J.D.M.: Stereoscopic atlas of macular disease: diagnosis and treatment, ed. 2, St. Louis, 1977, The C.V. Mosby Co.

22. Gifford, S.R., and Cushman, B.: Certain retinopathies due to changes in the lamina vitrea, Arch. Ophthalmol. **23:**60, 1940.

23. Goldberg, M.F.: Chorioretinal vascular anastomoses after blunt trauma to the eye, Am. J. Ophthalmol. **83:**892, 1976.

24. Goldzieher, W.: Über die Hutchinson'sche Veränderung des Augenhintergrundes, Wien. Med. Wochenschr. **37:**861, 1887.

25. Green, W.R., and Key, S.M.: Senile macular degeneration: a histopathological study, Trans. Am. Ophthalmol. Soc. **75:**180, 1977.

26. Hibbert, G.: A case of Greenblad-Strandberg syndrome with disciform degeneration of the maculae, Br. J. Ophthalmol. **32:**478, 1948.

27. Hilton, G.F.: Late serosanguineous detachment of the macula after traumatic choroidal rupture, Am. J. Ophthalmol. **79:**997, 1975.

28. Junius, P., and Kuhnt, H.: Die scheibenförmige Entartung der Netzhautmitte (Degeneratio maculae lateae disciformis), Berlin, 1926, S. Karger AG.

29. Kornzweig, A.L.: The eye in old age. V. Disease of the macula: a clinicopathologic study, Am. J. Ophthalmol. **60:**835, 1965.

30. Krill, A.E., and Archer, D.: Choroidal neovascularization in multifocal (presumed histoplasmic) choroiditis, Arch. Ophthalmol. **85:**595, 1970.

31. Marshall, J., Hamilton, A.M., and Bird, A.C.: Histopathology of ruby and argon laser lesions in monkey and human retina, Br. J. Ophthalmol. **59:**610, 1975.

32. Maumenee, A.E.: Serous and hemorrhagic disciform detachment of the macula, Trans. Pac. Coast Otoophthalmol. Soc. **40:**139, 1959.

33. Maumenee, A.E.: Clinical manifestations (symposium; macular disease), Trans. Am. Acad. Ophthalmol. Otolaryngol. **69:**605, 1965.

34. Maumenee, A.E.: Further advances in the study of the macula, Arch. Ophthalmol. **78:**151, 1967.

35. Maumenee, A.E., and Ryan, S.J.: Photocoagulation of disciform macular lesions in the ocular histoplasmosis syndrome, Am. J. Ophthalmol. **75:**13, 1973.

36. Neame, H.: Retinitis proliferans: clinical report, with illustrations of a case which developed after gunshot wound of orbit, pathological report with notes of other cases and review, Trans. Ophthalmol. Soc. U.K. **43:**296, 1923.

37. Oeller, J.: Atlas seltener ophthalmoskopischer Befunde, Wiesbaden, 1900-1905, J.F. Bergmann.

38. Pagenstecher, H., and Genth, C.: Atlas der pathologischen Anatomie des Augenapfels, Wiesbaden, 1875, C.W. Kriedel.

39. Paton, D., and Goldberg, M.F.: Management of ocular injuries, Philadelphia, 1976, W.B. Saunders Co.

40. Pau, H.: Die zentrale seröse Retinitis oder Chorioretinitis (Retinopathie oder Chorioretinopathie) und die zentrale hämorrhagische Chorioretinitis (juvenile disciforme Makulaablösung; fokale hämorrhagische Chorioiditis, presumed Histoplasmosis), Klin. Monatsbl. Augenheilkd. **175:**634, 1979.

41. Polyak, S.: The vertebrate visual system, Chicago, 1957, University of Chicago Press.

42. Ryan, S.J.: De novo subretinal neovascularization in the histoplasmosis syndrome, Arch. Ophthalmol. **94:**329, 1976.

43. Ryan, S.J.: The development of an experimental model of subretinal neovascularization in disciform macular degeneration, Trans. Am. Ophthalmol. Soc. **77:**707, 1979.

44. Ryan, S.J.: Subretinal neovascularization after argon laser photocoagulation, Albrecht von Graefes Arch. Klin. Ophthalmol. **215:**29, 1980.

45. Ryan, S.J., Mittl, R.N., and Maumenee, A.E.: The disciform response: an historical perspective, Albrecht von Graefes Arch. Klin. Ophthalmol. **215:**1, 1980.

46. Ryan, S.J. Mittl, R.N., and Maumenee, A.E.: Enzymatic mechanically induced subretinal neovascularization, Albrecht von Graefes Arch. Klin. Ophthalmol. **215:**21, 1980.

47. Sarks, S.H.: New vessel formation beneath the retinal pigment epithelium in senile eyes, Br. J. Ophthalmol. **57:**951, 1973.

48. Sarks, S.H.: Ageing and degeneration in the macular region: a clinicopathologic study, Br. J. Ophthalmol. **60:**324, 1976.

49. Shields, J.A., Federman, J.L., and Tomer, T.L.: Angioid streaks. I. Ophthalmoscopic variations and diagnostic problems, Br. J. Ophthalmol. **59:**257, 1975.

50. Small, M.L., Green, W.R., and Alpar, J.J.: Senile macular degeneration: a clinicopathologic correlation of two cases with neovascularization beneath the retinal pigment epithelium, Arch. Ophthalmol. **94:**601, 1976.

51. Smith, J.L., Gass, J.D.M., and Justice, J.: Fluorescein fundus photography of angioid streaks, Br. J. Ophthalmol. **48:**517, 1964.

52. Smith, R.E., Kelley, J.D., and Harbin, T.S.: Late macular complications of choroidal ruptures, Am. J. Ophthalmol. **77:**650, 1974.

53. Teeters, V.W., and Bird, A.C.: A clinical study of the vascularity of senile disciform macular degeneration, Am. J. Ophthalmol. **75:**53, 1973.

54. Teeters, V.W., and Bird, A.C.: The development of neovascularization of senile disciform macular degeneration, Am. J. Ophthalmol. **76:**1, 1973.

55. Verhoeff, F.H., and Grossman, H.P.: Pathogenesis of disciform degeneration of the macula, Arch. Ophthalmol. **18:**561, 1937.

56. Woods, A.C., and Wahlen, H.E.: The probable role of benign histoplasmosis in the etiology of granulomatous uveitis, Trans. Am. Ophthalmol. Soc. **57:**318, 1959.

57. Zauberman, H., Ivrey, M., and Sachs, U.: The macular vessels in predisciform and disciform senile macular degeneration, Am. J. Ophthalmol. **70:**498, 1970.

5

Treatment of neovascularization, vitreous hemorrhage, and retinal detachment in sickle cell retinopathy

Morton F. Goldberg
Lee M. Jampol*

If it were not for the neovascular and hemorrhagic sequelae of proliferative sickle cell retinopathy (PSR), this retinal disorder would be largely free of ocular symptoms. Occasionally, rigid, sickled erythrocytes occlude perifoveal arterioles or even the central retinal artery, and visual disability can occur suddenly in these ischemic circumstances. In most patients with sickle cell disease, however, visual loss is the net result of months and years of repetitive peripheral retinal vaso-occlusions, which eventuate in some cases in neovascular growth, hemorrhage into the vitreous, vitreous traction, and ultimately retinal detachment.

The purposes of this chapter will be to review briefly the pathogenesis, classification, and natural course of PSR and then to discuss treatment strategies for each of the following: retinal neovascularization, vitreous hemorrhage, retinal detachment, and combined hemorrhage and detachment.

PATHOGENESIS, CLASSIFICATION, AND NATURAL HISTORY

The initiating events in proliferative sickle cell retinopathy are attributable to the closure of small retinal arterioles, typically in the temporal periphery, though any retinal arteriole is at risk (Fig. 5-1). Often the occlusion occurs at a Y-shaped arteriolar bifurcation. Because of the lowered oxygen tension in retinal venules and the known propensity of sickling erythrocytes to adopt the rigid, sickle configuration under hypoxic circumstances, older ideas about the pathogenesis of PSR falsely implicated the retinal venules as the site for primary vaso-occlusion. Fluorescein angiography, however, unequivocally demonstrates that venules become obstructed after, rather than before, arterioles. Furthermore, it is decidedly rare (and probably fortuitous) in sicklers to observe the typical fundus appearance of either branch or central retinal vein occlusion. Whether

*M.D., Professor of Ophthalmology, Department of Ophthalmology, University of Illinois Eye and Ear Infirmary, Chicago, Illinois.

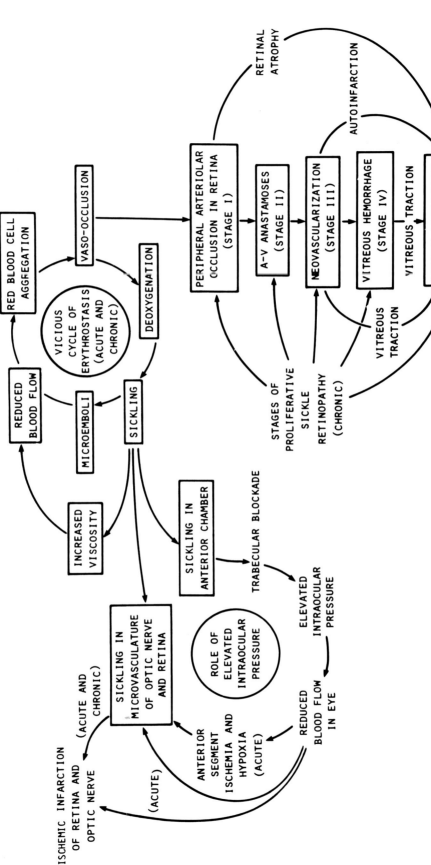

Fig. 5-1. Interpretation of pathogenetic events in sickle cell retinopathy and in sickle cell–induced ocular hypertension.

the cells responsible for the arteriolar occlusions become sickled locally or are derived from more proximal portions of the ocular or systemic circulation (and are thus acting as microemboli) has not been established.

In any event, arteriolar obstructions set off a chain of events that lasts months or years. Surprisingly, the pattern of the retinal vasculature does not necessarily remain constant, and substantial remodeling of the involved portions of the vascular tree occurs, both in the periphery and in the macula.

From the site of arteriolar obstruction in the periphery, runoff of blood into adjacent venules occurs through dilated capillaries, and functional arteriovenous anastomoses develop (Fig. 5-1). Flow through these anastomoses, some of which can occupy as much as 90 degrees of the fundus periphery, tends to be so slow that deoxygenation of blood during a single passage may be sufficient to induce further sickling in situ and additional vaso-occlusion.

As a result of these peripheral retinal vascular events, a border zone is created between central or perfused retina and peripheral or ischemic retina. Sprouts of neovascular tissue may arise from the arteriovenous anastomoses, break through the internal limiting membrane, and grow toward the ischemic zone, that is, toward the ora serrata. These neovascular growths frequently take a fan-shaped form that resembles marine sea fans, hence their name. "Sea fans" are highly characteristic but are not pathognomonic for PSR. They also occur in a variety of other diseases, including Eales' disease, sarcoid, rheumatic fever, chronic leukemia, incontinentia pigmenti, talc embolization, and others.[26]

Sea-fan neovascularization occurs in almost all electrophoretic varieties of sickle cell disease. It is most characteristic of sickle cell hemoglobin C (SC) disease but is almost as frequently observed in sickle cell B thalassemia (SB thal). To a lesser extent, sea fans are also observed in homozygous patients with sickle cell anemia (SS). They have even been seen, though uncommonly, in heterozygous carriers of sickle cell trait (AS). Their occurrence in these generally asymptomatic individuals may be fortuitous.

The discrepancy between ocular and systemic manifestations of the various sickle cell hemoglobinopathies is intriguing because it suggests the possibility of better understanding the pathogenesis of the retinal disease. To date, however, no clearly documented explanation has been provided for the repetitively observed lower incidence of PSR in the most systemically severe hemoglobinopathy type (namely SS). Possibilities include lower whole blood viscosity in the more anemic SS patients. Higher total hemoglobin levels and lower fetal hemoglobin levels have been implicated as high-risk factors, as have higher levels of irreversibly sickled cells, but their precise roles, if any, have not been elucidated.[24]

The onset of PSR may take place in the first decade of life but more typically occurs between the ages of 15 and 30 years.[3] Disability stemming from PSR thus affects individuals during formative and productive periods of life. In nonselected groups of patients, sea fans have been observed in about 33% of SC, 14% of SB thal, and 2.6% of SS individuals.[14] In older patients these percentages are higher, particularly in SS disease.

Individual sea fans appear as early as 8 months (average, 18 months) after the onset of arteriovenous anastomoses.[34] As the years pass, new sea fans develop and old ones enlarge. Vitreous adherence to the neovascular patch may result in tractional elevation of the sea fan when vitreous syneresis occurs. The collapse of the vitreous may be potentiated by the retinal ischemia and by the constant transudation of plasma occurring from the incompetent ("leaky") neovascular capillaries into the vitreous chamber.

Vitreous traction often induces hemorrhage from neovascular tissue into both liquid and gelatinous components of the vitreous chamber (Fig. 5-1). The presence of iron and other blood products probably accelerates vitreous degeneration, collapse, and ultimately further traction.

Additional traction, especially when coupled with thin atrophic retina, often results in retinal holes and tears, with development of rhegmatogenous retinal detachment. As might be expected, the incidence of such detachments roughly parallels that of neovascular tissue; that is, most retinal detachments in sickle cell hemoglobinopathies occur in SC disease. Patients with sickling hemoglobinopathies may, of course, develop rhegmatogenous retinal detachments even in the absence of PSR.

Not infrequently, the natural (untreated) course of PSR terminates in autoinfarction of the sea fans. Vitreous traction, retinal hole formation, and retinal detachment may still occur (Fig. 5-1), but the hemorrhagic propensity of the involved sea fan is greatly reduced. Autoinfarcted sea fans resemble white preretinal membranes. Most if not all of the red neovascular channels disappear or are converted to narrow white lines, sometimes maintaining the fan-shaped configuration. Fluorescein angiography shows either total nonperfusion or greatly diminished perfusion. Eventually, the autoinfarcted sea fan may completely tear away from the retina and remain adherent to the detached posterior vitreous.

The cause of autoinfarction has not been clearly established but could involve any or all of the following: repetitive sickling and thrombotic events in the sea fan; traction on the fan with kinking and decreased flow in its nutrient blood supply; total avulsion of the sea fan because of vitreous collapse[31]; cessation of production of an angiogenic factor; and other reasons.

Approximately 20% to over 60% of patients with PSR show autoinfarction.[3,31] This process may proceed in one portion of the fundus while progressive neovascularization is affecting another. Autoinfarction may occur quickly, over days or weeks, but it also may take years. The effect on visual prognosis is usually favorable, in that the chance of disabling vitreous hemorrhage is lessened. The overall rate of blindness associated with PSR is thus lower (approximately 12% to 14%)[3] than might be expected from the frequency of PSR and the rapidity of sea fan growth seen in some younger patients. The rate of blindness is, nonetheless, substantially higher in the sickling population than in the normal population.

Classification

Because of the foregoing sequence of events, it is possible to classify the clinical stages of PSR into five major subdivisions: (1) peripheral arteriolar occlusions, (2) arteriolovenular anastomoses, (3) neovascularization, (4) vitreous hemorrhage, and (5) retinal detachment.

This classification has several advantages. It is easily utilized and requires only the simple clinical techniques of indirect ophthalmoscopy and fluorescein angiography; it reflects the chronology of events; it emphasizes the initiating role of arteriolar occlusion; it is applicable to other proliferative retinopathies, such as talc retinopathy[26,40] and diabetic retinopathy; and it permits clinical staging for therapeutic purposes.

TREATMENT OF NEOVASCULARIZATION—PHOTOCOAGULATION OF PROLIFERATIVE SICKLE CELL RETINOPATHY
Historical review

Photocoagulation therapy has been utilized in an attempt to prevent visual loss from vitreous hemorrhage and retinal detachment in patients with sickling hemoglobinopathies. In 1970, Archer et al. reported their results in treating PSR in three patients with hemoglobin SC disease with recurrent vitreous hemorrhages.[1] Five eyes were treated using xenon arc photocoagulation after retrobulbar anesthesia. The authors found that photocoagulation was successful in eliminating areas of neovascularization. In 1971, Goldberg reported his results in treating PSR with the xenon arc.[13] Flat neovascular lesions were directly coagulated, whereas elevated lesions were treated with the feeder-vessel technique (see below). After treatment with xenon arc, the number of eyes with neovascularization was reduced from 100% to 55% and the presence of vitreous hemorrhage was reduced from 41% to 26%. With a short follow-up study, the only complication noted was the occurrence of vitreous hemorrhage.

With the development of the argon laser, attempts were made to utilize the feeder-vessel technique with this modality. Goldberg and Acacio treated 21 eyes of patients with sickling hemoglobinopathies who had proliferative retinopathy.[16] Again, small lesions were directly treated, whereas larger lesions were managed by use of the feeder-vessel technique. Angiographic studies showed that 97% of individual sea fans were successfully obliterated. Subsequently, Condon and Serjeant utilized similar techniques with the O'Malley Log II xenon arc photocoagulator to treat PSR.[2] These authors again found the xenon arc to be effective in obliterating sea-fan neovascularization by a combination of direct and feeder-vessel techniques. Complications in treated eyes included uveitis and small hemorrhages. Subsequent publications have also described photocoagulation of PSR.[4,10,25,35]

Indications for treatment

Sea-fan neovascularization varies from small, virtually invisible lesions to large, elevated fibrovascular lesions that can extend throughout the fundus periphery. A lesion may have a single feeding arteriole and draining venule or may have multiple nutrient blood vessels. Patients with large elevated lesions are much more at risk of vitreous hemorrhage or retinal detachment than those with small, flat lesions. However, some patients with early PSR may show rapid progression, with the development of large lesions in a relatively short period of time. Natural history studies have shown that some but not all patients with PSR will show vitreous hemorrhage and retinal detachment. Since autoinfarction also occurs and some patients do not show growth of lesions, the exact indications for therapeutic intervention are as yet uncertain. We now believe that patients with bilateral proliferative retinopathy should have one eye treated. Patients who have lose an eye previously to PSR are also logical candidates for treatment. In a patient with early sea-fan neovascularization in only one eye, follow-up study without therapy is reasonable, if the patient is reliable.

Special considerations related to proliferative sickle cell retinopathy

The proliferative retinopathy seen in association with sickle cell disease differs considerably from that seen in patients with diabetes and other posterior proliferative retinopathies. The neovascularization is almost invariably present in the periphery, usually anterior to the equator. Anterior to the sea-fan neovascularization, the retina is totally nonperfused. This retina is infarcted, and there is a loss of inner retinal elements. The retina posterior to the lesion is usually well perfused without major capillary bed abnormalities. The zone between the posterior perfused and anterior avascular retina would appear to be a hypoxic zone. The infarcted peripheral retina is thin and atrophic, and very intense retinal necrosis will result from photocoagulation, even at relatively low power settings. In addition, one should keep in mind that the vitreous is firmly adherent to sea-fan neovascularization, and thus the patient must be evaluated for evidence of traction on the retina. Treatment of the peripheral retina with photocoagulation requires skill in utilizing the three-mirror lens if a slitlamp delivery system is being used, or the direct ophthalmoscope if a xenon arc photocoagulator is being used.

TECHNIQUES OF PHOTOCOAGULATION

Sea-fan neovascularization can be treated by direct focal treatment, feeder-vessel technique, or scatter photocoagulation (Fig. 5-2).

Focal treatment

Very small sea fans can be directly treated by use of xenon arc or argon laser photocoagulation. Moderately intense burns will close such lesions. Since these lesions are flat on the retinal surface without much vitreous traction and very intense burns are not required, complications are minimal.

Feeder-vessel technique

Closure of feeding arterioles to sea-fan neovascularization can be accomplished by use of the xenon arc or argon laser. The xenon arc is utilized after retrobulbar anesthesia, whereas most patients can be treated with the argon laser and only topical anesthesia. The xenon arc can be delivered by use of a direct ophthalmoscopic attachment or the Fankhauser slitlamp delivery system.[33] Argon laser photocoagulation is performed with a slitlamp delivery system. The initial step in feeder-vessel technique requires that one obtain a moderately intense spot adjacent to the sea fan. This is a determination of a base-line energy. A typical base-line energy might be 200 mW at 0.2 second in a 500 μm spot size. A gray-white burn is the desired result. The feeding arteriole to the sea fan is then treated posterior to the sea fan in a flat retina with about 2.5 times the base-line energy (Figs. 5-2 and 5-3). All of our treatment presently utilizes a 500 μm spot size at durations of at least 0.1 or 0.2 second. A photocoagulation burn placed directly on the arteriole may induce complete interruption of the blood column (Fig. 5-4). If segmentation of the arteriolar blood column is not achieved by one or two well-placed spots, the power level is increased, usually in 50 or 100 mW increments, until segmentation is achieved. Alternatively, the duration of the burns is increased; this may induce pain and a retrobulbar anesthetic may be required.

If one places very intense white burns that still do not succeed in segmenting the blood column, two possible techniques are then utilized. One of us (M.F.G.) prefers to re-treat the arteriole within the previous photocoagulation burn using a 50 μm spot size at high-energy settings (Fig. 5-2). This will often achieve complete segmentation of the blood column in one photocoagulation session. The initially placed larger burn at the level of the retinal pigment epithelium protects Bruch's membrane and the choroid by

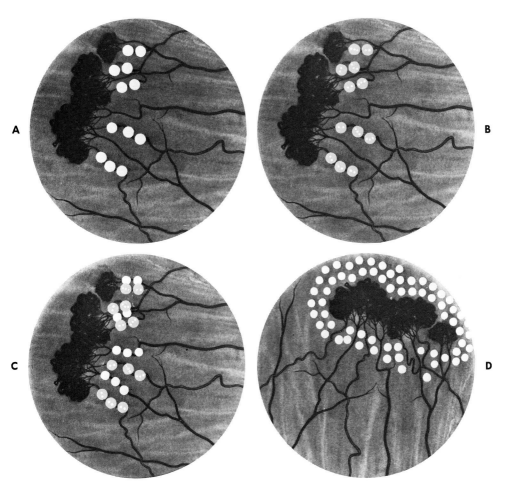

Fig. 5-2. Schematic view of different modalities for coagulating retinal neovascularization in sickle cell disease. **A,** Feeder-vessel technique: arteries treated first with large-diameter laser burns. **B,** Feeder-vessel technique: arteries next treated with small-diameter laser burns if initial coagulation did not interrupt their blood columns. **C,** Feeder-vessel technique: veins are finally coagulated with laser. **D,** Scatter technique of laser photocoagulation.

reflecting most of the incident light. Absorption of blue-green light continues to occur in the red blood column. However, perforation of Bruch's membrane may still occur if the energy density rises too high. Another technique is to have the patient return 2 weeks later, at which time the photocoagulation burn has become pigmented and the retina has thinned considerably. It is then relatively easy to obtain segmentation of the arteriolar blood column by re-treating the original photocoagulation burn site at a much lower energy setting with the 500 μm spot size setting. In patients with moderate to large neovascular lesions, particularly those that are elevated, treatment to the lesion itself should be avoided because this frequently causes vitreous hemorrhaging. Once all the arterioles are closed, the veins are similarly treated until complete segmentation of

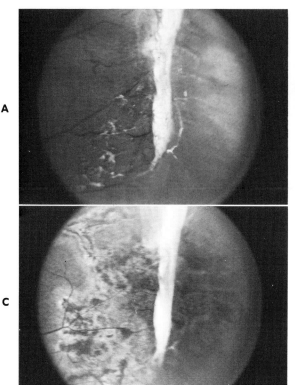
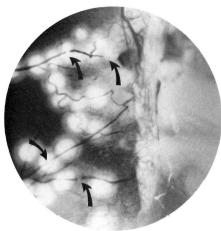

Fig. 5-3. Fundus photographs of feeder-vessel technique of laser photocoagulation. **A,** Ophthalmoscopic view of large sea fan with multiple nutrient arteries and veins (before treatment). **B,** Immediately after laser photocoagulation. Note interruption in blood columns, *arrows,* and plethoric appearance of neovascular tissue in sea fan. **C,** After infarction by feeder-vessel photocoagulation. Preretinal fibrous tissue no longer contains perfused vessels.

the venous blood column is obtained (Fig. 5-2). This is accomplished at lower energy densities than those used when the arterioles are treated. Fluorescein angiography should then be utilized to confirm vascular closure. If closure is achieved and persists for a day or two, subsequent reperfusion of the lesion is unusual. Occasionally, feeding vessels are missed at the time of treatment, but these can be detected during subsequent fluorescein angiography or angioscopy.

The present success rate with feeder-vessel photocoagulation in closing neovascularization is approximately 95%.[10] However, complications can be seen. Retinal hemorrhages can occur, but since we have been avoiding direct treatment of the sea fans, these are rare. Intense laser spots can cause breaks in Bruch's membrane, and they may be noted at the time of treatment. Breaks in Bruch's membrane should be avoided if possible. We have found that they are rare with the 500 μm spot size, whereas they are more common with 50 or 100 μm spot sizes. Breaks in Bruch's membrane may also be associated with choroidal hemorrhage or scattering of pigment. If a hemorrhage occurs, pressure on the contact lens and treatment at the base of the hemorrhage will usually result in cessation of bleeding. Permanent loss of vision from choroidal hemorrhaging is unusual but has been reported.

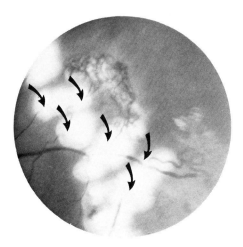

Fig. 5-4. Feeder-vessel technique of laser photocoagulation demonstrating occlusion of nutrient vessels, *arrows*, that had supplied sea fans.

A potentially serious complication of the feeder-vessel technique is choroidal neovascularization[5] (see Chapter 4). After intense photocoagulation with the argon laser or xenon arc, choroidal vascular ingrowth into the photocoagulation scar may occur, presumably because of breaks in Bruch's membrane and the retinal pigment epithelium. This choroidal neovascularization may remain flat in the plane of the retina (chorioretinal neovascularization) or may grow up into the vitreous (choriovitreal neovascularization). In general, eyes with chorioretinal neovascularization do not seem to be adversely affected. We have only rarely seen bleeding into the vitreous in these eyes. Some of these lesions, however, may spontaneously progress to choriovitreal neovascularization. Photocoagulation of chorioretinal neovascularization may convert it to choriovitreal neovascularization. Choriovitreal neovascularization can cause significant vitreous hemorrhages and, in some patients, tractional or rhegmatogenous retinal detachment. At present, we recommend no treatment for flat chorioretinal neovascularization. We also do not treat most eyes with choriovitreal neovascularization unless progressive vitreous hemorrhaging and retinal detachment are occurring. It is unclear whether the best therapy for choriovitreal neovascularization is photocoagulation, cryopexy, or diathermy. We have had difficulty in closing choriovitreal neovascularization with all these modalities. Since we have been utilizing the 500 μm spot size for argon laser photocoagulation and we have avoided being too aggressive at the time of the first treatment, we have seen a decrease in the incidence of choroidal neovascularization, but follow-up study is somewhat limited.

Another complication of feeder-vessel technique is peripheral choroidal ischemia.[9] The intense photocoagulation required by this technique closes underlying ciliary arteries. This results in the appearance of white wedge-shaped areas of choroidal ischemia within the first 24 hours after treatment. These have been noted to be present in about 35% of photocoagulated eyes. Over the next several weeks these lesions show gradual development of mild, mottled pigmentation. Since the lesions are peripheral, they result in only minimal if any constriction of the peripheral visual fields.

Another complication that we have observed with the argon laser, but not xenon arc, is retinal tear formation.[27] After closure of neovascularization and with the progression of vitreoretinal traction, tears may develop adjacent to the treated sea fan. In most of these cases we have been able to surround the tear with additional photocoagulation, and most of these eyes have not required scleral buckling surgery. Xenon arc photocoagulation does not appear to produce retinal tears frequently, perhaps because larger areas of the retina are treated, resulting in a rather broad adhesion of the retina to the choroid in the region of treatment.

Conclusions—feeder-vessel photocoagulation. It is apparent that feeder-vessel photocoagulation can close the majority of vasoproliferative lesions. However, this is a difficult technique to master and is associated with significant morbidity. To assess the efficacy of feeder-vessel photocoagulation compared to the natural history of proliferative sickle cell retinopathy (which includes autoinfarction in some patients), we have initiated a randomized trial of feeder-vessel photocoagulation in association with the Medical Research Council Laboratory in Kingston, Jamaica. A total of 167 eyes have been enrolled in this trial, which has been underway since 1978. Preliminary results from the study indicate that photocoagulation can definitely reduce the incidence of vitreous hemorrhaging in treated eyes. However, complications have occurred in treated eyes, including retinal tears and choroidal neovascularization. With longer follow-up observation, this study should indicate the risk-to-benefit ratio for the feeder-vessel technique.

Scatter photocoagulation for proliferative sickle cell retinopathy

Scatter treatment in the form of panretinal photocoagulation has proved to be of great value in patients with diabetic retinopathy or with rubeosis iridis diabetica. Because of this, we have utilized scatter photocoagulation in patients with PSR. We have recently reported a series of 21 eyes with 45 sea-fan lesions that were treated with argon laser scatter photocoagulation.[35] Scatter lesions were generally placed from 1.5 mm posterior to the lesion to 1.5 mm anterior to the lesion and one clock hour to each side of each lesion (Fig. 5-2). The burns were separated by approximately one burn diameter and were of light to moderate intensity. These were much less intense than the argon laser burns used in the feeder-vessel technique. We do not directly treat the lesion or its feeding vessels. Analysis of the data from this preliminary study shows that patients with flat neovascular lesions appear to respond very well to photocoagulation. Complete regression was noted in 24 of 28 such lesions. Elevated sea fans, especially large ones, responded poorly, however, with complete regression occurring in only four of 17 lesions. This preliminary study thus suggests that scatter photocoagulation is of value in patients with *early* but not advanced PSR (Fig. 5-5).

Complications were seen in only two of the 21 eyes. One patient developed a small choroidal hemorrhage from a burn that was too intense. There were no permanent sequelae from this treatment. Another patient developed anterior segment ischemia and choroidal and retinal arteriolar occlusions, which were seen in areas of the fundus not photocoagulated. This patient was subsequently determined to have severe carotid artery disease with a low ocular perfusion pressure. It appears that ocular compression with

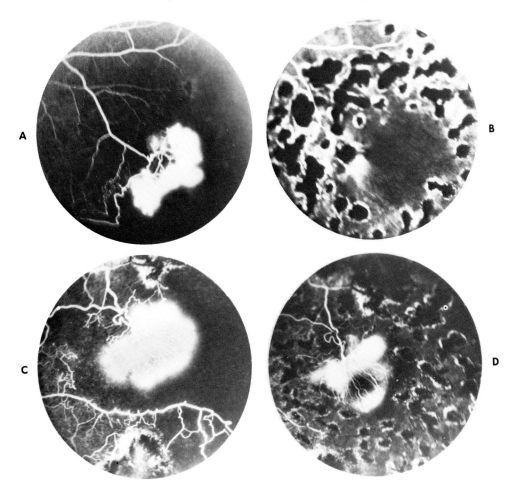

Fig. 5-5. Scatter photocoagulation technique. **A,** Sea fan before treatment. **B,** Virtually complete nonperfusion of sea fan after scatter photocoagulation. **C,** Another sea fan before scatter treatment. **D,** After scatter photocoagulation sea fan has only partially involuted.

the fundus contact lens was enough to compromise the vascular supply to this eye because of its decreased perfusion pressure. We have not seen ocular ischemia in any other treated eyes in this series.

Because of this preliminary success with scatter photocoagulation, we are planning a randomized trial comparing scatter photocoagulation with the natural history of the retinopathy and with our prior data utilizing the feeder-vessel technique.

Cryocoagulation

Opacities in the crystalline lens or in the vitreous may make visualization of sea fans difficult. Vitreous blood and the opaque white fibroglial mantle enveloping some sea fans are not infrequent. The delivery of therapeutic levels of photocoagulation energy is thereby compromised in some cases. Under these circumstances, closure of a sea fan by either xenon arc or argon laser may be impossible, and therapeutic recourse to transconjunctival cryotherapy may be necessary.

Even in the presence of moderately hazy ocular media, it is usually possible to visualize sea fans with binocular indirect ophthalmoscopy. When the media are even denser (because of, for example, repetitive bleeding into the vitreous), it is still sometimes possible to view the sea fans responsible for the hemorrhage by use of fluorescein angioscopy. The dose of fluorescein that is used routinely for angiography (such as 10 ml of 5% sodium fluorescein) is administered intravenously, and the fundus is inspected within 1 to 2 minutes. A Wratten 47 blue filter is placed over the illuminating source of the indirect ophthalmoscope. In the presence of perfused neovascular tissue, a characteristic and telltale green cloud emanates from the sea fan and can be seen through all but the densest of ocular media. This green cloud can be used for placement of the cryoprobe, but as the fluorescein disperses quickly throughout the vitreous chamber, cryocoagulation must be accomplished promptly (within minutes). If the media are clear, there obviously is no time limit on performing the treatment.

Cryocoagulation is moderately effective in closing retinal blood vessels and has been successfully employed, as in the therapy of von Hippel's angiomatosis retinae. We have studied the benefits and risks of transconjunctival cryotherapy of sea fans by utilizing both single-freeze and triple-freeze techniques. With a single freeze, approximately 70% of sea fans were completely eradicated. Fluorescein angioscopy or angiography has confirmed absence of perfusion for up to 3 years after such treatment.[29] About 30% of sea fans maintained some perfusion, but even in these cases the nutrient arterioles and draining venules became greatly attenuated, and parts of the neovascular tissue were obliterated. Leakage of fluorescein dye decreased substantially, and none of these sea fans has bled or caused important fundus complications over the years since the original report. Reduction of the hemorrhagic propensity of sea fans allows the vitreous to clear and, if vitrectomy or scleral buckling becomes necessary, also minimizes the risk of intraoperative bleeding.

In an effort to increase the benefits of cryocoagulation, a triple-freeze technique was also evaluated.[12] All sea fans were closed, but two of nine eyes developed rhegmatogenous retinal detachment, an unacceptably high complication rate. Creation of retinal breaks was apparently caused by persistent or exacerbated vitreous traction on areas of infarcted, thin retina that were made even more attenuated and fragile by the intense cryoinduced necrosis. Accordingly, we have abandoned this technique, and now use single-freeze cryocoagulation as an acceptable alternative to photocoagulation when opacities in the media prohibit the use of light energy or during scleral buckling or vitrectomy surgery.

If one is to perform single-freeze cryocoagulation, the following technique is recommended. Anesthesia is obtained topically or by subconjunctival injection of lidocaine in the quadrants to be treated. The subconjunctival technique is preferable to a retrobulbar injection because it permits the patient to rotate the eye in the direction of the lesion to be treated, thereby enhancing precise ophthalmoscopic localization of the cryoprobe.

The therapeutic end point is reached when the entire neovascularization is just barely enveloped by the white ice ball. Care must be exercised so that there is essentially no overlap of adjacent cryoapplications (Fig. 5-6). It may be advisable to encircle this sometimes heavily treated area by a circle of lighter cryotherapy (orange reaction in the

Fig. 5-6. Schematic view of cryocoagulation of sea fans.

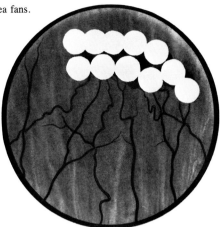

choroid). Cryotherapy to ischemic fundus zones anterior to the sea fans may possibly also have a beneficial effect.

Diathermy

Surface diathermy to the sclera overlying retinal sea fans was first reported by Hannon in 1956.[23] Sea fans were obliterated in two cases, and complications did not occur.

In 1974, Condon and Serjeant[2] reported results in 29 elevated fibrovascular proliferations in 13 patients. A lamellar scleral dissection technique was employed to encompass the entire area of retinal involvement. Diathermy was applied to the whole of the dissected area, and the end point was whitening of the retina. The average extent of the operated area was approximately one quadrant. Diathermy sealed off the feeder vessels in all eyes, and 12 of 13 patients maintained their preoperative level of visual acuity. One eye developed anterior segment ischemia after up to 180 degrees of the globe's circumference had been diathermized. Anterior uveitis developed in all cases, but resolved over 1 month with use of topical corticosteroids and mydriatics. In two patients systemic corticosteroid therapy was required for treatment of posterior uveitis.

Because of these complications and the necessity for operating-room techniques, diathermy has been supplanted by transconjunctival cryotherapy in some circumstances and by photocoagulation in the majority of instances.

TREATMENT OF VITREOUS HEMORRHAGE

With the advent of pars plana surgery in the 1970s, sickle cell patients with chronically disabling vitreous hemorrhage became candidates for visual rehabilitation.[11] Initial results of vitrectomy were far from uniformly successful (Table 5-1). Ryan, for example, reported four of seven eyes to be unsuccessfully operated on.[36] Iatrogenic retinal tears and detachments occurred secondarily to difficulty in cutting the equatorial vitreous. Treister and Machemer reported on three eyes,[39] two of which had retinal detachment in addition to vitreous hemorrhage. (These cases are discussed below.) The postoperative course of the eye with the isolated vitreous hemorrhage was complicated after vitrectomy by repeated hemorrhages, hyphema, secondary glaucoma, and ultimately no perception of light. At the Sickle Cell Eye Clinic of the University of Illinois Eye and

Table 5-1. Isolated vitreous hemorrhage in patients with sickle cell treated by vitrectomy (combined series)

Reference	Visual improvement	Complications
Ryan*	3 of 7 eyes	Possible artery occlusion in one eye
Treister and Machemer†	None in one eye	Hyphema and secondary glaucoma (no light perception) in one eye
Sickle Cell Eye Clinic, University of Illinois‡	4 of 5 eyes	Recurrent vitreous hemorrhage, secondary glaucoma, phthisis, and enucleation of one eye
Total	7 of 13 eyes	

*Ryan, S.J.: Trans. Ophthalmol. Soc. U.K. **95**:403, 1975.
†Treister, G., and Machemer, R.: Am. J. Ophthalmol. **84**:349, 1977.
‡Jampol, L.M., Green, J.L., Jr., Goldberg, M.F., and Peyman, G.A.: An update on vitrectomy surgery and retinal detachment repair in sickle cell disease, Arch. Ophthalmol. **100**:591, 1982.

Table 5-2. Eyes with isolated vitreous hemorrhage having vitrectomy at the Sickle Cell Eye Clinic, University of Illinois

Case number	Age (years)	Sex	Follow-up study (months)	Hemoglobin*	Operation	Visual acuity† Preoperatively	Last visit
1	25	M	61	SC	Vitrectomy	HM	NLP, enucleated
2	31	M	72	SC	Vitrectomy	HM	20/20 (6/6)
3	57	F	62	AS	Vitrectomy	HM	20/25 (6/7.5)
4	22	F	4	AS	Vitrectomy	HM	20/100 (6/30)
5	33	F	7	SC	Vitrectomy and lensectomy	HM	20/40 (6/12)

*SC, Sickle cell hemoglobin C; AS, heterozygous carriers of sickle cell trait.
†HM, Hand motions; NLP, no light perception.

Ear Infirmary, we have performed pars plana vitrectomy in five eyes with vitreous hemorrhage (and no simultaneous retinal detachment). Four of the five operations were successful.[28] One eye behaved similar to that reported by Treister and Machemer. It sustained recurrent vitreous hemorrhage and secondary glaucoma and eventually became phthisic and was enucleated. Visual improvement was substantial in our four successful cases (Table 5-2).

Indications for surgical removal of vitreous hemorrhage are, in general, somewhat more restrictive than those for patients without sickle cells in because the technique is more difficult and the chances of intraoperative and postoperative complications are higher. Approximately 6 months are allowed to elapse after onset of a visually disabling vitreous hemorrhage. During this time, transconjunctival cryotherpy or even photocoagulation, if the clarity of the media permits, may be employed to render sea fans less well perfused or totally closed. If acuity improves during this interval, vitrectomy is not performed. If visual functioning remains inappropriately low for the needs of the individual patient, vitrectomy is then suggested. If the media are too dense to allow visualization of the fundus, ultrasound evaluation is carried out monthly. If ultrasonic evidence of retinal detachment occurs, operative intervention is performed forthwith. The detached posterior hyaloid face is often very thickened, taut, and layered with erythrocytes in patients with sickle cells, however, and ultrasonically may mimic a retinal detachment inserting at the disc. Thus an ophthalmologist may intend to do a combined scleral buckling and vitrectomy only to find during surgery that a simple vitrectomy will suffice. On the other hand, iatrogenic retinal breaks or retinal detachment may rather easily occur during surgery, and it is wise for one to be prepared for an extensive operation, utilizing the preoperative anesthetic and intraoperative precautions discussed below.

The goals of vitrectomy surgery in the sickling patient include clarification and restoration of the media sufficiently well that the peripheral sea fans are relieved of traction and become amenable to coagulation, either intraoperatively or postoperatively. Two anatomic features unique to the sickling patient should be borne in mind by the surgeon who is considering intraoperative manipulations and their potential complications. First, the far peripheral (equatorial or preequatorial) location of sea fans often requires that the shaft of the vitrectomy instrument come dangerously close to the posterior pole of the crystalline lens (Fig. 5-7) as the tip of the instrument is directed toward the vitreous adherent to the neovascular tissue. Occasionally the crystalline lens must be sacrificed and removed through the pars plana during the procedure. One can sometimes avoid inadvertent striking of the lens by softening the eye (as by lowering the infusion bottle, which is safer than increasing the suction) and simultaneously indenting the sclera overlying the sea fans (Fig. 5-7). This maneuver brings the sea fans closer to the visual axis of the operating microscope and irrigated contact lens and also allows the vitrectomy instrument to remain posterior to the crystalline lens. The vitreous attached to the sea fan is then carefully removed piecemeal.

This surgical technique, however, also has two major potential complications. First, the vitreous may be so tightly adherent to the neovascular tissue that any tugging at all initiates fresh intravitreal bleeding, which may be difficult to control, even with the usual techniques of modern vitrectomy surgery, such as hydrostatic control of intraocular pressure, bipolar diathermy, and unipolar diathermy. Thus preoperative attempts to coagulate the sea fans, as discussed on p. 58, are worthwhile. The second problem relates to the extremely thin peripheral retina, to which vitreous may be attached by its base or by the sea fan itself. Removing the pre-equatorial cuff of vitreous is always a dangerous part of any vitrectomy procedure, but is even riskier (though usually more desirable) in the patient with sickle cell disease. In patients with sickle cells, repetitive ischemic infarction of the peripheral retina characteristically has rendered the retinal tissue even thinner than it ordinarily is. Thus any traction, however slight, may cause tears in the retina, thereby requiring a buckling procedure with its attendant, substantial risks (see p. 71). There is no infallible way of avoiding intraoperative hemorrhages or retinal tears under these circumstances, though it is wise to minimize both the power and duration of the suctioning components of the vitrectomy procedure. Generally the

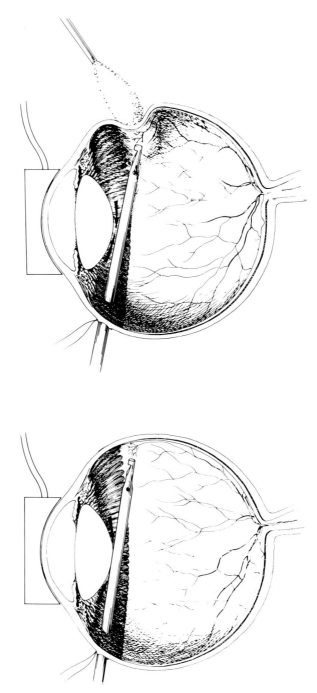

Fig. 5-7. Vitrectomy for proliferative sickle cell retinopathy and vitreous hemorrhage (blood not shown). *Left,* Shaft of instrument can easily traumatize posterior pole of lens, *arrows,* as it approaches retinal sea fan (compare diagram on right). *Right,* With sea fan indented, it can be visualized more easily and shaft of vitrectomy instrument is more likely to avoid striking posterior pole of lens, *arrows.*

suction is applied in repetitive, brief intervals, each lasting less than a second, to allow the sea fans and retina to be spared from prolonged traction. Furthermore, the oscillation frequency of the guillotine in the Vitrophage is increased to several cuts per second in order to reduce the duration of drag on intraocular structures. If the sea fans have undergone *documented* closure preoperatively by photocoagulation or cryocoagulation, one can avoid doing the far peripheral vitreous removal and thus minimize the risk of lens trauma and peripheral retinal breaks.

Once the sea fans are well visualized and the vitrectomy is completed, the sea fans are cryocoagulated with a single freeze-thaw cycle, as described above, or are closed with intravitreal photocoagulation. An alternative approach to coagulating sea fans is to perform photocoagulation in the immediate postoperative period. If the intraocular fluid becomes cloudy quickly, this may not be possible. If vitreous traction is completely released and no retinal breaks or detachments are uncovered, scleral buckling is not carried out routinely. The chance of postoperative anterior segment ischemia is thereby reduced (see discussion of scleral buckling, p. 73).

Another potential problem unique to the patient with sickle cells is the postoperative secondary glaucoma caused by sickled cells obstructing outflow channels of aqueous humor.[15,17-22] This form of glaucoma is analogous to but clinically worse than ghost cell glaucoma.[41] The problem is induced by rigid, sickled erythrocytes that are decidely less capable of traversing the outflow pathways than are nonsickled, pliable erythrocytes. The trabecular logjam is created by cells from the vitreous that enter the anterior chamber (Fig. 5-8). If the patient is aphakic or has been made aphakic during the operation, the chance for this complication to occur is increased because intravitreal erythrocytes have ready access to the trabecular meshwork.

Insofar as an erythrocyte containing hemoglobin S is concerned, the milieu of the anterior chamber is probably the most noxious of any compartment in the body. In comparison with circulating blood, human aqueous humor is characterized by low oxygen tension and low pH, high carbon dioxide tension, and a high concentration of ascorbic acid (a reducing agent). If the fluid is stagnant, further deoxygenation and acidification occur. The net effect of these metabolic conditions is to enhance sickling. The aqueous outflow is impeded, and the intraocular pressure (IOP) therefore rises.

A vicious cycle is induced, whereby elevated IOP reduces the vascular perfusion pressure (perfusion pressure equals mean arterial blood pressure minus IOP) in blood vessels of the anterior segment, thereby contributing to further deoxygenation, acidification, sickling within the blood vessels of the anterior segment (sometimes causing the anterior segment ischemia syndrome), further sickling within the cells suspended in the aqueous humor, additional obstruction to aqueous outflow, and exacerbation of the elevated IOP (Fig. 5-1).

An anatomically remote but clinically deleterious effect of the elevated IOP involves the small blood vessels of the optic nerve and retina. As the IOP increases, the perfusion pressure in these vessels falls. Infarction of the optic nerve and retina can occur at only moderately elevated levels of IOP (Fig. 5-1). Thus it appears desirable to maintain an IOP of less than 25 mm Hg whenever possible.

The usual pharmacologic mainstays for control of secondary glaucoma tend to have only minimal value in the patient with sickle cell disease. Acetazolamide (Diamox) and mannitol may be beneficial but, if given more than once a day, may cause hemoconcentration, increased viscosity of the circulating blood, and thus impaired flow through the eye's small blood vessels. Diamox may induce undesirable acidification of the blood. Methazolamide (Neptazane) may be a more valuable carbonic anhydrase inhibitor in this circumstance, since it contributes less to systemic acidification and raises the pH of aqueous humor more than does Diamox.

Topical epinephrine is contraindicated because of its vasoconstricting properties in the anterior segment. Timolol is virtually the only topical antiglaucomatous medication that would appear to be well tolerated. If it is unsuccessful in lowering the IOP quickly, paracentesis of the anterior chamber should be performed and, if necessary, repeated.[15]

Expandable gases are sometimes injected intravitreally in vitreous surgery and may have rather unpredictable effects on IOP. Because raised IOP in patients with sickle cell disease is so deleterious, ordinary air is preferred. Expandable gases are reserved for selected cases with retinal breaks that require combined vitrectomy and buckling. Postoperatively, the IOP must be monitored several times a day.

Because vitrectomy may require removal of the lens (with possible migration of

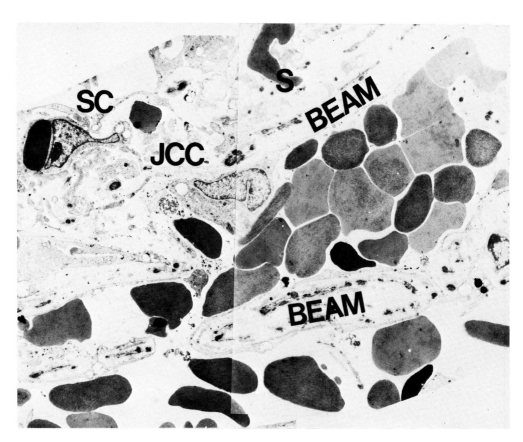

Fig. 5-8. Electron micrograph of sickle-shaped erythrocytes becoming jammed in intertrabecular space. *SC,* Schlemm's canal; *S,* sickle-shaped red blood cell; *JCC,* juxtacanalicular connective tissue; *BEAM,* trabecular beam. (From Goldberg, M.F., and Tso, M.O.M.: Ophthalmic Surg. **10:**89, 1979.)

sickling cells from the vitreous into the trabecular meshwork) or scleral buckling (with possible anterior segment ischemia), preoperative and intraoperative anesthetic and surgical manipulations should be chosen so that hypoxia and ischemia of ocular tissues are minimized (p. 73). In caring for the vitrectomized eye postoperatively, the routine measures employed for the eye after a scleral buckling procedure for sickle cell disease should be followed (pp. 75 and 76), including continuous administration of oxygen by face mask for the first 48 hours postoperatively.

TREATMENT OF RETINAL DETACHMENT

The complexity of performing retinal detachment surgery on the eyes of patients with hemoglobin S has been known for about a decade. In comparison with nonsickling cases, intraoperative and postoperative complications are more severe. Some of the complications (both ocular and systemic) are unique to the sickling population and can be sight- or life-threatening. Because of these considerations, buckling surgery is not performed for tractional retinal detachments unless progression is documented. Even in rhegmatogenous retinal detachment, where the indication for surgery is obvious, the potential for ocular and systemic complications of surgery in patients with sickle cell disease is great enough that any black patient with a retinal detachment should have appropriate laboratory tests performed preoperatively to rule out the sickling condition. The absence of typical proliferative sickle retinopathy should not lull the unwary observer into a false sense of security. A patient with sickle cell disease and a conventional rhegmatogenous retinal detachment is more prone to surgical complications than is the patient with normal hemoglobin who has the same type of detachment.

Scleral buckling for rhegmatogenous retinal detachment has been performed with a variety of techniques. Most of them have been modifications of basic procedures using segmental or encircling methods and explants or implants. Ryan and Goldberg reported on 10 eyes in 1971[37]; four eyes were visually improved, but four eyes became phthisic or prephthisic. The major complication was anterior segment ischemia. Subsequently, we have obtained improved results and up to now have not experienced the anterior segment ischemia syndrome whenever we have preoperatively replaced about half the circulating sickle cell blood with transfused blood from normal donors. Six patients have recently been treated in this fashion, and all had successful results[28] (Table 5-3).

Table 5-3. Eyes with rhegmatogenous retinal detachment having scleral buckling at the Sickle Cell Eye Clinic, University of Illinois

Case number	Age (years)	Sex	Follow-up study (months)	Hemoglobin*	Visual acuity	
					Preoperative	Last visit
1	32	M	32	SC	6/7.5 (20/25)	6/6 (20/20)
2	36	F	27	SS	6/7.5 (20/25)	6/6 (20/20)
3	23	F	6	SC	6/7.5 (20/25)	6/6 (20/20)
4	47	F	6	SS	6/9 (20/30)	6/9 (20/30)
5	55	M	4	SC	6/60 (20/200)	6/24 (20/80)
6	40	F	3	SS	6/6 (20/20)	6/6 (20/20)

*SC, Sickle cell hemoglobin C; SS, homozygous patients with sickle cell disease.

Table 5-4. Scleral buckling for retinal detachment in sickle cell patients (combined series)

Reference	Successful reattachment	Comments
Ryan and Goldberg*	4 of 10 eyes	Four eyes developed phthisis or became prephthisic; major complication was anterior segment ischemia (no special precautions taken)
Sickle Cell Eye Clinic, University of Illinois†	All 6 eyes	Preoperative partial-exchange blood transfusion (no anterior segment ischemia)
Freilich and Seelenfreund‡	All 11 eyes	Surgery performed in hyperbaric chamber (no anterior segment ischemia)
Zinn§	One eye	Surgery performed in hyperbaric chamber (no anterior segment ischemia) in this one case

*Ryan, S.J., and Goldberg, M.F.: Am. J. Ophthalmol. **72**:35, 1971.
†Jampol, L.M., Green, J.L., Jr., Goldberg, M.F., and Peyman, G.A.: An update on vitrectomy surgery and retinal detachment repair in sickle cell disease, Arch. Ophthalmol. **100**:591, 1982.
‡Freilich, D.B., and Seelenfreund, M.H.: Mod. Probl. Ophthalmol. **18**:368, 1977.
§Zinn, K.M.: Mt. Sinai J. Med. **48**:79, 1981.

Table 5-5. Scleral buckling in hyperbaric chamber[7]

Eye number	Hemoglobin*	Visual acuity†	
		Preoperative	Postoperative
1	SC	HM at 1 ft	6/90 (20/300)
2	SS	HM at 2 ft	6/9+ (20/30+)
3	SS	6/12 (20/40)	6/7.5 (20/25)
4	SC	HM at 1 ft	6/12 (20/40)
5	SC	CF at 1 ft	6/90 (20/300)
6	AS	6/9 (20/30)	6/7.5 (20/25)
7	AS	6/6 (20/20)	6/6 (20/20)
8	AS	HM at 6 in	6/120 (20/400)
9	AS	HM at 1 ft	6/60 (20/200)
10	SC	6/7.5 (20/25)	6/7.5 (20/25)
11	AS and diabetes	HM at 6 in	6/60 (20/200)
12	AS and diabetes	HM at 6 in	6/60 (20/200)

*AS, Heterozygous carriers of sickle cell trait; SC, sickle cell hemoglobin C; SS, homozygous patients with sickle cell disease.
†HM, Hand motions; CF, count fingers.

Similar buckling procedures performed in a hyperbaric chamber at two atmospheres of oxygen pressure have yielded excellent results (Tables 5-4 and 5-5).[7,43] Unfortunately, this complex equipment is not generally available. The favorable results, however, and the absence of postoperative anterior segment ischemia underscore the necessity for maximizing oxygenation of ocular tissues during scleral buckling surgery.

Anterior segment ischemia

The postoperative syndrome of anterior segment ischemia has been well characterized in the past. Striate keratopathy and corneal edema often make their appearance on the second or third postoperative day and may be harbingers of progressive necrotic changes that lead eventually to phthisis. The anterior chamber may have a heavy flare and cells, and infectious endophthalmitis may be mimicked. Iris necrosis may be severe or mild, in which case irregularity of pupillary dilatation may be the only finding. Rubeosis iridis and ectropion uveae may be seen. Hypotony is often pronounced, and the anterior chamber may become shallow. In one hemoglobin SC case studied at autopsy 1 week after scleral buckling, thrombosis of the major arterial circle of the iris was documented histologically and appeared to be the cause of anterior segment necrosis.[6]

The importance of this operative complication should not be underestimated. Once it occurs, it is largely untreatable. Prophylaxis is far more effective than therapy after the fact. If full-blown anterior segment necrosis occurs, it may nullify an otherwise successful buckling procedure. Even though the retina may remain attached, the vision may not improve and may even worsen because of the anterior segment changes. This clinical situation is akin to winning the battle but losing the war. Anterior segment ischemia and necrosis are disproportionately common in patients with sickle cell disease after retinal detachment surgery. Ryan and Goldberg estimated its incidence to be about 70% in their patients with sickle cell disease (when special precautions were not taken), but only about 3% in normal patients undergoing similar buckling procedures.

The anterior segment ischemia syndrome can be induced clinically or experimentally by a variety of surgical insults, including interruption of blood flow in the anterior ciliary arteries, the long posterior ciliary arteries, or the major arterial circle of the iris. Insufficient perfusion of these vessels may be caused or exacerbated by tenotomy of a rectus muscle, prolonged traction on rectus muscles, heavy diathermy or cryotherapy overlying the long posterior ciliary artery, a tight encircling band, a high buckle requiring excessive tightening of scleral sutures, ocular hypertension, and systemic hypotension. Faulty perfusion of the blood vessels in the anterior segment of the eye exacerbates the preexisting ischemia that ordinarily characterizes the ocular tissues in the patient with sickle cell disease. Furthermore, the ischemia induces the so-called vicious cycle of erythrostasis because it leads to hypoxia, which, in turn, causes sickling. The sickled cells increase the viscosity of the blood in the small vessels of the eye, leading to slowing of flow, further ischemia and deoxygenation, additional sickling, and so on, until tissue death occurs. The astute therapist will attempt to prevent or break the vicious cycle by doing everything possible to maximize blood flow and oxygenation.

The goals of the buckling procedure in patients with sickle cell disease are similar to those employed for patients with normal hemoglobin. All retinal breaks must be sealed, an adhesive chorioretinitis created, and vitreous traction relieved. In eyes with proliferative sickle retinopathy, however, breaks may be obscured by blood or sea fans, and the vitreous traction may be extensive. It may be believed desirable, therefore, to create a broad, high buckle with a tight encircling band (Fig. 5-9). Because sea fans are commonly located in the temporal quadrants and lead to vitreous traction and retinal breaks in their immediate vicinity, it is often necessary to apply cryotherapy (or diathermy) over the temporal long posterior ciliary artery, immediately under the lateral rectus

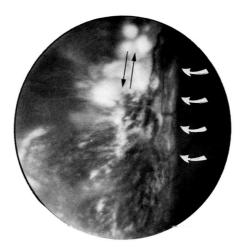

Fig. 5-9. High-circumferential scleral buckle, *curved arrows,* in patient with sickle cell retinal detachment. Fresh laser burns, *straight arrows,* were applied postoperatively to coagulate a persistently perfused sea fan on crest of buckle.

muscle. Any of these technical maneuvers can initiate or contribute to the vicious cycle of erythrostasis and anterior segment ischemia.

In an attempt to minimize these dangers, a large number of prophylactic preoperative and intraoperative measures have been proposed. Most of them have not been substantiated by rigorous clinical trials, but their use appears logical and reasonably free of complications. Preoperatively, the pupil is dilated with only two to three instillations of topical phenylephrine hydrochloride (Neo-Synephrine) in an attempt to minimize anterior segment vasoconstriction. In addition, six instillations of 5% homatropine, 15 minutes apart, $1\frac{1}{2}$ to 2 hours before surgery, are given. When feasible, local anesthesia is preferred to general anesthesia in an effort to avoid systemic hypotension. Epinephrine is withheld from the retrobulbar solution. Single doses of a carbonic anhydrase inhibitor and intravenous mannitol are utilized to soften the eye and maximize intraocular perfusion pressure. Repeated dosages, however, may lead to potentially dangerous acidosis, hemoconcentration, or both.

Partial-exchange blood transfusion has been the mainstay of our preoperative management in hemoglobin SS and hemoglobin SC patients. The goal of this therapy is to replace about 50% to 60% or more of the circulating erythrocytes with normal-donor red blood cells. The chances of substantial intravascular sickling, sludging, hyperviscosity, and erythrostasis in the ocular and systemic circulations are presumably reduced.

Because sickle trait blood (hemoglobin AS) requires considerably more severe conditions of deoxygenation and acidosis for induction of sickling to occur, preoperative partial-exchange transfusion is rarely necessary in these cases for the prevention of anterior segment necrosis. Sickle trait erythrocytes, however, rather frequently became sickled in the anterior chamber[15,17-22] and can clog the trabecular meshwork and induce secondary glaucoma just as easily as red blood cells with SS or SC hemoglobins. (Refer to the section on vitrectomy for a discussion of management of this serious complication.) The surgeon should also remember that general anesthesia can increase the risk of inducing sickle cell crisis even in patients with sickle cell trait.

Preoperative partial exchange blood transfusion is performed over a 3- to 5-day interval and usually requires about six units of transfusion blood for a normal-sized adult. Whole blood is removed by phlebotomy and discarded. Simultaneously, washed packed erythrocytes from normal volunteer donors are infused. The procedure is repeated until over 50% of the circulating blood is normal, as determined by repetitive hemoglobin electrophoresis (more than 50% hemoglobin A; less than 50% hemoglobin S or C, or both). The hematocrit, however, should not exceed about 39% because hemoconcentration can raise whole blood viscosity and impair blood flow.

Recently, the technique of erythropheresis, utilizing an automatic blood cell separator, has been advocated as a means of quickly replacing sickle cells with normal cells.[42] The major advantage of this procedure is its speed (approximately 90 minutes).

Both erythropheresis and partial-exchange blood transfusion induce systemic risks, such as septicemia, transfusion reaction, and, most importantly, hepatitis of the non-A non-B variety.[38] The attack rate of non-A non-B hepatitis among recipients of blood from volunteer donors is about 7%.[38] The rate increases to 40% or more if commercially derived blood is used. Because the majority of patients with posttransfusion hepatitis are anicteric, the ophthalmologist must maintain a high index of diagnostic suspicion well into the postoperative period (6 to 12 months or more[38]). There is a distressing tendency of some of these patients to develop chronic or progressive courses, including the development of cirrhosis.[38] Up to now we have not observed any clear-cut instances of anterior segment necrosis when partial-exchange blood transfusion was used as described. One of our patients did develop hepatitis, however. This resolved without sequelae. From our limited experience it would appear that the benefits outweigh the risks, but the patient should be aware of the potential dangers of transfusion therapy and those of anterior segment ischemia. It is essential to obtain properly informed consent before undertaking this form of therapy.

Intraoperatively oxygen is maintained at as high a level as possible; systemic hypotension is avoided or treated; and ocular hypertension is prevented. Specifically, we recommend elimination of rectus muscle detachment or prolonged traction; avoidance, if possible, of cryotherapy to the long posterior ciliary arteries; avoidance of diathermy altogether because it shrinks the sclera and raises the IOP; and minimization of the height and extent of the buckle, if possible, though vitreous traction may require doing just the opposite.

Most importantly we recommend drainage of subretinal fluid in every case, unless the amount of fluid is so small that retinal perforation would be likely to occur. Drainage of subretinal fluid softens the eye, thereby raising the arterial perfusion pressure and maximizing blood flow. Drainage of fluid, furthermore, allows creation of a higher buckle, with relief of vitreous traction. Despite the well-known dangers inherent in drainage of subretinal fluid, it is probably one of the most valuable components of the buckling procedure in the patient with sickle cell hemoglobin.

Postoperatively we advocate continuous use of supplemental oxygen by face-mask inhalation. This is carried out with a portable tank of oxygen while the patient is being transferred from operating room to recovery room and from recovery room to the hospital bedroom. If there are no complications, oxygen is discontinued 48 hours later.

Because anterior segment necrosis can cause severe uveitis and miosis, intensive efforts are made to maintain maximum mydriasis postoperatively. Again, sympathomimetics are minimized, and parasympatholytics are emphasized.

If anterior segment necrosis occurs postoperatively, there is little one can offer except additional oxygenation and mydriasis. Rheologic enhancers, such as dextran and anticoagulants, and corticosteroids have their advocates, but their therapeutic efficacy has not been substantiated.

In addition to the prophylactic measures just considered, it is worth attempting to close perfused sea fans before the actual buckling procedure. This can only be accomplished quickly by use of the feeder-vessel technique of photocoagulation. The media must be clear, and the sea fans must lie in regions of the retina that are still attached. If sea fans are located in detached portions of the retina, as is often the case, they cannot be closed preoperatively. It is helpful to place sea fans, particularly if still perfused, on a buckle, either with a segmental explant or implant or with an encircling strap. This will loosen the invariably present vitreous traction bands attached to the vascular tissue. Single-freeze cryocoagulations can be performed on the sea fans during surgery, or focal, scatter, or feeder-vessel photocoagulation can be carried out postoperatively.

Monitoring perfusion of sea fans, or the lack thereof, is rather easily achieved by fluorescein angioscopy, and photocoagulation is repeated until neovascular perfusion has ceased. The chances of postoperative vitreous hemorrhage are thereby reduced substantially.

TREATMENT OF COMBINED RETINAL DETACHMENT AND VITREOUS TRACTION OR HEMORRHAGE

In preceding sections of this chapter, the operative and postoperative complications that characterize either vitrectomy or scleral buckling in the patient with sickle cell disease have been described. That they may be severe and blinding has been demonstrated. When vitrectomy and scleral buckling are combined in a single operation, the risks to the eye are intensified. Expandable gas, with its tendency for postoperative ocular hypertension, is a particular hazard, and it must be used with discretion and with close postoperative monitoring of IOP. If IOP increases to a level as low as 25 to 30 mm Hg, arterial perfusion pressure within the eye may be seriously compromised. Early and, if necessary, repetitive paracentesis of the anterior chamber may be required.

With these particular problems in mind, it is essential that the surgeon choose a combined vitrectomy and scleral buckling only when convinced that neither procedure alone will suffice. This usually means that, in the surgeon's judgment, the media are too dense or the traction is too severe to allow simple buckling to be successful.

Experience, to date, with combined vitrectomy and scleral buckling has been somewhat limited. Treister and Machemer reported two cases in 1977.[39] In one case the retina was attached, but anterior segment ischemia occurred, the IOP dropped to zero, and the ultimate visual acuity was worse than that preoperatively. The late results in the second case included a total tractional retinal detachment necessitating a second vitrectomy and buckling. The final acuity was 6/48 (20/160), and the retina was attached.

At the Sickle Cell Eye Clinic of the University of Illinois, we have performed combined vitrectomy and scleral buckling on 11 eyes.[28] The success rate was 45%. Five

Table 5-6. Eyes having combined vitrectomy and scleral buckling at the Sickle Cell Eye Clinic, University of Illinois

Case number	Age (years)	Sex	Follow-up study (months)	Hemoglobin*	Visual acuity	
					Preoperative	*Last visit*
1	26	F	13	SC	Light perception	6/120 (20/400)
2	26	F	53	SC	Light perception	6/9 (20/30)
3	29	M	34	SC	Count fingers	Light perception
4	25	M	1	SC	6/60 (20/200)	Count fingers
5	22	F	43	SC	6/24 (20/80)	6/9 (20/30)
6	29	F	36	SC	6/60 (20/200)	Hand motions
7	48	F	12	SC	Count fingers	Light perception
8	22	F	20	SC	6/7.5 (20/25)	6/6 (20/20)
9	49	F	6	AS	Hand motions	Light perception
10	29	M	8	SS	Hand motions	6/7.5 (20/25)
11	49	F	9	SC	Light perception	No light perception

*AS, Heterozygous carriers of sickle cell trait; *SC*, sickle cell hemoglobin C; *SS*, homozygous patients with sickle cell disease.

Table 5-7. Combined vitrectomy and scleral buckling in patients with sickle cell disease (combined series)

Reference	Visual improvement	Comments
Treister and Machemer*	1 of 2 eyes	One eye with anterior segment ischemia (prephthisic); one eye with repeat retinal detachment
Michels†	1 of 2 eyes	One eye developed postoperative rhegmatogenous retinal detachment and lost all vision
Sickle Cell Eye Clinic, University of Illinois‡	5 of 11 eyes	Five eyes with iatrogenic retinal breaks; one eye with anterior segment ischemia (prephthisic); no partial-exchange blood transfusion in this one case

*Treister, G., and Machemer, R.: Am. J. Ophthalmol. **84:**394, 1977.
†Michels, R.G.: Vitreous surgery, St. Louis, 1981, The C.V. Mosby Co.
‡Jampol, L.M., Green, J.L., Jr., Goldberg, M.F., and Peyman, G.A.: An update on vitrectomy surgery and retinal detachment repair in sickle cell disease, Arch. Ophthalmol. **100:**591, 1982.

eyes sustained iatrogenic retinal breaks. One developed anterior segment ischemia and became prephthisic (Tables 5-6 and 5-7). Preoperative partial-exchange blood transfusion was not used in this case.

The preoperative, intraoperative, and postoperative management of these eyes is highly complex and represents an amalgam of the techniques employed with vitrectomy or scleral buckling alone. It is apparent, however, that these eyes are very fragile and that potentially devastating complications affect all the major technical manipulations that are required in such cases.

SYSTEMIC FACTORS

Complications stemming from the vicious cycle of erythrostasis can cause serious and sometimes irreversible tissue damage throughout the body as well as in the eye. Relatively healthy individuals have been admitted for surgery only to sustain severe or even lethal pulmonary embolus, pulmonary infarction, and the like.[6,8,28] Considerable attention must be paid to the details before, during, and after operative systemic management. Consultation with a hematologist and an anesthesiologist is desirable. The patient should be in optimal cardiovascular and hematologic condition before surgery. Any intercurrent disease, such as an infectious process, that could initiate a sickle cell crisis must be ameliorated quickly. Premedication is kept to a minimum, and respiratory depressants are avoided. During induction of general anesthesia, breath-holding, laryngeal spasm, and struggling are prevented, if possible.[32]

During surgery, oxygenation, blood pressure, and the status of circulating blood volume must be assessed repeatedly. Oxygen is provided during local anesthesia by nasal catheter or face mask. If cautery or diathermy is to be used, the oxygen should be switched temporarily to room air so that sparks or ignited tissue or drape fragments do not induce a fire or explosion. As soon as possible, the oxygen inhalation is resumed. With endotracheal anesthesia, the anesthetist maintains as high a level of tissue oxygenation as possible and avoids the use of any drug tending to lower systemic blood pressure. Hemoconcentration, hypoxia, hypercapnia, and acidosis must be assiduously avoided. Arterial blood gas and pH levels should be obtained as necessary.

Postoperatively, early recovery of consciousness and of upper respiratory tract reflexes is important, as stressed by Oduro and Searle.[32] As noted previously, postoperative oxygen is administered by face mask for the first 48 hours. Early ambulation is encouraged if the ocular status permits. If not, elastic stockings and leg exercises in bed are utilized as prophylaxis against pulmonary embolus.

There is controversy surrounding the prognosis for patients with sickle cell trait. Ordinarily, this condition has no morbidity. Extreme conditions, however, such as hypoxia, systemic hypotension, or ocular hypertension, can induce sickling of sickle trait erythrocytes either in the eye or in other organs. Great care should be taken with these patients whenever they undergo ocular surgery, general anesthesia, or both.

CONCLUSIONS

Sickle cell retinopathy is characterized in its advanced form by preretinal neovascularization, vitreous hemorrhage, and retinal detachment. Neovascularization can be treated by focal, feeder-vessel, and panretinal photocoagulation. Visually threatening complications include retinal breaks, retinal detachment, and choriovitreal neovascularization. Whether the benefits of photocoagulation outweigh its risks is currently under scrutiny.

Cryocoagulation is a useful means of attenuating or obliterating sea-fan neovascularization and is reserved for eyes with media too hazy to permit photocoagulation. It is also employed during scleral buckling and vitrectomy procedures.

In the presence of prolonged and dense vitreous hemorrhage, pars plana vitrectomy can be curative, but in the aphakic eye, secondary glaucoma caused by a logjam of sickled erythrocytes in the trabecular meshwork can be a serious threat to vision in the postoperative period.

For rhegmatogenous retinal detachment and clear media, conventional scleral buckling is indicated, but postoperative anterior segment ischemia may cause sufficient corneal, lenticular, and uveal necrosis that visual improvement does not occur, even though the retina may have been reattached. A combination of preoperative and postoperative measures designed to maximize oxygenation and blood flow may serve to protect the eye. Included in this prophylactic regimen is partial-exchange blood transfusion, erythropheresis, or use of a hyperbaric operating room. Also included are a group of medical and surgical maneuvers designed to keep intraocular pressure as low as possible and arterial perfusion pressure as high as possible.

For eyes with retinal detachment characterized by both cloudy media and severe vitreous traction, combined scleral buckling and vitrectomy can be performed. The present success rate is approximately 50%, indicating the fragility of these eyes and their propensity for severe intraoperative and postoperative complications.

REFERENCES

1. Archer, D., Krill, A.E., and Newell, F.W.: Fluorescein angiographic evaluation of the effects of photocoagulation in three retinal vascular diseases, Trans. Ophthalmol. Soc. U.K. **90:**677, 1970.
2. Condon, P.I., and Serjeant, G.R.: Photocoagulation and diathermy in the treatment of proliferative sickle retinopathy, Br. J. Ophthalmol. **58:**650, 1974.
3. Condon, P.I., and Serjeant, G.R.: Behaviour of untreated proliferative sickle retinopathy, Br. J. Ophthalmol. **64:**404, 1980.
4. Condon, P.I., and Serjeant, G.R.: Photocoagulation in proliferative sickle cell retinopathy: results of a 5-year study, Br. J. Ophthalmol. **64:**832, 1980.
5. Dizon-Moore, R.V., Jampol, L.M., and Goldberg, M.F.: Chorioretinal and choriovitreal neovascularization, Arch. Ophthalmol. **99:**842, 1981.
6. Eagle, R.C., Yanoff, M., and Morse, P.H.: Anterior segment necrosis following scleral buckling in hemoglobin SC disease, Am. J. Ophthalmol. **75:**426, 1973.
7. Freilich, D.B., and Seelenfreund, M.H.: Long-term follow-up of scleral buckling procedures with sickle cell disease and retinal detachment treated with the use of hyperbaric oxygen, Mod. Probl. Ophthalmol. **18:**368, 1977.
8. Galinos, S.O., Smith, T.R., and Brockhurst, R.J.: Angioma-like lesion in hemoglobin sickle cell disease, Ann. Ophthalmol. **11:**1549, 1979.
9. Goldbaum, M.H., Galinos, S.O., Apple, D., Asdourian, G.K., Nagpal, K., Jampol, L.M., Woolf, M.B., and Busse, B.: Acute choroidal ischemia as a complication of photocoagulation, Arch. Ophthalmol. **94:**1025, 1976.
10. Goldbaum, M.H., Goldberg, M.F., Nagpal, K., Asdourian, G.K., and Galinos, S.O.: Proliferative sickle retinopathy. In L'Esperance, F.A., editor: Current diagnosis and management of chorioretinal diseases, St. Louis, 1977, The C.V. Mosby Co.
11. Goldbaum, M.H., Peyman, G.A., Nagpal, K.C., Goldberg, M.F., and Asdourian, G.K.: Vitrectomy in sickling retinopathy: report of five cases, Ophthalmic Surg. **7:**92, 1976.
12. Goldbaum, M.H., Fletcher, R.C., Jampol, L.M., and Goldberg, M.F.: Cryotherapy of proliferative sickle retinopathy. II. Triple freeze-thaw cycle, Br. J. Ophthalmol. **63:**97, 1979.
13. Goldberg, M.F.: Treatment of proliferative sickle retinopathy, Trans. Am. Acad. Ophthalmol. Otolaryngol. **75:**532, 1971.
14. Goldberg, M.F.: Retinal neovascularization in sickle cell retinopathy, Trans. Am. Acad. Ophthalmol. Otolaryngol. **83:**409, 1977.
15. Goldberg, M.F.: Sickled erythrocytes, hyphema, and secondary glaucoma. I. The diagnosis and treatment of sickled erythrocytes in human hyphemas, Ophthalmic Surg. **10:**17, 1979.

16. Goldberg, M.F.: Sickled erythrocytes, hyphema, and secondary glaucoma. IV. The rate and percentage of sickling of erythrocytes in rabbit aqueous humor, in vitro and in vivo, Ophthalmic Surg. **10:**62, 1979.

17. Goldberg, M.F.: Sickled erythrocytes, hyphema, and secondary glaucoma. V. The effect of vitamin C on erythrocyte sickling in aqueous humor, Ophthalmic Surg. **10:**70, 1979.

18. Goldberg, M.F., and Acacio, I.: Argon laser photocoagulation of proliferative sickle retinopathy, Arch. Ophthalmol. **90:**35, 1973.

19. Goldberg, M.F., Dizon, R., and Moses, V.K.: Sickled erythrocytes, hyphema, and secondary glaucoma. VI. The relationship between intracameral blood cells and aqueous humor pH, P_{O_2}, and P_{CO_2}, Ophthalmic Surg. **10:**78, 1979.

20. Goldberg, M.F., Dizon, R., and Raichand, M.: Sickled erythrocytes, hyphema, and secondary glaucoma. II. Injected sickle cell erythrocytes into human, monkey, and guinea pig anterior chambers: the induction of sickling and secondary glaucoma, Ophthalmic Surg. **10:**32, 1979.

21. Goldberg, M.F., Dizon, R., Raichand, M., Goldbaum, M.H., and Jampol, L.M.: Sickled erythrocytes, hyphema, and secondary glaucoma. III. Effects of sickle cell and normal human blood samples in rabbit anterior chambers, Ophthalmic Surg. **10:**52, 1979.

22. Goldberg, M.F., and Tso, M.O.M.: Sickled erythrocytes, hyphema, and secondary glaucoma. VII. The passage of sickled erythrocytes out of the anterior chamber of the human and the monkey eye: light and electron microscopic studies, Ophthalmic Surg. **10:**89, 1979.

23. Hannon, J.F.: Vitreous hemorrhages associated with sickle cell hemoglobin-C disease, Am. J. Ophthalmol. **42:**707, 1956.

24. Hayes, R.J., Condon, P.I., and Serjeant, G.R.: Haematological factors associated with proliferative retinopathy in homozygous sickle cell disease, Br. J. Ophthalmol. **65:**29, 1981.

25. Jampol, L.M.: New techniques in treating proliferative sickle cell retinopathy. In Fine, S., editor: Current concepts in management of retinal vascular and macular diseases, Baltimore, The Williams & Wilkins Co. (In press.)

26. Jampol, L.M., and Goldbaum, M.H.: Peripheral proliferative retinopathies, Surv. Ophthalmol. **25:**1, 1980.

27. Jampol, L.M., and Goldberg, M.F.: Retinal breaks after photocoagulation of proliferative sickle cell retinopathy, Arch. Ophthalmol. **98:**676, 1980.

28. Jampol, L.M., Green, J.L., Jr., Goldberg, M.F., and Peyman, G.A.: An update on vitrectomy surgery and retinal detachment repair in sickle cell disease, Arch. Ophthalmol. **100:**591, 1982.

29. Lee, C.B., Woolf, M.B., Galinos, S.O., Goldbaum, M.H., Stevens, T.S., and Goldberg, M.F.: Cryotherapy of proliferative sickle retinopathy. I. Single freeze-thaw cycle, Ann. Ophthalmol. **7:**299, 1975.

30. Michels, R.G.: Vitreous surgery, St. Louis, 1981, The C.V. Mosby Co.

31. Nagpal, K.C., Patrianakos, D., Asdourian, G.K., Goldberg, M.F., Rabb, M.F., and Jampol, L.M.: Spontaneous regression (autoinfarction) of proliferative sickle retinopathy, Am. J. Ophthalmol. **80:**885, 1975.

32. Oduro, K.A., and Searle, J.F.: Anaesthesia in sickle-cell states: a plea for simplicity, Br. Med. J. **4:**596, 1972.

33. Peyman, G.A., Wyhinny, G.J., and Goldberg, M.F.: Optical radiation and Zeiss short-pulsed xenon photocoagulators. I. Clinical considerations of articulation with the Fankhauser slit-lamp delivery system, Arch. Ophthalmol. **92:**341, 1974.

34. Raichand, M., Goldberg, M.F., Nagpal, K.C., Goldbaum, M.H., and Asdourian, G.K.: Evolution of neovascularization in sickle cell retinopathy, Arch. Ophthalmol. **95:**1543, 1977.

35. Rednam, K.R.V., Jampol, L.M., and Goldberg, M.F.: Scatter retinal photocoagulation for proliferative sickle cell retinopathy, Am. J. Ophthalmol. **93:**594, 1982.

36. Ryan, S.J.: Role of the vitreous in the haemoglobinopathies, Trans. Ophthalmol. Soc. U.K. **95:**403, 1975.

37. Ryan, S.J., and Goldberg, M.F.: Anterior segment ischemia following scleral buckling in sickle cell hemoglobinopathy, Am. J. Ophthalmol. **72:**35, 1971.

38. Simons, E.R., editor: Clinical conferences at the Johns Hopkins Hospital, Johns Hopkins Med. J. **149:**45, 1981.

39. Treister, G., and Machemer, R.: Results of vitrectomy for rare proliferative and hemorrhagic diseases, Am. J. Ophthalmol. **84:**394, 1977.

40. Tse, D.A.D., and Ober, R.R.: Talc retinopathy, Am. J. Ophthalmol. **90:**624, 1980.
41. Wilensky, J.T., Goldberg, M.F., and Alward, P.: Glaucoma after pars plana vitrectomy, Trans. Am. Acad. Ophthalmol. Otolaryngol. **83:**114, 1977.
42. Wilhelm, J.L., Zakov, Z.N., and Hoeltge, G.A.: Erythropheresis in treating retinal detachments secondary to sickle-cell retinopathy, Am. J. Ophthalmol. **92:**582, 1981.
43. Zinn, K.M.: Vitreoretinal surgery in a patient with sickle cell retinopathy, Mt. Sinai J. Med. **48:**79, 1981.

6

Observations on retinal neovascularization

Arnall Patz

Retinal neovascularization can be conveniently defined as an abnormal growth of retinal vessels in a pattern different from that of the normal retinal vessels and lying anterior to the plane of the normal retinal vessels. These new vessels frequently extend through the internal limiting membrane into the vitreous cavity. They show a loss of the normal blood-retinal barrier so that on fluorescein angiography retinal neovascularization almost always shows significant leakage of fluorescein. Gross abnormalities in permeability are associated with hemorrhage. Where longitudinal studies have been done, patients subsequently developing proliferative retinopathy, such as diabetics, virtually always have areas of capillary nonperfusion, which can be demonstrated on fluorescein angiography. In general, the more capillary nonperfusion is present, the greater is the likelihood for the development of neovascularization.

THEORY OF A RETINAL ANGIOGENIC SUBSTANCE

Michaelson[12], in his classic paper on the development of the retinal vessels, first suggested that in the mammalian retina there was a factor or factors in the substance of the retina that affected the growth of vessels. Michaelson stated that the factor has the following characteristics:

1. It is present in the extravascular tissue of the retina.
2. It is present in a gradient of concentration such that it differs in arterial and venous neighborhoods.
3. Its action is on the retinal veins predominantly.
4. The factor initiating the capillary growth from a vein probably determines the distance to which that growth will extend, with initiation and cessation depending on variations and concentration of the factor.

Michaelson presented evidence from human pathology to support the existence of a factor capable of stimulating vessel growth in the retina. He cited the examples of diabetic retinopathy, retinal venous occlusion, and the retinal vasculitis of young adults (Eales' disease) in which neovascularization developed. Michaelson postulated that common to these pathologic conditions, which had a chronic course, altered metabolism resulted and the "accession of vessels being directed toward insufficiently or nonvascularized situations" was responsible for the new vessel formation. This is the first reference in the literature relating the association of retinal neovascularization with "nonvascularized situations."

Ashton et al.[3] utilizing the observations from his elegant experiments on oxygen in retrolental fibroplasia, stated that the retinal tissue, when in a state of metabolic embarrassment, liberates a factor with vasoformative (angiogenic) properties that is able to diffuse into vitreous and stimulate the growth of new capillaries on the surface of the retina.

George N. Wise's[18] thesis on retinal neovascularization published in 1956 provided a thorough review of the literature at that time. Wise made a point of not distinguishing between simple dilatation of preexisting channels and actual newly formed vessels. Wise coined the term for the extravascular intraretinal factor postulated by Michaelson as "factor X." He commented, based on Michaelson's observations, that there is an orderly evolvement of the definitive retinal blood supply suggesting a gradient of factor X in the developing retina. The capillary-free zone noted by Michaelson about the arteries was one example. "Furthermore, the capillary-free zone of approximately the same dimensions which is present at the ora, at the fovea, and in the outer retinal layers suggested that factor X varies in degree in arterial and venous vicinities, being more potent in the latter."

Michaelson suggested that the choroid's capacity to nourish the outer layers of the retina affected the vessel growth and development in the retina. Michaelson pointed out that up to the third month of fetal life the choroid was capable of nourishing the retina. As the retina thickens, the choroidal nutrition becomes inadequate and vessels grow into the retina from the optic disc with the "capillaries appearing first in the portion of the retina farthest from the choroid, i.e., the nerve fiber layer, and only later in the inner nuclear layer." Michaelson attributed this retinal vascularization pattern to the accumulation in the retina of a factor or factors associated with retinal metabolism whose requirements were not fully met after the third month by the choroid's nutritional supply. Michaelson further stated that in certain regions, such as the fovea, periphery of the retina, and the outer layers of the retina, the nutritional needs are completely met by the choroidal circulation and these portions remain avascular.

RECENT OBSERVATIONS ON THE RETINAL ANGIOGENESIS HYPOTHESIS

The observations of retinal capillary closure with presumed ischemia followed by neovascularization is consistent with the hypothesis just discussed.[13] There is increasing evidence consistent with the theory that retinal ischemia leads to the production of a substance, an "angiogenic or vasoproliferative factor," that may diffuse from the areas of retinal ischemia. Since the tissue adjacent to the area of ischemia would most likely have the highest concentration of the hypothetical angiogenic factor, the neovascularization that occurs adjacent to the nonperfused areas is logically explained. Furthermore, studies on the diffusion pathway through the vitreous have demonstrated a predilect pathway of diffusion toward the optic disc from the peripheral portions of the vitreous (Gärtner 1968).[5] The accumulation of the hypothetical angiogenic factor in the disc area might then explain the predilection for the development of neovascularization at the disc. Lastly, the diffusion of this presumed substance or substances forward to stimulate vessels on the iris is consistent not only with the findings of diabetic retinopathy, where extensive capillary closure in proliferative retinopathy is frequently associated with iris

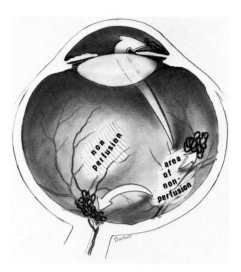

Fig. 6-1. Schematic diagram showing areas of retinal capillary closure (with nonperfusion) resulting in retinal ischemia. An angiogenesis or vasoproliferative factor is postulated to stimulate neovascularization in the retina, at the disc, or on the iris.

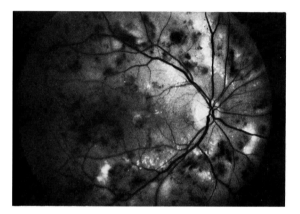

Fig. 6-2. Sixty-five-year-old white female with history of diabetes of 20 year's duration. The patient showed evidence of preproliferative retinopathy with beaded veins. Also extensive intraretinal edema, hemorrhages, and hard exudates are present. (Red-free 60 degree field.)

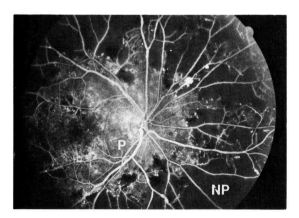

Fig. 6-3. Midtransit of the fluorescein angiogram showing retinal perfusion essentially intact in the posterior pole, but severe capillary closure with nonperfusion involving the entire midperiphery. *P*, Perfused retina; *NP*, nonperfused retina.

neovascularization, but also with the observations noted in patients with central retinal vein occlusion (Fig. 6-1 to 6-3). Studies by Laatikainen and Blach[10] and by others showed very strikingly in patients with central retinal vein occlusion that those with severe nonperfusion had a high incidence of iris neovascularization. These investigators reported that in patients with extensive capillary closure, 58% developed iris neovascularization and many of the 58% went on to develop neovascular glaucoma. On the other hand, in the patients who have central retinal vein occlusion with relatively good capillary perfusion, based on fluorescein angiography, only 4% developed iris neovascularization and none of these progressed to neovascular glaucoma.

The hypothesis of a diffusible angiogenic factor being liberated by ischemic retina has received circumstantial support in the treatment of neovascularization by panretinal photocoagulation, a technique whereby the retina is coagulated in a large area with the resolution of the retinal neovascularization in a highly significant number of cases. It is of interest that the photocoagulation treatment need not be directed specifically toward the abnormal retinal neovascularization itself, but directed rather to the surrounding, presumably ischemic, retinal tissue. It is presumed that the photocoagulation utilizing the panretinal technique destroys, or alters, ischemic retina tissue that may be producing a neovascularization stimulating factor so that the production of the stimulating factor is eliminated or significantly reduced.

It is appropriate to point out that the mechanism of panretinal photocoagulation for the treatment of retinal neovascularization in diabetic retinopathy may be explained on other mechanisms than the elimination of an angiogenic stimulant. Wolbarsht et al.[19] have suggested that neovascularization may develop from oxygen deprivation without the intermediary of a diffusible angiogenic factor. Their studies, utilizing oxygen electrodes in the animal model, have demonstrated that the oxygen tension measured with a polarographic electrode at the internal limiting membrane of the retina is increased after photocoagulation therapy. This alternative hypothesis is of interest because the principal tissue that is altered by the photocoagulation consists of the retinal pigment epithelium and outer portions of the retina with only minimal absorption of energy in the inner "presumed ischemic" areas in the inner retina. Since the photoreceptors are immediately adjacent to the pigment epithelium, they are largely destroyed in the selective damage to the outer portion of the retina. Weiter and Zuckerman[17] have also pointed out the large oxygen consumption of the photoreceptors. The destruction of the photoreceptors would diminish the total oxygen extracted from the choroidal circulation allowing greater diffusion of unused oxygen to the inner layers, which are now closer to the choriocapillaries after destruction of the outer retinal layers.

Foulds[4] has suggested a possible mechanism for the effect of photocoagulation through the role of the retinal pigment epithelial barrier between the choriocapillaris-choroidal circulation and the retina. Conceivably, a vasoproliferative or angiogenic factor could be accumulating in the vitreous and in the retina, and photocoagulation, which has been demonstrated by Peyman et al.[16] to break the retinal pigment epithelial barrier, might enable the diffusion of angiogenic substances out of the retina and vitreous reservoir into the choroidal circulation. This latter hypothesis is gaining further credibility by the recent observations that the retinal pigment epithelium may play a role in the production of retinal edema, either by virtue of breaks in the zonular occludents or by diffusion across the pigment epithelium cell that has lost its barrier effect.

In addition to diabetic retinopathy, there are several disease entities that support the working hypothesis that ischemic retina produces an angiogenesis or vasoproliferative material. These other diseases include retrolental fibroplasia and branch vein occlusion, both of which have suggested through their clinical appearance other features of the hypothesized angiogenic mechanisms. It is this clinical background that has supported the concept of an angiogenic factor since the original suggestion of Michaelson[12] and Ashton et al.[2] was postulated over 25 years ago. With this clinical background in mind, investigators at several laboratories have begun a biochemical and physiologic search for possible retinal angiogenic substances.

Studies on retinal neovascularization at the Wilmer Institute date back to the early 1950s, when the proliferative stage of retrolental fibroplasia was produced in experimental animals.[15] These laboratory studies paralleled a controlled nursery investigation of the role of oxygen in retrolental fibroplasia.[14] The oxygen model of retinal neovascularization, which was developed in Ashton's laboratories in London and in our laboratories in Baltimore, proved to be an excellent model to study the early proliferative stages of retrolental fibroplasia, and it is still the most predictable and reproducible model now available for the experimental investigation of retinal neovascularization. The mechanism of oxygen action is discussed in Chapter 16. It is appropriate to summarize briefly the mechanism of oxygen action on the premature retina as it relates to our current thoughts on retinal ischemia, a presumed angiogenic factor, and retinal neovascularization.

OXYGEN MODEL OF RETINAL NEOVASCULARIZATION

The experimental counterpart of early proliferative human retrolental fibroplasia was first produced in kittens by Ashton and co-workers,[3] in mice, kittens, and puppies in our laboratory;[15] and in mice by Gyllensten and Hellström[7] in Stockholm. Ashton's elegant India ink injection studies demonstrated the mechanism of oxygen effect on the premature retina and clarified the understanding of retrolental fibroplasia pathogenesis; our production of the lesions in three different species demonstrated the broad susceptibility of the premature retina to oxygen.

When the oxygen exposure is relatively minor, such as 30 hours at 50% concentration, capillary closure occurs only in the anterior part of the retina. On return to room air, the neovascularization is limited to the far periphery, possibly from an angiogenic material liberated by the peripheral ischemic tissue. As the initial oxygen exposure is increased, vascular closure occurs more posteriorly. With prolonged exposure to oxygen, such as 96 hours at 85% concentration, some of the capillary bed near the disc is also permanently closed and disc neovascularization results. The relationship of the vascular closure and presumed retinal ischemia to the locus of secondary retinal neovascularization has analogies to the neovascularization noted in the clinical retinopathies. It also is significant that the oxygen itself in these experiments is probably not directly involved in the neovascular response, but simply a method of inducing vascular closure. For example, Ashton and Henkind[1] produced retinal neovascularization in young kittens after the carotid arterial injection of Ballotini glass microspheres into them and suggested that the vascular closure is the key ingredient rather than the oxygen exposure.

LABORATORY STUDIES ON ANGIOGENESIS

We have reported an inhibitor of tumor-induced neovascularization in an extract prepared from adult vitreous. After Glaser and co-workers[6] demonstrated stimulation of experimental neovascularization from an extract obtained from retina, it was logical to test the vitreous extract for its possible inhibitory effect on the retinal material. Lutty and co-workers[10] performed a series of experiments in our laboratory where the chick chorioallantoic membrane system was used to test this question. Fertilized chicken eggs were implanted with pellets containing the extract derived from bovine retina. A coverslip containing either an extract from adult vitreous or a control substance was placed over the treated area of the membrane. The neovascular response was graded on a daily basis. There was a striking difference in the mean growth scores for the neovascularization between the vitreous-treated chick membranes and the controls. The inhibition of the retinal extract was dose dependent and increased as the concentration of bovine vitreous material was further concentrated. This was of considerable interest because the extract prepared from retinal tissue may have relevance to a presumed substance postulated to stimulate neovascularization in the human proliferative retinopathies.

CURRENT CLINICAL CONCEPTS

Capillary nonperfusion with resultant retinal ischemia is common to the major proliferative retinopathies. An angiogenic or vasoproliferative factor or combination of factors, which remains to be documented has been postulated to stimulate the development of neovascularization in the retina or at the optic disc or by diffusion forward on the iris. In diabetic retinopathy, the more severe the capillary nonperfusion in general, the more severe the ensuing proliferative retinopathy will be (Fig. 6-3).

Although the exact mechanism of photocoagulation remains to be documented, it is widely recognized that panretinal photocoagulation, which involves the treatment of presumed ischemic areas of the retina, will arrest the progression of retinal neovascularization in diabetic retinopathy. Not only is the continued growth of the abnormal new vessels stopped, but the vessels that have already proliferated undergo atrophic changes and disappear. Fluorescein angiography after successful panretinal photocoagulation in the patient with proliferative diabetic retinopathy will show no residum of the neovascularization and no evidence of leakage whatsoever at the sites of previous new vessels, whereas before treatment these new vessels leaked fluorescein profusely. The early treatment diabetic retinopathy collaborative study that is now in progress will investigate the feasibility of earlier treatment in the management of mild retinal neovascularization. The role of scatter photocoagulation in the involved sector of nonperfusion in patients with branch vein occlusion is being investigated in a collaborative branch vein occlusion study, and we will await the results of this study to develop better guidelines for the management of these patients.

Refer to comprehensive recent reviews of retinal neovascularization. The first is the Krill Memorial Lecture published by Henkind[8] and the review on peripheral retinal neovascularization by Jampol and Goldbaum.[9]

SUMMARY AND CONCLUSION

Retinal vascular closure, which presumably leads to retinal ischemia, is generally observed in all the proliferative retinopathies. The association of capillary closure with development of proliferative diabetic retinopathy is well documented. It has been proposed that a factor resulting from the retinal ischemia stimulates the formation of retinal new vessels (angiogenic or vasoproliferative factor). Although the concept that retinal ischemia is associated with the liberation of an angiogenic substance remains to be proved, the theory is consistent with the findings in virtually all the proliferative retinopathies. Recent experimental studies open new avenues for investigation and exploration of the underlying pathogenesis of the neovascularization that occurs in diabetic and other proliferative retinopathies.

REFERENCES

1. Ashton, N., and Henkind, P.: Experimental occlusion of retinal arterioles using graded glass Ballotini, Br. J. Ophthalmol. **49**(5):225-234, 1965.
2. Ashton, N., Ward, B., and Serpell, G.: Role of oxygen in the genesis of retrolental fibroplasia: preliminary report, Br. J. Ophthalmol. **37**:513, 1953.
3. Ashton, N., Ward, B., and Serpell, G.: Effects of oxygen on developing retinal vessels with particular reference to the problem of retrolental fibroplasia, Br, J. Ophthalmol. **38**:397, 1954.
4. Foulds, W.S.: The role of photocoagulation in the treatment of retinal disease, Trans. Ophthalmol. Soc. N.Z. **32**:82, 1980.
5. Gärtner, J.: Importance of the perivascular space of the central vessels in vitreopapillar drainage: electron microscopic observations on the normal mouse eye and on the human eye under pathological conditions, Albrecht von Graefes Arch. Klin. Ophthalmol. **175**:13-27, 1968.
6. Glaser, B.M., D'Amore, P.A., Michels, R.G., Patz, A., and Fenselau, A.: Demonstration of vasoproliferative activity from mammalian retina, J. Cell Biol. **84**:298, 1980.
7. Gyllensten, L.J., and Hellström, B.E.: Experimental approach to the pathogenesis of retrolental fibroplasia: changes of eye induced by exposure of new-born mice to concentrated oxygen, Acta Paediatr. **43**:131, 1954.
8. Henkind, P.: Ocular neovascularization, The Krill Memorial Lecture, Am. J. Ophthalmol. **85**:287, 1978.
9. Jampol, L.M., and Goldbaum, M.H.: Peripheral proliferative retinopathies, Survey Ophthalmol. **25**:1, 1980.
10. Laatikainen, L., and Blach, R.K.: Behaviour of the iris vasculature in central retinal vein occlusion: a fluorescein angiographic study of the vascular response of the retina and the iris, Br. J. Ophthalmol. **61**:272-277, 1977.
11. Lutty, G.A., Thompson, D.C., Gallup, J.G., and Patz, A.: Inhibition of neovascularization by bovine vitreous in the CAM assay, Invest. Ophthalmol. Vis. Sci. **19**(suppl.):138, 1980.
12. Michaelson, I.C.: The mode of development of the vascular system of the retina, with some observations on its significance for certain retinal diseases, Trans. Ophthalmol. Soc. U.K. **68**:137, 1948.
13. Patz, A.: The Friedenwald Memorial Lecture. I. Studies on retinal neovascularization, Invest. Ophthalmol. **19**:1127-1149, 1980.
14. Patz A., Hoeck, L.E., and de La Cruz, E.: Studies on the effect of high oxygen administration in retrolental fibroplasia: nursery observations, Am. J. Ophthalmol. **35**:1248, 1952.
15. Patz, A., Eastham, A., Higgenbotham, D.H., and Kleh, T.: Oxygen studies in retrolental fibroplasia: production of the microscopic changes of retrolental fibroplasia in experimental animals, Am. J. Ophthalmol. **36**:1511, 1953.
16. Peyman, G.A., Spitznas, M., and Straatsma, B.R.: Peroxidase diffusion in the normal and photocoagulated retina, Invest. Ophthalmol. **10**(3):181-189, 1971.
17. Weiter, J.J., Zuckerman, R.: The influence of the photoreceptor-RPE complex on the inner retina: an explanation for the beneficial effects of photocoagulation, Ophthalmology **87**(11):1133-1139, 1980.
18. Wise, G.N.: Retinal neovascularization. Trans. Am. Ophthalmol. Soc. **54**:729, 1956.
19. Wolbarsht, M.L., and Landers, M.B.: The rationale of photocoagulation therapy for proliferative diabetic retinopathy: a review and a model, Ophthalmol. Surg. **11**:235, 1980.

7

Presumed histoplasmosis syndrome

Robert C. Watzke

I present here the state of knowledge of the pathogenesis and treatment of the presumed ocular histoplasmosis syndrome. Much of our knowledge is speculative, but during the last few years we have learned a great deal about this enigmatic disease. Treatment, however, remains unproved.

HISTOPLASMA SPOT ("HISTO SPOT")

Clinicians are familiar with the appearance of the so-called typical *Histoplasma* spot ("histo spot"). It is an atrophic chorioretinal scar, usually circular with a dot of pigment in or near the center. It occurs in groups, clusters, or sometimes tracks (Fig. 7-1).

However, there is a more characteristic and subtle choroidal lesion that is the basic form of the disease. This is a yellow, round lesion just under the pigment epithelium. It is unpigmented and varies in size from 50 to 300 μm. It may be so subtle as to be invisible on clinical examination and visible only on fluorescein angiography. It has slightly indistinct borders, and the overlying pigment epithelium and retina appear normal. On fluorescein angiography it may be hypofluorescent early and hyperfluorescent in later stages.

The characteristics of these choroidal spots were first described by Schlaegel, and their significance was emphasized by Krill, who also demonstrated that these lesions change in appearance over time.[10,18] They may enlarge, they may almost disappear, but they usually become more evident and finally more atrophic and pigmented (Fig. 7-1). This remodeling occurs completely asymptomatically. To document it, one must follow a large number of patients over a period of at least 10 to 15 years.[23]

The incidence of typical spots in individuals inhabiting an endemic area is 2.8%.[6] Although we do not know the incidence of these choroidal lesions in nonendemic areas, we do know that such lesions exist.[1,3-5]

If one practices in an endemic area, one would expect occasionally to see a patient in whom the choroidal lesions appear in fundi that were previously normal. I believe that many clinicians have seen such patients and are reluctant to report them since the diagnosis of ocular histoplasmosis is difficult to prove and a prolonged follow-up study would be required to demonstrate the entire course of the disease. During the past 25 years of practice in an endemic area I have seen seven patients in whom I believe the choroidal lesions began. I now describe an example.

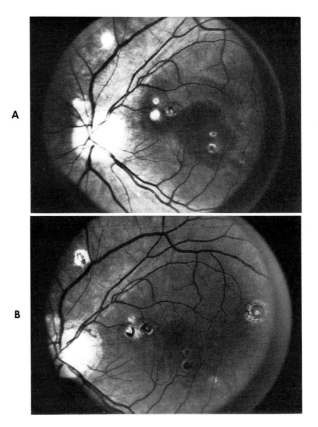

Fig. 7-1. A, Opposite eye of a patient with ocular histoplasmosis syndrome. Atrophic pigmented and unpigmented *Histoplasma* spots involve the posterior pole. **B,** Seven years later, the spots are larger and more pigmented.

A 21-year-old medical student was first seen for refraction on October 18, 1973. She was approximately −7.00 myopic in each eye, and on the fundus examination there were no abnormalities noted except for a small chorioretinal scar inferotemporal to the fovea in the left eye. The patient had previously been seen by an ophthalmologist in 1969, 1971, 1972, and 1973 and was reported by him to have had a completely normal fundus.

On September 5, 1974, she noted two brightly lighted scotomas just nasal and temporal to fixation in the left eye. Vision was 20/20 in each eye. there were no aqueous or vitreous cells. A group of yellow, choroidal infiltrates were noted about the left fovea (Fig. 7-2, *A*). One spot, about 1 disc diameter temporal to the left fovea, was quite atrophic. There were two very small spots approximately 200 μm in diameter just temporal to the fovea and a larger spot in the maculopapular bundle. All spots appeared to be at the level of the pigment epithelium. The only exception to this was the larger inferotemporal spot where choriocapillaris atrophy had occurred.

On fluorescein angiography the lesions neither perfused with fluorescein nor transmitted choroidal fluorescence (Fig. 7-2, *B* and *C*). An additional spot temporal to the

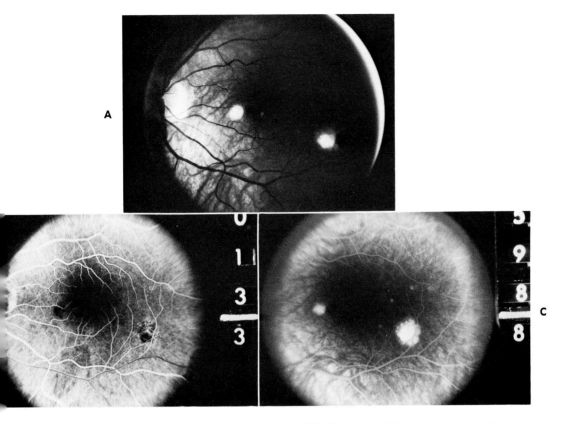

Fig. 7-2. A, Left fundus of a 21-year-old woman in October 1975. Four choroidal lesions have appeared since an examination 6 months ago. The spot just below the center of the fovea is an artifact. Vision 20/20. **B** and **C,** On fluorescein angiography, the lesions are hypofluorescent with late staining except for the large atrophic spot inferotemporal to the fovea.

fovea was present but was not visible on clinical examination. The inferotemporal atrophic spot demonstrated some larger choroidal vessels. All spots showed faint, late staining.

By February 20, 1975, an obvious subretinal neovascular membrane appeared from the spot under the maculopapular bundle (Fig. 7-3). The other spots appeared more atrophic and pigmented, and a new choroidal lesion had appeared in the temporal macula. On February 28, 1975, xenon photocoagulation of the subretinal neovascular membrane in the maculopapular bundle was performed. Subsequently, the subretinal neovascular membrane appeared to be completely obliterated. Vision remained 20/30 despite a progressively more pigmented and enlarging scar in the maculopapular bundle. The rest of the lesions also became atrophic and pigmented.

On September 14, 1976, a new subretinal neovascular membrane appeared at the superior margin of the light coagulation scar. Over the next 8 months the membrane enlarged but did not involve the fovea. Vision dropped to 20/200, however, because of progressive involvement of the foveolar pigment epithelium by the enlarging photocoagulation scar.

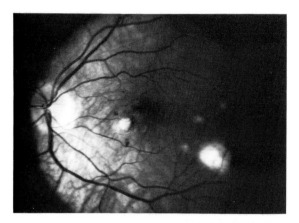

Fig. 7-3. Six months later, all spots are larger and more prominent. A subretinal neovascular membrane has appeared from the spot in the maculopapillary bundle. A new spot has also appeared temporally.

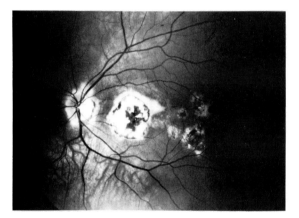

Fig. 7-4. Five years later, all spots are larger and more pigmented. The spot in the maculopapillary bundle has been photocoagulated. Vision 20/400.

By November 1977, a new subretinal neovascular membrane had started from a new spot temporal to the fovea. Remodeling and increased pigmentation of all macular lesions continued (Fig. 7-4). The patient was last seen in January 1982. There was extensive pigmentation and atrophy of all choroidal scars. Numerous new choroidal scars had also appeared in the posterior pole. The right eye stayed normal.

Chest film was negative except for small calcified right lower lobe granulomas and left hilar granulomas. A PPD of tuberculin skin test was positive (it was negative in 1971), and a histoplasmin skin test was negative. The hemogram was normal. A histoplasmin, blastomycosis, and coccidioidomycosis complement-fixation titer was negative at less than 1:2 dilution at the time of appearance of the choroidal infiltrates. However, on April 9, 1980, a lymphocyte transformation test showed a strong lymphocytic response to mitogen PHA, histoplasmin, PPD, SK-SD, and *Candida* antigens.*

SOURCE OF CHOROIDAL SPOTS

One hypothesis of the source of choroidal scars is that they are acquired early in life during the first two decades in an asymptomatic fashion, presumably by inhalation of yeast forms of *Histoplasma* organisms.[6] Small granulomatous abscesses occur in various organs because of a *Histoplasma* fungemia.[19] These abscesses usually heal, and in the eye the person is left with small choroidal scars. Choroidal lesions may be visible only on fluorescein angiography or on clinical examination, depending on the cellular morphology, the degree of atrophy of the pigment epithelium, and the presence of neovascular tissue.

A second hypothesis recognizes that these choroidal lesions appear in clinically normal areas of the fundus progressively over a patient's life and that the longer patients are followed, the more frequent is such an event.[11,23] Thus early choroidal lesions may consist of a cellular infiltrate under an intact pigment epithelium, and the infiltrate becomes visible over the years as remodeling occurs. An alternative explanation is continual seeding into the choroid by some organism and from some focus as yet unknown.

Histoplasma spots vary from the most subtle choroidal infiltrates to a large, deeply pigmented and almost confluent chorioretinal scar. They appear to become more pigmented and atrophic with age, but there are no long-term studies to prove this. In fact, most spots do not change over 1 to 5 years. However, in a recent study of 40 patients followed for at least 10 and up to 15 years, it was common to see spots appear from a clinically normal retina and become more pigmented and atrophic[23] (Fig. 7-1).

Histoplasma spots vary in number from one to fundi that are so studded with them that it appears inconceivable that they could have developed asymptomatically. Occasionally, they have a track or branching streak configuration.

Two reports of pathologic studies of *Histoplasma* spots described lymphocytes and giant cells in the choroid with atrophy of the overlying pigment epithelium and photoreceptors.[12] Other reports, however, have demonstrated atrophic chorioretinal scars with none or few inflammatory cells.[14,16] A recent study demonstrated new blood vessels under the retina or between Bruch's membrane and the pigment epithelium in all histoplasmotic spots whatever their appearance.[24] These vessels were very subtle and could be found only in serial, ultrathin sections in lesions from an eye fixed with glutaraldehyde and not paraffin.

DISC SCARRING

Our concepts of the evolution of peripapillary scars and subsequent subretinal neovascular membranes is even more tentative than those of *Histoplasma* spots. Disc scarring is seen in about 85% of patients with this syndrome.[17] Presumably, a subclinical papillitis occurs at the time of first exposure, but no one has really explained or demonstrated this, either by clinical observation or primate experiments.

---

*PHA, Phytohemagglutinins; PPD, purified protein derivative of tuberculin; SK-SD, streptokinase-streptodornase.

There has been reported only one patient who could represent an acquired peripapillary scarring of the histoplasmosis type.[8]

TWOFOLD EVOLUTION OF CHOROIDAL SCARS

There are two types of symptomatic activity that can be observed in perifoveal *Histoplasma* spots over a long period.

First is a very subtle alteration in the appearance of the perifoveal choroidal infiltrates. Symptoms are subtle and are usually noticed only by patients who have lost vision in one eye and are extremely fearful of loss in their remaining eye. These patients will describe a very subtle pericentral scotoma or, if the choroidal lesion is subfoveal, very slight blurring of vision. On examination one sees a yellow, choroidal spot usually within one disc diameter of the fovea and having a very slight serous detachment of the overlying retina. The serous detachment is restricted to the choroidal infiltrate and does not extend beyond its margins. On contact-lens examination the margins of the choroidal infiltrate are somewhat blurred. On fluorescein angiography one sees a slight hyperfluorescence of these spots, but no evidence of a subretinal neovascular membrane, pigmentation or hemorrhage.

This type of activity usually has a benign prognosis. Within 2 or 3 weeks, the patient is asymptomatic and the choroidal scar has assumed its usual morphology. Lesions usually do not progress to a frank, subretinal neovascular membrane.

Some clincans treat this inflammatory or "choroiditis" activity with oral steroids. I have not found this necessary and usually observe the patients closely until they become asymptomatic.

The second evolution of a perifoveal *Histoplasma* spot is progression into a subretinal neovascular membrane. The incidence of this complication is probably about 4.5%.[21] Of patients who have this complication in one eye and demonstrate clinically evident perifoveal *Histoplasma* spots in the second eye, approximately 1 in 5 will develop such a subretinal neovascular membrane over an ensuing 5-year period.[11] This proportion suggests that these patients with a disciform lesion are different from the average patient with perifoveal *Histoplasma* spots.

There are two theories proposed to explain these two types of activity.

First is the concept that these choroidal foci are formed at the time of first exposure to histoplasmosis and occur by hematogenous spread. A variety of choroidal lesions are formed. These lesions vary from small choroidal foci of inflammatory cells with an intact overlying pigment epithelium to small foci with atrophy of the overlying pigment epithelium visible as small, yellow subretinal nodules or clinically obvious atrophic pigmented chorioretinal scars. The type of choroidal lesion depends on the size of the inoculum and resistance othe host. Eventually, these lesions heal and all organisms are destroyed so that only a few sensitized lymphocytes are left in these scars.

Years after the initial exposure, an unknown event, perhaps a recurrent fungemia from healed lesions in the spleen or liver or exposure to the same etiologic agent, causes these sensitized lymphocytes to recruit other cells and develop a clinically evident inflammatory choroiditis with a serous overlying detachment. With repeated activity Bruch's membrane is damaged and subretinal neovascularization from the choriocapillaris occurs. Eventually a few patients will develop a progressive fibrovascular scar.

Evidence for this is the presence of lymphocytes in *Histoplasma* spots.[9,12] Another bit of clinical evidence is the fact that one never sees a disciform process develop from a perifoveal, atrophic pigmented chorioretinal scar. They always seem to develop from the more subtle choroidal nodules. Further evidence is the statistically higher incidence of certain HLA antigens in patients with the disciform syndrome and the model of ocular histoplasmosis in primate eyes by Smith and co-workers.[2,7,15] Smith has produced histoplasmotic spots by intracarotid injection of yeast forms of *Histoplasma* organisms. Many of these choroidal infiltrates with time became clinically and angiographically invisible. Several years later a repeat challenge by killed yeast-phase *Histoplasma* organisms produced the reappearance of the same choroidal lesions.[20]

A second theory is suggested by the finding that all *Histoplasma* spots in one eye examined by meticulously prepared thin sections contained a subretinal or subpigment epithelial neovascular membrane.[24] It may be that these membranes are simply a natural evolution of the remodeling that all such spots undergo over a long time. No reexposure to an endogenous or exogenous antigen is necessary. The clinical activity involved in some spots with overlying serous detachment may be attributable to leakage from subretinal vessels already in place. The pigment rim seen around the clinically obvious subretinal neovascular membrane in the disciform stage is caused by blood seeping under the retinal pigment epithelium from such vascular tissue. This theory assumes no immunologic basis for the two types of activity involved in such choroidal scars. It also explains the appearance of new spots over time as the normal remodeling that such lesions undergo.

Subretinal neovascular membranes occur in chorioretinal scars of many diverse origins. The development of the disciform process may be only a chance occurrence or may be related to the variable response to trauma seen in all individuals.

Our knowledge of the presumed ocular histoplasmosis syndrome is hampered by the lack of pathologic tissue at various stages of the disease and, when such tissue is obtained, failure to examine portions of the fundus without clinical *Histoplasma* spots. Correlation of ocular findings with presence of *Histoplasma* foci in other organs such as lungs, liver, and spleen would also be most valuable.

TREATMENT

Presently, treatment involves the decision to do nothing but counsel a patient or perform photocoagulation. If the decision is photocoagulation, one must decide whether to use either the argon or krypton mode. All studies, including the ongoing macular photocoagulation study, have so far failed to confirm the superiority of photocoagulation therapy over no treatment for membranes outside the foveal avascular zone. Until this controlled prospective clinical trial is concluded, ophthalmologists not in the study and in areas where it is not feasible to send patients to study centers for recruitment are free to counsel such patients according to their own inclination.

Krypton photocoagulation certainly makes treatment of membranes within the foveal avascular zone safer and more feasible.[13] It is even more evident here that an early controlled prospective clinical trial of this laser treatment is necessary before the proliferation of a new and unproved laser system has become widespread. Fortunately this trial has begun.

I do not recommend either steroid or antifungal treatment of the disciform process. Evidence previously cited indicates that by the time a disciform process has occurred, one is dealing with the consequences of a subretinal neovascular membrane. Such disciform fibrovasular tissue has neither organisms in it, nor inflammatory components.

Patients with a perifoveal disciform process should be given a complete explanation of present concepts of this disease, the chance of visual loss, the rationale of photocoagulation therapy, and the lack of absolute proof of its efficacy. After such a discussion, most patients can make an informed decision and learn to live with the eventual result.

REFERENCES

1. Archer, D.B., Maguire, C.J.F., and Newell, F.W.: Multifocal choroiditis, Trans. Ophthalmol. Soc. U.K. **95:**184, 1975.
2. Braley, R.E., Meredith, T.A., Aaberg, T.M., Koethe, S.M., and Witkowski, J.A.: The prevalence of HLA-B7 in presumed ocular histoplasmosis, Am. J. Ophthalmol. **85:**859, 1978.
3. Braunstein, R.A., Rosen, D.A., and Bird, A.C.: Ocular histoplasmosis syndrome in the United Kingdom, Br. J. Ophthalmol. **58**(11):893-898, 1974.
4. Craandijk, A.: Focal macular choroidopathy, The Hague, 1979, Dr. W. Junk bv Publishers.
5. François, J., de Laey, J.J., and Dakir, M.: Choroïdopathic maculaire hémorragique chez les sujets jeunes, Ophthalmologica **170:**977, 1975.
6. Ganley, J.P.: Epidemiologic characteristics of presumed ocular histoplasmosis, Acta Ophthalmol. (Suppl.) **119:**1-63, 1973.
7. Godfrey, W.A., Sabates, R., and Cross, D.E.: Association of presumed ocular histoplasmosis with HLA-B7, Am. J. Ophthalmol. **85:**858, 1978.
8. Husted, R.C., and Schock, J.P.: Acute presumed histoplasmosis of the optic nerve head, Br. J. Ophthalmol. **59:**409-412, 1975.
9. Irvine, A.R., Spencer, W.H., Hogan, M.J., Meyers, R.L., and Irvine, S.R.: Presumed chronic ocular histoplasmosis syndrome: a clinical-pathologic case report, Trans. Am. Ophthalmol. Soc. **74:**91-106, 1976.
10. Krill, A.E., Chishti, M.I., Klein, B.A., Newell, F.W., and Potts, A.M.: Multifocal inner choroiditis, Trans. Am. Acad. Ophthalmol. Otolaryngol. **73:**222-242, 1969.
11. Lewis, M.L., Van Newkirk, M.R., and Gass, J.D.M.: Follow-up study of presumed ocular histoplasmosis syndrome. Am. J. Ophthalmol. **87:**390-399, 1980.
12. Makley, T.A., Jr., Craig, E.L., and Long, J.W.: Histopathology of presumed ocular histoplasmosis, Palestra Oftamológica Pan-Americana **1:**72-82, 1977.
13. Marshall, J., and Bird, A.C.: A comparative histopathological study of argon and krypton laser irradiations of the human retina, Br. J. Ophthalmol. **63:**657, 1979.
14. Meredith, T.A., Green, W.R., Key, S.N., Dolin, G.S., and Maumenee, A.E.: Ocular histoplasmosis: clinicopathologic correlation of 3 cases, Surv. Ophthalmol. **22:**189-205, 1977.
15. Meredith, T.A., Smith, R.E., and Duquesnoy, R.: Association of HLA-DRw2 antigen with presumed ocular histoplasmosis, Am. J. Ophthalmol. **89:**70-76, 1980.
16. Scheffer, A., Green, W.R., Fine S.L., and Kincaid, M.: Presumed ocular histoplasmosis syndrome: a clinicopathologic correlation of a treated case, Arch. Ophthalmol. **98:**335-340, 1980.
17. Schlaegel, T.F., Jr., and Kenney, D.: Changes around the optic nervehead in presumed ocular histoplasmosis, Am. J. Ophthalmol. **62:**454-458, 1966.
18. Schlaegel, T.F., Jr., Weber, J.C., Helveston, E., and Kenney, D.: Presumed histoplasmic choroiditis, Am. J. Ophthalmol. **63:**919-925, 1967.
19. Schwartz, J.: Histoplasmosis, New York, 1981, Praeger Publishers.
20. Smith, R.E.: Long term follow-up of primate experimental histoplasmosis, Presented at the Ocular Histoplasmosis Conference, Department of Ophthalmology, Indiana University, School of Medicine, Indianapolis, Indiana, January 22-23, 1982.
21. Smith, A.E., and Ganley, J.P.: An epidemiologic study of presumed ocular histoplasmosis, Trans. Am. Acad. Ophthalmol. Otolaryngol. **75:**994, 1971.
22. Smith, R.E., Macy, J.I., Parett, C., and Irvine, J.: Variations in acute multifocal histoplasmic choroiditis in the primate, Invest. Ophthalmol. Vis. Sci. **17:**1005, 1978.
23. Watzke, R.C., and Claussen, R.W.: The long-term course of multifocal choroiditis (presumed ocular histoplasmosis), Am. J. Ophthalmol. **91:**750-760, 1981.
24. Weingeist, T.A., and Watzke, R.C.: Ocular involvement by *Histoplasma capsulatum,* Arch. Ophthalmol. (In press.)

8

Acute herpetic thrombotic retinal angiitis and necrotizing neuroretinitis (''acute retinal necrosis syndrome'')

J. Donald M. Gass

Acute retinal necrosis (ARN) is one of several names used to describe a recently recognized clinical syndrome characterized by the development in one or both eyes of typically healthy individuals of all ages of an initially mild anterior uveitis, followed within a few days by vitreous inflammation, pain, occasionally glaucoma, and usually a rapid decline in visual function caused by vitreous opacificaton and a rapidly progressing necrotizing retinitis, thrombotic retinal vasculitis, and optic neuritis[1,3,6-13,16-18] (Figs. 8-1 and 8-2). Typically, multiple foci of necrotizing retinitis begin in the peripheral fundus, become concentrically confluent, and spread into the posterior fundus within a matter of days or a few weeks. The necrosis is accompanied by perivascular retinal hemorrhages, narrowing, sheathing, and occlusion of the major retinal vessels, particularly the arteries. In some cases, the walls of the major arteries and veins in the posterior fundus become thickened and opaque causing a picture resembling massive embolic occlusion of the central retinal artery (Fig. 8-3). Fluorescein angiography demonstrates reduced perfusion and in areas occlusion of the retinal vasculature, as well as evidence of choroidal inflammatory cell infiltration and pigment epithelial damage (Fig. 8-2). In some patients the necrosis progresses to involve the entire fundus, in others vitreous inflammation obscures the fundus before this happens. In some patients progression of the disease may spontaneously stop before reaching the posterior fundus (Fig. 8-1). The white necrotic retina may disappear in some patients within a few days as its crumbled remnants shed into the vitreous. In others the areas of white retinitis may persist for longer periods of time. A sharply outlined pattern of usually mild pigment mottling is left in the areas of previous retinal necrosis. Even as the areas of retinitis are clearing, the patient may experience further sudden and profound loss of vision caused by thrombotic arterial occlusion within or near the optic nerve head (Fig. 8-3).

In approximately 75% of cases, large irregular retinal holes develop in the necrotic retina, and vitreous organization and traction cause extensive retinal detachments that are amenable to surgery in only a small percentage of cases.

The second eye becomes involved in approximately one third of patients, usually within 6 weeks of onset in the first eye.

97

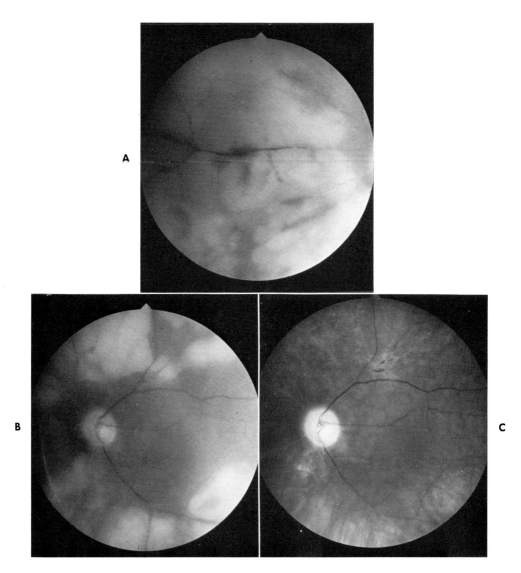

Fig. 8-1. Case 1. Acute retinal necrosis, or necrotizing retinitis. **A** and **B,** December 5, 1980. **C,** January 20, 1981. Visual acuity 20/30.

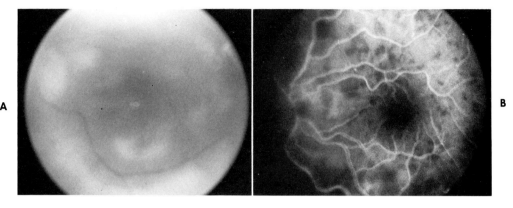

Fig. 8-2. Case 2. **A,** Widespread acute necrotizing retinitis 1 week before enucleation. Visual acuity was light perception only. **B,** Angiography showing hypofluorescent defects caused by multifocal choroiditis.

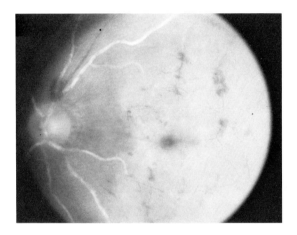

Fig. 8-3. Case 3. Acute necrotizing retinitis misdiagnosed as central retinal artery occlusion caused by embolization from atheromatous carotid artery disease.

Of the approximately 50 patients reported up to now with this syndrome, approximately two thirds have been males. In only a few cases has any evidence of systemic disease been incriminated. In two cases the development of aphthous ulcers was interpreted as possible evidence of Behçet's disease. In one patient seen at the Bascom Palmer Eye Institute and another I have seen elsewhere, the onset of the ocular symptoms was preceded by a history of intravenous injection of cocaine One patient (Fig. 8-2) developed abdominal pain and fever 1 week before the onset of ocular symptoms. His diagnosis was probable acute cholecystitis. There are reports in the literature of immunosuppressed patients with Hodgkin's disease,[7] and central nervous system toxoplasmosis,[14] who had an ophthalmoscopic picture and clinical course identical to that of the acute retinal necrosis syndrome.

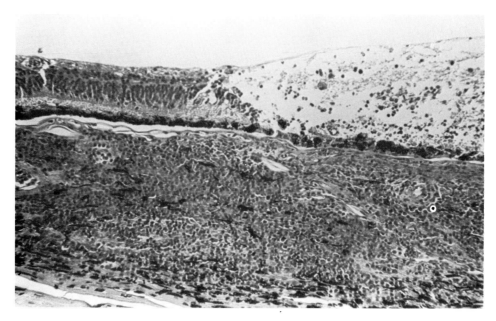

Fig. 8-4. Case 2. Focal retinal necrosis overlying diffuse choroiditis. (From Culbertson, W.W., et al.: Ophthalmology **89:**1317, Dec. 1982.)

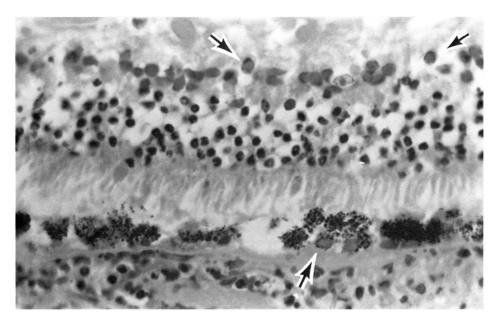

Fig. 8-5. Case 2. Eosinophilic intranuclear viral inclusions in retinal and pigment epithelial cells, *arrows.* (From Culbertson, W.W., et al.: Ophthalmology **89:**1317, Dec. 1982.)

HISTOPATHOLOGY

The eye depicted in Fig. 8-2 was enucleated during the acute phase of the disease and was studied histopathologically (Figs. 8-4 to 8-12).[3] The primary findings were (1) full-thickness necrotizing retinitis caused by a virus with light and electron microscopic features of a herpetic type of virus (Figs. 8-4, 8-5, and 8-12), (2) a thrombosing retinal arteritis (Figs. 8-6 and 8-7), (3) segmental necrotizing optic neuritis (Fig. 8-8), and (4) a panuveitis and vasculitis (Figs. 8-9 and 8-10). In those areas where the white necrotizing retinitis had faded from view clinically, only the partly thrombosed major retinal vessels remained histologically (Fig. 8-11). The electron microscopic study of this eye is still incomplete, but up to now virus and typical intranuclear inclusions have been identified only in the retina, pigment epithelium, and optic nerve (Fig. 8-12).

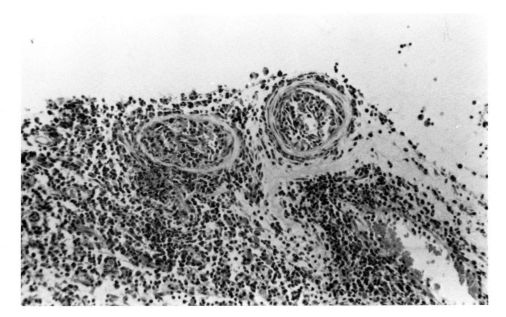

Fig. 8-6. Case 2. Thrombotic occlusive retinal arteritis, optic nerve head. (From Culbertson, W.W., et al.: Ophthalmology **89:**1317, Dec. 1982.)

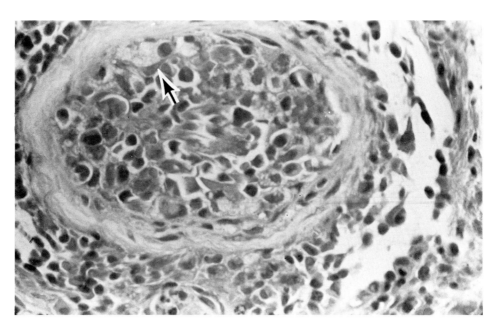

Fig. 8-7. Case 2. Note vacuolization of endothelial cells, *arrow,* in this occluded retinal artery. (From Culbertson, W.W., et al.: Ophthalmology **89:**1317, Dec. 1982.)

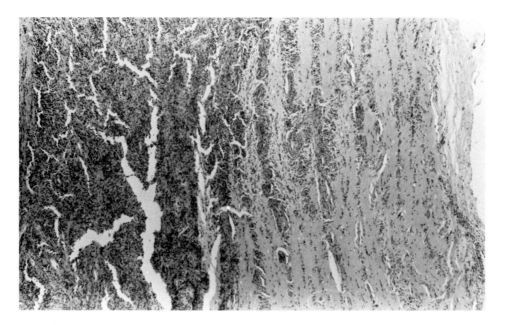

Fig. 8-8. Case 2. Segmental infarction and inflammation of nasal half of optic nerve. (From Culbertson, W.W., et al.: Ophthalmology **89:**1317, Dec. 1982.)

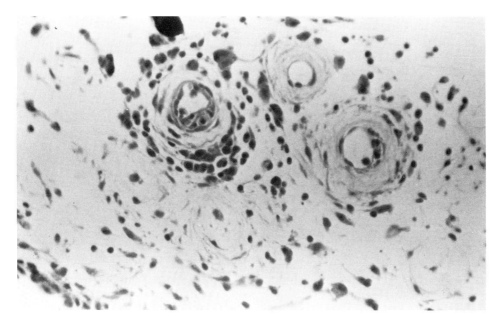

Fig. 8-9. Case 2. Partial occlusion of inflamed iris artery. (From Culbertson, W.W., et al.: Ophthalmology **89:**1317, Dec. 1982.)

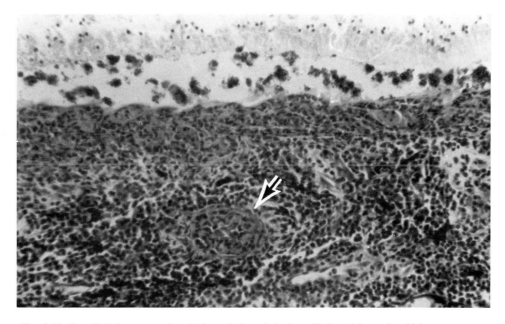

Fig. 8-10. Case 2. Inflammatory thrombotic occlusion of choriocapillaris and large choroidal artery, *arrow.* (From Culbertson, W.W., et al.: Ophthalmology **89:**1317, Dec. 1982.)

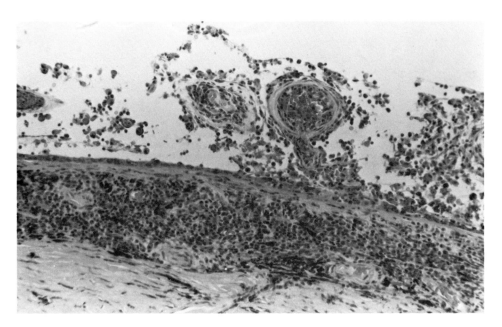

Fig. 8-11. Case 2. Network of thrombosed retinal arteries remaining after retinal necrosis. (From Culbertson, W.W., et al.: Ophthalmology **89**:1317, Dec. 1982.)

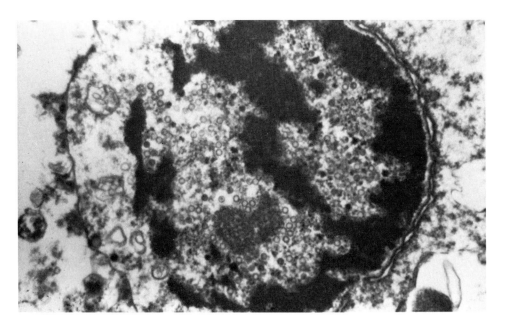

Fig. 8-12. Case 2. Electron micrograph showing intranuclear viral particles in retinal cell. (From Culbertson, W.W., et al.: Ophthalmology **89**:1317, Dec. 1982.)

PATHOGENESIS AND ETIOLOGY

Attempts to culture the virus from fresh retinal and vitreous specimens in the above-mentioned eye were unsuccessful. Attempts here and elsewhere to culture virus from aspirated vitreous in these patients have failed uniformly. This suggests the possibility that the herpetic type of virus may be zoster, since simplex and cytomegalovirus are usually easy to culture. None of the reported cases of this syndrome have had evidence of herpes zoster. At the recent Macula Society meeting, Dr. Lee Jampol cited a patient who approximately 1 year after developing the typical ocular findings of ARN developed herpes zoster ophthalmicus on the same side. Schwartz et al.[15] have reported eye findings similar to ARN caused by herpes zoster. Diddie et al.[5] studied histologically the eyes of an immunosuppressed patient who developed the clinical picture of bilateral acute retinal necrosis 1 year after acquiring Hodgkin's disease and 3 months after an episode of herpes zoster.[5] Light and electron microscopic evidence of the Herpetoviridae family was found. Reese reported a nonimmunosuppressed patient who developed the typical picture of ARN in both eyes followed by fever, loss of consciousness, and a Sabin-Feldman titer of 1:512.[14] Her systemic disease cleared promptly after therapy for toxoplasmosis. She was apparently blind in both eyes when she later died of an unrelated disease. *Toxoplasma* organisms were found in the brain, but no organisms were found in the eye in which virtually no retinal tissue remained. Examination of the herpetoviral titers in patients with ARN have been unrewarding in establishing any one of these as the cause of ARN. Although the clinical appearance of the sharply defined areas of acute necrotizing retinitis and the perivascular hemorrhages in this syndrome are similar to that seen in cytomegalic inclusion disease in immunosuppressed individuals[4] and in primary herpes simplex in newborns,[2] the clinical course of patients with these three syndromes is usually quite different. Although there is good evidence to suggest that at least some cases of ARN are caused by a herpetic type of virus, its precise identification is unknown. Other puzzling questions concerning ARN are, Why are there no reports of this devastating and blinding disease before 1971? Why does the disease attack primarily healthy individuals? Why does it not spread posteriorly to involve the brain?

Thus far we have identified the virus only in the retina and optic nerve where it appears to be responsible for full-thickness necrosis of the retina similar to that seen in cytomegalic inclusion disease and in herpes simplex retinitis. It is not known whether the underlying choroiditis and iridocyclitis is caused by direct infection by the virus or is a secondary response to the retinitis.

None of the large blood vessels in the preceding case has been examined yet by electron microscopy. The clinical and light microscopic findings suggest that the retinal vessels, particularly the arteries, are directly involved with the virus that probably causes endothelial damage and massive inflammatory cellular thrombosis. Retinal death in this disease appears to be caused primarily by intraneuronal replication of the virus and by retinal arterial occlusion. It is possible, however, that the intense choroidal vasculitis and infiltration may also play an important role in causing infarction of the outer retina (Fig. 8-9). It was not possible to determine by light microscopy whether the intense inflammatory reaction and vasculitis in the area of segmental necrosis of the optic nerve was a secondary response to ganglion cell death or a primary cause of the necrosis.

SPECTRUM OF ARN

Up to now our knowledge of this syndrome is based on approximately 50 patients. As we study more patients, undoubtedly the clinical spectrum of the syndrome will broaden. Although these patients are typically healthy, we can expect to identify the disease in immunosuppressed or otherwise abnormal individuals. Although the necrotizing retinitis typically begins in the peripheral fundus, we have seen several patients whose initial lesions were in the posterior fundus. Although progression of the disease is usually rapid, in some it progresses at a much slower pace and, in such cases, may be difficult to differentiate from other diseases, such as toxoplasmosis or reticulum cell sarcoma that cause retinal necrosis. In most patients with the early stages of ARN, peripheral necrotizing retinitis is the predominant fundus finding. In others, however, widespread retinal arteritis may precede the development of large areas of retinal necrosis. Two such patients seen at the Bascom Palmer Eye Institute were initially misdiagnosed as having carotid artery obstruction and the ischemic ocular syndrome. In one the fundus picture suggested central retinal artery occlusion caused by massive embolization from the carotid artery (Fig. 8-3).

DIFFERENTIAL DIAGNOSIS

During the acute stages of the disease, the white necrotizing retinitis and vitritis may simulate that seen in a variety of diseases, including cytomegalic inclusion disease in immunosuppressed individuals; primary herpes simplex in infants; bacterial or fungoid retinitis; reticulum cell sarcoma (non-Hodgkin's lymphoma), usually in elderly patients; diffuse toxoplasmosis, usually in elderly immunosuppressed individuals; Behçet's disease; sarcoidosis; retinoblastomas in infants and young children; pars-planitis and nematode endophthalmitis in children and young adults; traumatic retinopathy (commotio retinae); and central retinal artery occlusion in association with severe carotid artery disease (ischemic ocular syndrome). During the healed stage of this disease, the pigmentary changes, chorioretinal atrophy, and severe vascular narrowing and sheathing simulate that seen in ophthalmic artery occlusion, severe diffuse unilateral subacute neuroretinitis, and posttraumatic chorioretinopathy.

DIAGNOSIS

The diagnosis of ARN is based primarily on the clinical picture and exclusion of other causes of retinal whitening and retinal vascular occlusion. There are no consistent laboratory findings of diagnostic importance. Vitreous biopsy specimens are unlikely to show evidence of intranuclear inclusions, and viral cultures up to now have been negative. The histopathologic findings in the one eye examined to date suggest that in vivo retinal biopsies in this disease have a significant chance of missing those limited areas where the diagnostic intranuclear inclusions are present in viable but inflamed retina. A biopsy specimen that includes the edge of a recently developed white area of retinitis and its apparently normal surrounding retina probably has the best chance of revealing the viral inclusions.

TREATMENT

No treatment including systemic corticosteroids, or antimetabolites, have proved successful. Most of the patients have received systemic corticosteroids. In view of the experience that discontinuance of corticosteroid therapy in immunosuppressed individuals with cytomegalic inclusion retinitis is of benefit, it is probably prudent to avoid corticosteroid therapy in patients with ARN. The value of antiviral agents such as acyclovir and adenine arabinoside in the treatment of this disease is unknown.

REFERENCES

1. Bando, K., and Kinoshita, A.: Six cases of so-called "Kirisawa type" uveitis, Jpn. J. Clin. Ophthalmol. **33:**1515-1521, 1979.
2. Cibis, G.W., Glynn, J.T., and Davis, E.B.: Herpes simplex retinitis, Arch. Ophthalmol. **96:**299-302, 1978.
3. Culbertson, W.W., Blumenkranz, M., Haines, H., Gass, J.D.M., Mitchell, K.B., and Norton, E.W.D.: The acute retinal necrosis syndrome. Part II. Histopathology and etiology, Ophthalmology **89:**1317, Dec. 1982.
4. DeVenecia, G., ZuRhein, G.M., Pratt, M.V., and Kisker, W.: Cytomegalic inclusion retinitis in an adult, Arch. Ophthalmol. **86:**44-57, 1971.
5. Diddie, K.R., Schanzlin, D.J., Mausolf, F.A., Minckler, D.S., and Trousdale, M.D.: Necrotizing retinitis caused by opportunistic virus infection in a patient with Hodgkin's disease, Am. J. Ophthalmol. **88:**668-673, 1979.
6. Fisher, J.P., Lewis, M.L., Blumenkranz, M., et al.: The acute retinal necrosis syndrome. Part I. Clinical manifestations, Ophthalmology **89:** 1309, Dec. 1982.
7. Gorman, B.D., Nadel, A.J., and Coles, R.S.: Acute retinal necrosis, Presented at the American Academy of Ophthalmology, Atlanta, Nov. 1981.
8. Hayreh, S.S., Kreiger, A.E., Straatsma, B.R., et al.: Acute retinal necrosis: ARVO Abstracts, Invest. Ophthalmol. Vis. Sci. (suppl):48, 1980.
9. Martenet, A.C.: Nécrose rétinienne périphérique et décollement rétinien total d'origine vasculaire. Fifth Congress of the Société Européenne d'Ophtalmologie, Hamburg, 1976, Stuttgart, 1978, Ferdinand Enke Verlag.
10. Martenet, A.C.: Fréquence et aspects cliniques des complications rétiniennes de l'uvéite intermédiaire, Bull. Mem. Soc. Fr. Ophtalmol. **92:**40-42, 1980.
11. Kometani, J., and Asayama, T.: A case of specific uveitis occurring acutely in the right eye, Folia Ophthalmol. Jpn. **29:**1397-1401, 1978.
12. Okinami, S., and Tsukahara, I.: Acute severe uveitis with retinal vasculitis and retinal detachment, Ophthalmologica **179:**276-285, 1979.
13. Price, F.M., and Schlaegel, T.F.: Bilateral acute retinal necrosis, Am. J. Ophthalmol. **89:**419-424, 1980.
14. Reese, L.T., Shafer, D.M., and Zweifach, P.: Acute acquired toxoplasmosis, Ann. Ophthalmol. **13:**467-470, 1981.
15. Schwartz, J.N., Cashwell, F., Hawkins, H.K., and Klintworth, G.K.: Necrotizing retinopathy with herpes zoster ophthalmicus, Arch. Pathol. Lab. Med. **100:**386, 1976.
16. Urayama, A., Yamada, N., Sasaki, T., et al.: Unilateral acute uveitis with periarteritis and detachment, Jpn. J. Clin. Ophthalmol. **25:**607-619, 1971.
17. Willerson, D., Aaberg, T.M., and Reeser, F.H.: Necrotizing vaso-occlusive retinitis, Am. J. Ophthalmol. **84:**209-219, 1977.
18. Young, N.J.A., and Bird, A.C.: Bilateral acute retinal necrosis, Br. J. Ophthalmol. **62:**581-590, 1978.

9

Ocular toxoplasmosis

G. Richard O'Connor

Toxoplasmosis, caused by the obligate intracellular protozoan parasite *Toxoplasma gondii,* is a common infestation of man and other warm-blooded animals in the temperate and tropical zones of the world. Fortunately, a great number of those infested have no symptoms at all. The major symptoms of the disease are connected with lesions of the retina and of the brain, and unless one of these two tissues is affected symptomatically, the disease generally does not come to the attention of a physician. The minor symptoms of the disease consist of mild fever, myalgias, swelling of the lymph nodes, and occasionally a morbilliform skin rash. These minor symptoms, which are characteristically seen in the acute, acquired lymphadenopathic form of the disease in adult life, are often mistaken for the initial complex of infectious mononucleosis.

The major ocular disease caused by *Toxoplasma gondii* is a focal retinochoroiditis, occurring mainly in the posterior pole of the eye, but also affecting the peripheral retina in some individuals. *Toxoplasma* is believed to be the causative agent of 30% to 50% of all posterior uveitis.[11] These estimates vary from institution to institution, depending on the geographic location, the eating habits of the affected population, and the referral pattern of the reporting ophthalmologist. At the University of California in San Francisco 30% of all cases of posterior uveitis seen within the past 5 years were attributed to toxoplasmosis. Higher estimates of the incidence of toxoplasmic retinochoroiditis come from various clinical centers in South America and from France. It is believed that the habit of eating raw or barely cooked meats in some of these areas may contribute to the higher incidence of the disease. It is known that systemic toxoplasmosis can be transmitted by the ingestion of undercooked beef,[12] and other animals commonly used for domestic meat production also harbor the parasite in their skeletal muscle. Therefore the possibility of transmission of the disease by the ingestion of undercooked meat appears to be very strong.

The disease can also be transmitted by the ingestion (or possibly the inhalation) of the oocysts of the parasite, which are passed in the feces of domestic or feral cats. Recently, a minor epidemic of acquired systemic toxoplasmosis was described as affecting 37 patrons of a riding stable near Atlanta, Georgia.[31] Oocysts of *Toxoplasma* were found in the loose dirt covering one corner of the floor of this stable, and this appeared to be the only factor of importance in the transmission of the disease. Of particular interest was the fact that one patient who acquired the systemic, lymphadenopathic form of toxoplasmosis in this stable later developed a focal retinochoroiditis typical of ocular toxoplasmosis 3½ years after the onset of her systemic illness. This case, recently reported by Akstein,[1] is the only known case of eye disease transmitted by the oocysts of *Toxoplasma* to man.

It has been widely assumed, and correctly so, that the most ocular toxoplasmosis is a late manifestation of congenitally acquired disease. Prospective mothers who have not been previously exposed to the infection are believed to acquire toxoplasmosis through the ingestion of undercooked meat or through contact with *Toxoplasma* oocysts contained in the feces of domestic cats. The disease acquired during pregnancy may be very mild, producing symptoms no more serious than those of a mild cold. Occasionally, a morbilliform rash has been produced during this stage of the disease. Generally, however, the prospective mother is completely unaware that she has acquired the infection. Toxoplasmosis may be acquired during any stage of pregnancy. When it is acquired during the first trimester of pregnancy, the chances of doing damage to the fetus are greatest. Fetuses are often aborted during this period. If the fetus survives, it may be severely brain damaged and may have profound signs of congenital ocular toxoplasmosis. Later in pregnancy, particularly during the third trimester, the efficiency of transmission of the organism from the mother to the fetus is increased, but the damage done to the fetus is likely to be considerably less severe. During the third trimester of pregnancy, the fetal tissues are in a much more mature state of development, and the fetus has begun to develop its own immunologic defense system. Such babies may appear completely normal at the time of birth, but a considerable proportion of them may develop ocular toxoplasmosis as the only manifestation of congenital disease later in life. Longitudinal studies, performed by Desmonts et al.[3], have shown that, overall, a prospective mother stands a 40% chance of transmitting toxoplasmosis to her fetus if she acquires the disease during pregnancy. Prospective mothers having antibodies, even in low titer, are protected against the transmission of toxoplasmosis to their fetuses. This situation is analogous to that of rubella. Previous exposure to the disease, no matter how symptomatic, appears to confer permanent protection against the transmission of toxoplasmosis to the fetus. It is clear then that a female patient who has ocular toxoplasmosis will not transmit toxoplasmosis to any child that she wishes to procreate. It is similarly clear that if a woman has given birth to one child with congenital toxoplasmosis, she will not transmit the disease to subsequent children.

Perkins[20] is largely responsible for the promulgation of the theory that all, or nearly all, ocular toxoplasmosis represents a late manifestation of congenital disease. He could account for no more than 3% of all cases of ocular toxoplasmosis as manifestations of acquired disease. The number of case reports of ocular toxoplasmosis as a sequela of acquired toxoplasmosis is small. Nevertheless, the reports of Wising,[35] Saari,[25] Michelson,[15] Masur,[14] and Hoerni[10] deserve special scrutiny. Wising's case showed a monocular lesion occurring after a febrile lymphadenopathic illness in a young woman. Saari's description was concerned with the development of monocular toxoplasmosis in an agricultural worker who was holding a sick calf by the nostrils at the time that it was receiving an injection for a febrile, undiagnosed illness. The calf was later shown to have systemic toxoplasmosis. Michelson's case was concerned with a young woman who developed a disease resembling infectious mononucleosis soon after visting a mink farm. She, too, had in one eye a single, monofocal lesion that had all the characteristics of ocular toxoplasmosis. A lymph node biopsy performed on this woman yielded highly valuable results. It showed the typical histologic picture of toxoplasmic lymphadenopathy,[5] and *Toxoplasma* organisms were isolated from a minced lymph node. Masur's case occurred in a small family epidemic of toxoplasmosis in which five members of a family group became ill with systemic toxoplasmosis. The disease was acquired through the ingestion of undercooked lamb. Only one member of the family, a 56-year-old man, developed a monocular eye lesion compatible with the diagnosis of toxoplasmosis. Hoerni's cases were concerned with two patients suffering from Hodgkin's disease. One of these patients is known to have had a negative dye test before the onset of the ocular lesion. Therefore it seems quite certain that her disease was not a late manifestation of congenital toxoplasmosis. In all the other cases serum specimens had not been obtained before the onset of the ocular disease, and so one cannot determine with certainty that their ocular lesions were manifestations of acquired toxoplasmosis. In Michelson's case the presence of high titers of IgM antibodies to *Toxoplasma* indicated very strongly that her lymphadenopathic disease was recently acquired.

SIGNS AND SYMPTOMS OF OCULAR TOXOPLASMOSIS

The initial symptoms of ocular toxoplasmosis consist mainly of floating spots and blurred vision. These symptoms are generally insidious in onset, but occasionally there is an explosive onset. Occasionally the patients may also experience flashes of light. The diminution in visual acuity is usually caused by infiltration of the vitreous body with cells and strands of inflammatory debris. However, if the opacities in the vitreous are composed strictly of fine cells, visual acuity is generally retained at a fairly high level. When chorioretinal lesions impinge upon the macula, the papillomacular bundle, or the optic nerve head itself, there is generally serious loss of visual function.

Pain is almost never experienced by patients suffering from ocular toxoplasmosis unless there is an associated iridocyclitis. Iridocyclitis may be accompanied by serious degrees of secondary glaucoma, and this may produce extensive edema of the corneal epithelium. Iridocyclitis, with or without secondary glaucoma, is generally not a feature of initial attacks of toxoplasmic retinochoroiditis but frequently accompanies the recurrent attacks.

The principal signs of the disease are in the posterior segment of the eye and consist of a focal, necrotizing retinochoroiditis (Fig. 9-1). Such lesions are yellowish white and are often about the size of the optic disc. For the most part, they occur in and around the posterior pole of the eye, but they may also affect the periphery of the retina in certain individuals. The active lesions characteristically cast off large amounts of cellular debris into the overlying vitreous body. These exudative materials reduce the visibility of the lesion and, together with the associated retinal edema, produce the blurred appearance of the lesions. The lesions may appear as monofocal patches of retinochoroiditis in one eye, particularly in what is believed to be acute, acquired toxoplasmosis in adult life. Much more often, the active lesion is seen in the company of older, pigmented, atrophic scars, which are referred to as "satellites."

The retinal vessels in the near vicinity of an active chorioretinal lesion may show cuffs of exudate surrounding the external surface of the vessel (Fig. 9-2). Although many authors in the past have referred to this as a periphlebitis, I have found that arteries are much more often involved than veins. Schwartz[26] has also confirmed these observations in retinal arteries.

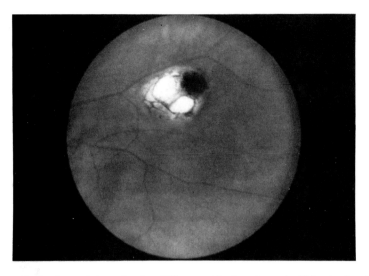

Fig. 9-1. Scar of a focal necrotizing retinochoroiditis caused by toxoplasmosis. Note atrophy of retina and choroid caused by necrosis.

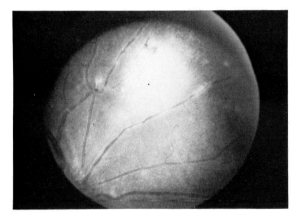

Fig. 9-2. Acute retinal vasculitis in the vicinity of a focus of active retinochoroiditis.

Peripapillary lesions are often seen in ocular toxoplasmosis. Although Jensen originally attributed these juxtapapillary lesions to tuberculosis, it is likely that many of the lesions that he had observed were actually caused by toxoplasmosis. This is not surprising, since tuberculosis was the popular disease of his day. Nevertheless, with the increasing acquisition of knowledge about infectious agents that can cause retinochoroiditis, it has become apparent that many judgments that were formerly made concerning the cause of certain forms of chorioretinitis were wrong. As a matter of fact, the very same tissue preparations that were formerly used at the Armed Forces Institute of Pathology to demonstrate the histopathologic findings of ocular tuberculosis were later found by Wilder to contain *Toxoplasma* organisms.[34]

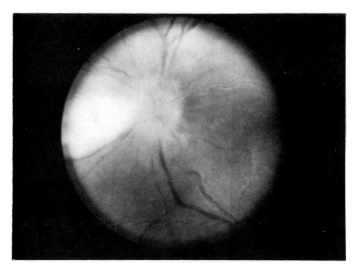

Fig. 9-3. Juxtapapillary lesion of ocular toxoplasmosis.

Juxtapapillary lesions are often confused with a primary optic neuritis (Fig. 9-3). During the acute phase of the lesion the adjacent optic nerve head may be swollen, and its edges may be obscured. Later, when the acute inflammatory lesion subsides, a distinction can be made between a normal optic nerve head and the adjacent chorioretinal lesion. Juxtapapillary lesions may be seen in patients who experience signs and symptoms of toxoplasmic meningoencephalitis. One such case has recently been described by Uchida et al.[33] In this patient, who had a typical toxoplasmic retinochoroiditis, *Toxoplasma* organisms were isolated from the cerebrospinal fluid. This may indicate that *Toxoplasma* organisms gain access to the peripapillary retina at a time when infective organisms are present in the subarachnoid space. Thus the sheaths of the optic nerve may serve to conduct organisms to the eye.

The vitreous opacity of ocular toxoplasmosis may be very extensive. It generally consists of cells and "snowball clumps," but it may also contain long strands of fibrin and other inflammatory debris. In the more severe cases an ophthalmoscopic view of the fundus is completely precluded. Organization of this vitreous debris, followed by subsequent contraction of collagenous elements, may produce traction on the retina and, ultimately, a retinal tear. This in turn may produce bleeding into the vitreous body. Recurrent flashes of light in the late phases of the disease may signal an incipient retinal detachment and should be taken seriously by the examining ophthalmologist.

As mentioned on p. 110, the iridocyclitis accompanying exacerbations of posterior disease may be of a severe nature. Both Koeppe and Busacca nodules may form on the iris. Synechia formation is common, and with recurrent attacks, the entire pupil may become secluded. Iris bombé may then occur, giving rise to secondary glaucoma of a severe degree.

PATHOGENESIS

The essential lesion of ocular toxoplasmosis is a focal necrotizing retinochoroiditis. When such a lesion occupies a structure important for vision (such as the macula, the papillomacular bundle, or the optic nerve) serious loss of visual acuity may result. By contrast, peripheral lesions, particularly those of the nasal portion of the retina, are generally of less importance. However, when such lesions become very large, they may cast off enormous amounts of inflammatory material into the overlying vitreous, sometimes causing permanent vitreous opacities. If the vitreous exudates subsequently become invaded by fibroblasts containing contractile elements, rhegmatogenous detachments of the retina may occur as a result of retinal tears. In view of the potential gravity of the lesions of toxoplasmic retinochoroiditis, it seems important to examine their pathogenesis.

Clearly, the invasion of retinal cells and the subsequent multiplication of the parasite within these cells are of the greatest importance. There is now abundant evidence that *Toxoplasma gondii* invades retinal cells and destroys these cells by its multiplicative activities. It should be pointed out that the retina is the primary target of attack. The inflammatory responses to parasitic invasion may well involve the subjacent choroid or even the sclera, but it is the retina itself, particularly the ganglion cell layer and the nerve fiber layer, that is under the most severe attack.

The method by which *Toxoplasma* attacks a cell and gains entrance to it has recently been the subject of intense study. The conoid of the parasite is extended, as if in search for a suitable host cell. When the extended conoid makes contact with a potential host cell membrane, it indents the host cell membrane slightly and releases a substance from the rhoptries (or toxonemes) that is presumably a phospholipase. This seems to permit the digestion of a small amount of substance in the host cell membrane and permits hole formation to take place. Once a hole has been made in the host cell membrane the parasite extends its conoid through that hole and squeezes its way into the cytoplasm of the host cell. After entrance has been gained to the host cell, the rhoptries can be seen to be emptied of material that was present before entry. The conoid also becomes retracted after entry. Within a few seconds after entry the parasite becomes surrounded by a parasitophorous vacuole. The wall of this vacuole appears to resist fusion with lysosomes that are present in the nearby host cytoplasm. The reason for this is not clearly understood, but it may be related to the fact that the parasite spews out large amounts of a tubular material that comes to line the inner wall of the vacuole. In any case, the parasite is not destroyed within the host cell unless macrophages, working in concert with lymphokines secreted by T lymphocytes, enter the tissue site. Failing this, the parasite is free to multiply within the host cell and does so until the host cell is actually ruptured. When the host cell is burst in this manner, it releases its charge of intracytoplasmic parasites. These in turn swim away to nearby, previously uninvolved retinal cells and attack them in the same manner. During their passage from one cell to another, the parasites attract considerable inflammatory reaction, particularly in hosts that have been previously sensitized. This inflammatory reaction consists mainly of lymphocytes, macrophages, and plasma cells. The last, whose only known function is to secrete antibody, may coat *Toxoplasma* parasites with immunoglobulins, a process that facilitates phagocytosis and ultimately aids in the destruction of the parasite. The walls of parasitophorous vacuoles that contain antibody-coated parasites fuse readily with lysosomes, allowing digestive enzymes to be poured into the vacuole. This, in turn, allows for digestion of the parasite and ultimate elimination of the breakdown products of the organism. Macrophages in the act of engulfment of parasites liberate lytic enzymes that have the power to injure normal bystander cells, as well as parasitized cells.[16] This may partly account for the enormous destruction that takes place in and around the lesion site. The liberation of enzymes by activated macrophages is to some extent limited by corticosteroids, and this may provide some rationale for treating patients with active lesions with corticosteroids. From the considerations discussed above it would seem that the inflammatory lesion represents a combination of damage inflicted by direct invasion of the parasite, on the one hand, and by the activities of mononuclear cells, particularly macrophages, on the other.

Within the past 2 years yet another important element has been discovered in the pathogenesis of the inflammatory lesions. On the basis of the work of Wyler, Blackman, and Lunde[37] it appears certain that chronic, recurrent *Toxoplasma* lesions result in the stimulation of the central lymphoreticular system of the body by retinal autoantigens. For the most part, these probably consist of S antigens, soluble antigens derived from the outer segments of the photoreceptors. It can be shown that the T lymphocytes of patients subjected to recurrent attacks of ocular toxoplasmosis show excessive levels of lymphocytoblast formation when stimulated with S antigens or other crude retinal extracts in tissue culture. The work of Nussenblatt et al.[17] has confirmed this. Thus it would appear that the retinal inflammatory lesion characteristic of ocular toxoplasmosis may represent a combination of microbial damage and of hypersensitivity directed against both *Toxoplasma* antigens and retinal autoantigens.

What role does antibody play in the lesions? It appears almost certain that circulating antibody, which is present in the retinal blood vessels, contributes to the formation of patchy retinal vasculitis, particularly in the near vicinity of active toxoplasmic lesions. Cuffs of exudate, appearing mainly around arterioles, but also affecting venules, are often seen in connection with active retinochoroiditic lesions. It is believed that antigen diffusing out of the lesions into nearby retinal vessels may stimulate a type of Arthus reaction in these vessels. Although this reaction usually occurs in the immediate vicinity of active lesions, it has also been observed in remote areas of the retina. This finding may indicate, though without proof, that the vitreous acts like a sponge for both retinal and autoimmune antigens, keeping them in contact with the surfaces of retinal vessels in various locations of the fundus.

Plasma cells in the lesion site may also contribute to the transformation of the proliferative form of *Toxoplasma gondii* into the encysted form. The secretion of antibody by plasma cells appears to influence this conversion both in the retina and in tissue culture systems, where the influence of invading mononuclear cells can be eliminated. This has been graphically demonstrated by Shimada et al.,[27] who showed that antibody, working in concert with complement, could convert the proliferative forms of *Toxoplasma* (tachyzoites) to the encysted forms (bradyzoites). This may be one of nature's ways of protecting the affected tissues, for cysts of *Toxoplasma* ordinarily attract very little inflammatory reaction and may be tolerated in the tissues for months or years without any dangerous sequelae.

Sections of the healed scars of toxoplasmic retinochoroiditis frequently show the presence of *Toxoplasma* cysts. In older lesions these may be present in various stages of degeneration, as shown by Rao and Font.[23] It is postulated that cysts containing viable *Toxoplasma* organisms periodically break down in the affected tissue. When this happens, antigens are released into the immediate environment of the cyst, and viable organisms may be released. These organisms have the ability to attack nearby, previously uninvolved retinal cells. This is believed to be the basis of the recurrent lesions of ocular toxoplasmosis. It should be pointed out, however, that the spontaneous rupture of *Toxoplasma* cysts has never been documented in the human eye or elsewhere. The theory that *Toxoplasma* cysts rupture spontaneously comes largely from the work of Frenkel.[7] who observed the spontaneous rupture of *Besnoitia* cysts in the hamster eye by means of direct ophthalmoscopic examination. The *Besnoitia* cyst is large enough to see under these circumstances, but the *Toxoplasma* cyst is not. In any case, Frenkel believes that there is very little invasion of new, previously uninvolved retinal cells when a cyst ruptures. He believes that most of the damage that is seen in recurrent focal retinochoroiditis comes about as a result of hypersensitivity.

Our group, working at the Proctor Foundation, has taken issue with this theory. By injecting soluble antigens of *Toxoplasma* into areas of the retina contiguous to old, previously active lesions, we have been unable to produce necrotizing focal retinitis of the type that is characteristically seen in recurrences of human toxoplasmic disease.[19] For this reason we believe that all, or nearly all, recurrent lesions represent at least a limited proliferation of *Toxoplasma* organisms in nearby retinal cells.

Inflammation of the anterior segment of the eye, manifested mainly as a granulomatous iridocyclitis, is believed to be attributable entirely to hypersensitivity. There is no convincing evidence of the presence of proliferating *Toxoplasma* organisms in the anterior uvea in the human eye. Previous work on this subject,[21] claiming the isolation of *Toxoplasma* parasites from the eye of a patient who had been affected by iridocyclitis alone, failed to segregate the anterior segment of the eye from the posterior segment when attempts were made to isolate *Toxoplasma* parasites. Thus, although proliferating *Toxoplasma* organisms appear to be able to cause active lesions in the anterior segments of animal eyes.[22] no proliferating *Toxoplasma* organisms have as yet been isolated from the human eye. Furthermore, experimental evidence, obtained by the inoculation of soluble *Toxoplasma* antigens into the vitreous of a previously sensitized rabbit eye, indicates that an iridocyclitis precisely analogous to that seen in the human eye can be produced in the experimental animal. These findings have implications for the therapy of ocular toxoplasmosis, for it is generally believed that since toxoplasmic iridocyclitis is a hypersensitivity phenomenon, local corticosteroid therapy may be administered freely without allowing the additional proliferation of the organism in the affected tissues.

The secondary glaucoma that so often accompanies exacerbations of toxoplasmic retinochoroiditis may be very severe in its intensity. It is generally connected with a severe, recurrent iridocyclitis. When this glaucoma occurs in an open-angle situation, it is believed to represent the congestion of the trabecular meshwork by inflammatory cells and other inflammatory products, including fibrin. This secondary glaucoma may be enormously helped by the use of both locally applied and systemically administered corticosteroids. Sometimes this is the only treatment that provides relief for the patient because standard antiglaucoma medications fail to lower the intraocular pressure to acceptable levels.

DIAGNOSIS

The diagnosis of ocular toxoplasmosis is based on (1) the presence of a focal, necrotizing retinochoroiditis, (2) the presence of antibodies, even in low titer, in the circulating blood of the patient, and (3) a reasonable exclusion of other diseases that might produce granulomatous lesions of the eye. The morphology of the lesion is an important criterion of diagnosis. Although the focal, necrotizing retinochoroiditis so characteristic of ocular toxoplasmosis may be present as a single lesion, much more often the active lesion is seen in the presence of older, healed, atrophic lesions, some of which may have extensive pigmentation. It should be emphasized that the primary lesion of ocular toxoplasmosis is a *retinal* lesion. In this way, the lesions of ocular toxoplasmosis can be differentiated from conditions such as disseminated choroiditis. The spectrum of retinal conditions that can be included in the diagnosis of ocular toxoplasmosis is wide. Thus Friedman and Knox[8] have shown that a deep punctate form of retinochoroiditis, often accompanied by hemorrhage, can be included in the spectrum of disease represented by ocular toxoplasmosis. This form of the disease causes very little clouding of the overlying vitreous body, at least during the early phases of the inflammation. Sooner or later, every toxoplasmic lesion of the fundus causes some clouding of the vitreous, and this is a diagnostic feature of the disease. Other forms of focal chorioretinitis that are sometimes confused with ocular toxoplasmosis include the early lesions of *Candida* retinitis, luetic chorioretinitis, and tuberculous chorioretinitis. The last is extremely rare, but it is being seen with ever greater frequency among patients who have recently emigrated to the United States from Southeast Asia. Occasionally, masquerade lesions, such as those of histiocytic lymphoma or angioid streaks, may be mistaken for the lesions of ocular toxoplasmosis. One should never consider a lesion that is strictly anterior in location as a candidate for ocular toxoplasmosis. Although iridocyclitis is sometimes said to be caused by ocular toxoplasmosis, one should not consider this as a valid diagnosis until the retinal periphery has been carefully screened for evidence of focal, necrotizing retinochoroiditis.

The serologic diagnosis of toxoplasmosis is important. The *Toxoplasma* dye test of Sabin and Feldman is still the mainstay of our serologic diagnosis. However, because this test requires the use of living organisms and it presents some danger of laboratory infection, it has been replaced in many medical centers by alternative testing procedures. These include the hemagglutination test, the indirect fluorescent antibody (IFA) test, and the newly developed ELISA test for toxoplasmosis. The last is one of many enzyme-linked immunosorbent assays (ELISA) for antibodies to microbial pathogens. It has been shown to have the same sensitivity and specificity as the *Toxoplasma* dye test and has the additional advantage of being able to be performed on very small fluid samples (such as 10 μl). Thus a single sample of aqueous humor could yield adequate fluid for 10 tests.

Occasionally the titers of positive serologic tests are extremely low, and the ophthalmologist is moved to doubt whether the test results are significant. It has now been shown repeatedly that low titers of anti-*Toxoplasma* antibody are significant so long as lesions are present in the fundus that are morphologically compatible with ocular toxoplasmosis. Thus a positive serologic test *at any titer* is significant so long as the patient has morphologic evidence of ocular toxoplasmosis. One does not need to show rising titers to document the presence of toxoplasmic eye disease, and one should not judge the activity of a given lesion by fluctuations in the titer of serum antibodies. This is an important point, but it is often neglected by ophthalmologists and internists alike. Zscheile[38] has shown without question that an ocular lesion from toxoplasmosis could be detected in a patient whose serum dye-test titer was only 1:1. Undeniable histologic evidence of ocular toxoplasmosis was found in this patient at autopsy.

In certain cases where the morphology of the fundus lesion is not absolutely characteristic or the presence of more than one type of serum antibody suggests two or more possible causes, some tests on the aqueous humor may be useful. Under these circumstances, the amount of specific antibody per unit of immunoglobulin in the aqueous humor is compared with the amount of specific antibody per unit of immunoglobulin in the serum. This is done so as to exclude the possibility that antibody present in the anterior segment is merely there as a result of increased blood-aqueous permeability. Under conditions of inflammation the blood-aqueous barrier could conceivably be lowered, permitting excessive amounts of antibody from the bloodstream to enter the eye. If there is more specific antibody per unit of immunoglobulin than could be expected on the basis of altered blood-aqueous permeability, it seems plausible to assume that there is local antibody formation in the uveal tract. Witmer[36] has produced ample evidence of this formation in his work with experimental leptospiral uveitis. Furthermore, in the case of toxoplasmosis, O'Connor[18] has shown that more specific antibody to *Toxoplasma* was present in the aqueous humor of patients with presumptive toxoplasmosis than was found in the simultaneously sampled serum. A newly developed ELISA technique for the detection of antibody to *Toxoplasma* is readily adaptable to tests of the blood and aqueous humor. Because the ELISA technique requires only a very small volume of fluid, multiple tests can be performed on the same sample of aqueous humor.[13]

Rollins et al.[24] have recently shown that *Toxoplasma* antigen could be detected in the vitreous humor of rabbits recently subjected to experimentally produced toxoplasmic retinochoroiditis. It appears that antigen diffuses from the retinochoroiditic lesion into the overlying vitreous and remains in the vitreous for a period of up to 6 weeks. This finding is in harmony with the finding of free antigen in the serum of patients in the early course of systemic toxoplasmic infections.[2] Thus another possibility is opened for the specific diagnosis of ocular toxoplasmosis.

TREATMENT

The primary goal of treatment is the preservation of visual acuity. Retinochoroiditic lesions that threaten the macula, the papillomacular bundle, or the optic nerve itself require immediate treatment. Peripheral lesions, particularly if they are small and on the nasal side of the optic nerve head, are best treated by observation alone. Occasionally a lesion, though peripheral in location, will require active treatment because of the large amount of exudate that this lesion is casting off into the overlying vitreous.

New lesions, particularly those that have been present for 10 days or less, require antimicrobial therapy. The time-honored treatment for these lesions is with pyrimethamine and sulfonamides. These agents disrupt the nuclear metabolism of the parasite and paralyze its replication in the ocular tissues. If a decision is made to treat with these agents, a high loading dose should be administered initially to achieve adequate levels of medication in the retina. For an average patient weighing 70 kg, it is recommended that 75 mg of pyrimethamine be administered orally on each of the first two days of therapy. The dosage is than reduced to 25 mg per day for the following 30 days. Likewise, a loading dose of 6.0 g of either sulfadiazine or trisulfapyrimidine is recommended, followed by a daily dosage of 1.5 g 4 times a day. The patient should be urged to force fluid intake and to take one teaspoonful of sodium bicarbonate at mealtimes in order to alkalinize the urine. Folinic acid, at a dosage of 3 mg, should be taken at least once a week. Although this material is produced only as a sterile injectable solution, the solution may be taken by mouth. The rationale of folinic acid therapy is that the parasite must form folinic acid from certain precursors such as folic acid, whereas man may utilize exogenous folinic acid. In practice, the administration of folinic acid is often omitted in otherwise normal individuals. Patients with a familial history of macrocytic anemia, on the other hand, should certainly receive this therapy as a means of protecting their hematopoietic tissues.

Other forms of antimicrobial therapy for ocular toxoplasmosis appear to be promising and possibly less toxic than pyrimethamine and sulfonamide therapy. These include therapy with clindamycin, a 7-chloro derivative of lincomycin. Clindamycin is an inhibitor of protein synthesis at the ribosomal level. Its antimicrobial spectrum includes certain protozoan parasites such as *Plasmodium,* as well as a large number of anaerobic and gram-positive bacteria. Thiermann[32] has shown that clindamycin functions synergistically with sulfonamides in the eradication of *Toxoplasma* from infected mice. Tabbara and O'Connor[29] have shown that this combination was effective in treating human ocular toxoplasmosis when administered at dosages of 300 mg of clindamycin every 6 hours by mouth, coupled with 1.5 g of sulfonamides 4 times a day. This treatment is generally continued for a period of 1 month though lesions generally show signs of improvement within 10 days. There is a significant risk for the development of pseudomembranous colitis when clindamycin is administered orally. This condition is now known to be attributable to the liberation of toxins by *Clostridium difficile,* an intestinal organism that tends to overgrow in the presence of certain antibiotic agents. Pseudomembranous colitis has not been observed among any of our patients treated with the combination of clindamycin and sulfonamides. It may well be that the simultaneous administration of sulfonamides prevents the overgrowth of *Clostridium difficile.* Furthermore it has now been demonstrated clinically that vancomycin administered orally will satisfactorily treat the pseudomembranous colitis caused by overgrowth of *Clostridium difficile,* and so the danger of complications from clindamycin therapy is now considerably reduced over what it once was.

A newly developed tetracycline derivative, minocycline, appears to offer great promise in the treatment of ocular toxoplasmosis. This agent also interrupts protein synthesis in the cytoplasm of the parasite by combining with the ribosomes. It has the theoretical advantage that it penetrates the blood-brain barrier better than any other tetracycline derivative. Therefore the possibility that it will be delivered to retinal lesions after oral administration is relatively good. An initial paper by Tabbara et al.[30] shows the efficacy of this agent in curing mice injected intraperitoneally with large inocula of the virulent RH strain of *Toxoplasma* organisms. It has yet to be evaluated in higher animals.

Corticosteroid therapy should be considered whenever toxoplasmic lesions appear to threaten areas of the retina that are important for vision. Occasionally, the vitreous body will be so infiltrated by cells thrown off from a peripheral lesion that corticosteroid therapy must also be considered, despite the fact that the basic lesion does not pose a threat to vision. Corticosteroid therapy is best given orally in doses of 100 to 150 mg of prednisone per day in the initial treatment period. This is most efficacious when given in divided doses throughout the day in the initial 7 days of treatment. Thereafter, systemic corticosteroids should be given as a large single dose at 8:00 in the morning on either a daily or an alternate-day basis. Under no circumstances should corticosteroid therapy be given without antimicrobial coverage. At least one agent, possibly sulfon-amides alone, should always be administered whenever corticosteroid therapy is being taken.

Periocular injections of corticosteroids, though they sometimes produce an immediate and dramatic result, are fraught with considerable danger. This is particularly true of the repository forms of corticosteroids, such as methylprednisolone acetate (Depo-Medrol) or Depo-Kenalog. Injections of these substances may deliver amounts of corticosteroids to the internal eye that are not only anti-inflammatory, but immunosuppressive as well. Under these conditions, the causative organism, *Toxoplasma gondii,* may be free to proliferate in an unchecked manner. This danger is probably minimized if antimicrobial agents are administered simultaneously, but the margin of safety is relatively narrow.

Other forms of therapy for ocular toxoplasmosis include surgical modalities such as photocoagulation, cryotherapy, and vitrectomy. Photocoagulation has been useful mainly as a prophylactic agent. Spalter et al.[28] have demonstrated the efficacy of laser coagulation in preventing the recurrences of toxoplasmic retinochoroiditis at the edges of previously active lesions. Statistically the greatest number of cysts of *Toxoplasma* will be found in areas immediately adjacent to healed, recently active lesions. The thermal energy generated by photocoagulation has the power to destroy *Toxoplasma* cysts, and it may also denature *Toxoplasma* antigens and retinal autoantigens that may be liberated at the lesion site. This form of treatment has been used mainly in prophylaxis. However, Ghartey and Brockhurst[9] have recently suggested that photocoagulation may be used to expedite the healing of chronically active lesions that have resisted all conventional modes of therapy. Treatment of active lesions by photocoagulation is still highly controversial, for it may result in burning a hole in Bruch's membrane or other undesirable disturbances.

Cryotherapy, as popularized by Dobbie,[4] may kill encysted organisms by rapid freezing. It may also stimulate the formation of a gliotic barrier around previously active lesions. Cryotherapy must generally be applied by means of a posteriorly placed cryoprobe, and this requires operative intervention. It has occasionally been useful in inducing the healing of a chronically active lesion.

Most recently Fitzgerald[6] has described the use of vitrectomy in the treatment of chronically active chorioretinal lesions caused by toxoplasmosis. This therapy is mainly aimed at the removal of vitreous debris, some of which may be organized in the form of strands and sheets. These strands and sheets have contractile potential and have sometimes been found to be responsible for retinal tears. Vitrectomy also has the potential advantage of clearing the visual axis so that good visual acuity is restored to patients whose macular apparatus is still intact. This mode of therapy also has the theoretical advantage of removing *Toxoplasma* antigens and retinal autoantigens that may be retained in the vitreous. It is known that the vitreous acts like a sponge for the retention of antigens. Such a sponge, constantly kept in contact with the retinal vasculature, may contribute to the chronicity of inflammation in some cases. Although Fitzgerald claims to have produced beneficial effects from vitrectomy, it is noteworthy that several of her patients developed exacerbations of retinochoroiditis as a result of this therapy. At the present time, therefore, it should be reserved only for the most stubborn of cases.

REFERENCES

1. Akstein, R.B., Wilson, L.A., and Teutsch, S.M.: Acquired toxoplasmosis, Ophthalmology **89:**1299, Dec. 1982.
2. Araujo, F.G., and Remington, J.S.: Antigenemia in recently acquired, acute toxoplasmosis, J. Infect. Dis. **141:**144, 1980.
3. Desmonts, G., and Couvreur, J.: Congenital toxoplasmosis: a prospective study of 378 pregnancies, N. Engl. J. Med. **290:**1110, 1974.
4. Dobbie, J.G.: Cryotherapy in the management of *Toxoplasma* retinochoroiditis, Trans. Am. Acad. Ophthalmol. Otolaryngol. **72:**364, 1968.
5. Dorfman, R.F., and Remington, J.S.: Value of lymph-node biopsy in the diagnosis of acute acquired toxoplasmosis, N. Engl. J. Med. **289:**878, 1973.
6. Fitzgerald, C.R.: Pars plana vitrectomy for vitreous opacity secondary to presumed toxoplasmosis, Arch. Ophthalmol. **98:**321, 1980.
7. Frenkel, J.K.: Pathogenesis of toxoplasmosis with consideration of cyst rupture in *Besnoitia* infection, Surv. Ophthalmol. **6:**799, 1961.
8. Friedmann, C.T., and Knox, D.L.: Variations in active toxoplasmic retinochoroiditis, Arch. Ophthalmol. **81:**481, 1969.
9. Ghartey, K.N., and Brockhurst, R.J.: Photocoagulation of active toxoplasmic retinochoroiditis, Am. J. Ophthalmol. **89:**858, 1980.
10. Hoerni, B., Vallat, M., Durand, M., and Pesme, D.: Ocular toxoplasmosis and Hodgkin's disease: report of two cases, Arch. Ophthalmol. **96:**62, 1978.
11. Jacobs, L., Naquin, H., Hoover, R., and Woods, A.C.: A comparison of the *Toxoplasma* skin tests, the Sabin-Feldman dye tests, and the complement fixation tests for toxoplasmosis in various forms of uveitis, Bull. Johns Hopkins Hosp. **99:**1, 1956.
12. Kean, B.H., Kimball, A.C., and Christenson, W.N.: An epidemic of acute toxoplasmosis, J.A.M.A. **208:**1002, 1969.
13. Lin, T.M., Halbert, S.P., and O'Connor, G.R.: Standardized quantitative enzyme-linked immunoassay for antibodies to *Toxoplasma gondii*, J. Clin. Microbiol. **11:**675, 1980.
14. Masur, H., Lempert, J.A., and Cherubini, T.D.: Outbreak of toxoplasmosis in a family and documentation of acquired retinochoroiditis, Am. J. Med. **64:**396, 1978.
15. Michelson, J.B., Shields, J.A., McDonald, P.R., Manko, M.A., Abraham, A.A., and Federman, J.L.: Retinitis secondary to acquired systemic toxoplasmosis with isolation of the parasite, Am. J. Ophthalmol. **86:**548, 1978.
16. Myrvik, Q.N., Kohlweiss, L.A., and Harpold, D.: Pathological potential of exaggerated immunological reactions. In Schlessinger, D., editor: Microbiology 1975, Washington D.C., 1975, American Society for Microbiology.
17. Nussenblatt, R.B., Gery, I., Ballintine, E.J., and Wacker, W.B.: Cellular immune responsiveness of uveitis patients to retinal S-antigen, Am. J. Ophthalmol. **89:**173, 1980.
18. O'Connor, G.R.: Precipitating antibody to *Toxoplasma:* a follow-up study on findings in the blood and aqueous humor, Am. J. Ophthalmol. **44**(Part II):75, 1957.
19. O'Connor, G.R.: The influence of hypersensitivity on the pathogenesis of ocular toxoplasmosis, Trans. Am. Ophthalmol. Soc. **68:**501, 1970.
20. Perkins, E.S.: Ocular toxoplasmosis, Br. J. Ophthalmol. **57:**1, 1973.
21. Pillat, A., and Thalhammer, O.: Herdförmige Iridocyclitis als (einzige) Manifestation einer erworbenen Toxoplasmose, ätiologisch gesichert durch Titerkurve und Tierversuch, Graefe Arch. Ophthalmol. **158:**403, 1957.
22. Piper, R.C., Cole, C.R., and Shadduck, J.A.: Natural and experimental toxoplasmosis in animals, Am.J. Ophthalmol. **69:**662, 1970.
23. Rao, N.A., and Font, R.L.: Toxoplasmic retinochoroiditis: electronmicroscopic and immunofluorescence studies of formalin-fixed tissue, Arch. Ophthalmol. **95:**273, 1977.
24. Rollins, D.F., Tabbara, K.F., O'Connor, G.R., Araujo, F.G., and Remington, J.S.: Detection of *Toxoplasma* antigen and antibody in ocular fluids in experimental ocular toxoplasmosis, Arch. Ophthalmol. (In press.)
25. Saari, M., Vuorre, I., Neiminen, H., and Raisanen, S.: Acquired toxoplasmic chorioretinitis, Arch. Ophthalmol. **94:**1485, 1976.

26. Schwartz, P.L.: Segmental retinal periarteritis as a complication of toxoplasmosis, Ann. Ophthalmol. **9:**157, 1977.

27. Shimada, K., O'Connor, G.R., and Yoneda, C.: Cyst formation by *Toxoplasma gondii* (RH strain) in vitro, Arch. Ophthalmol. **92:**496, 1974.

28. Spalter, H.F., Campbell, C.J., Noyori, K.S., et al.: Prophylactic photocoagulation of recurrent toxoplasmic retinochoroiditis: a preliminary report, Arch. Ophthalmol. **75:**21, 1966.

29. Tabbara, K.F., and O'Connor, G.R.: Treatment of ocular toxoplasmosis with clindamycin and sulfadiazine, Ophthalmology **87:**129, 1980.

30. Tabbara, K.F., Sakuragi, S., and O'Connor, G.R.: Minocycline in the chemotherapy of murine toxoplasmosis, Parasitology **84:**297, 1982.

31. Teutsch, S.M., Juranek, D.D., Sulzer, A., Dubey, J.P. and Sikes, R.K.: Epidemic toxoplasmosis associated with infected cats, N. Engl. J. Med. **300:**695, 1979.

32. Thiermann, E., and Werner, A.: A comparative study of some combined treatment regimens in acute toxoplasmosis in mice, Am. J. Trop. Med. Hyg. **27:**747, 1978.

33. Uchida, Y., Kakehashi, Y., and Kameyama, K.: Juxtapapillary retinochoroiditis with a psychiatric disorder possibly caused by *Toxoplasma:* a case report, Am. J. Ophthalmol. **86:**791, 1978.

34. Wilder, H.C.: *Toxoplasma* chorioretinitis in adults, Arch. Ophthalmol. **48:**127, 1952.

35. Wising, P.: Akut adult toxoplasmos med lymfadenopathi och chorioretinit, Nord. Med. **47:**563, 1952.

36. Witmer, R.H., Experimental leptospiral uveitis in rabbits, Arch. Ophthalmol. **53:**547, 1955.

37. Wyler, D.J., Blackman, H.J., and Lunde, M.N.: Cellular hypersensitivity to toxoplasmal and retinal antigens in patients with toxoplasmal retinochoroiditis, Am. J. Trop. Med. Hyg. **29:**1181, 1980.

38. Zscheile, F.P.: Recurrent toxoplasmic retinitis with weakly positive methylene blue dye test, Arch. Ophthalmol. **71:**645, 1964.

10

Experimental model of posterior penetrating injury

Stephen J. Ryan
Philip E. Cleary*

Prognosis after penetrating injury to the anterior segment of the eye has greatly improved in recent years.[17,36,41,47,49] Unfortunately, however, there has been little improvement in prognosis of injuries involving the posterior segment[17,29,44,48,50] and injuries involving both the anterior and posterior segments continue to result in blindness or enucleation in all but a few rare cases.[7,17,29,44] In many of these severely injured eyes, the disruption of intraocular contents and the extent of suprachoroidal hemorrhage are so great that restoration is not even attempted.[17,37] However, in other cases, loss of vision is not attributable to the primary injury but rather to complications resulting from that injury. In injuries confined to the posterior segment, for example, the most common cause of loss of vision is traction retinal detachment.[17,18,28,29]

Numerous posttrauma natural history and histopathologic studies have demonstrated that the vitreous traction and resultant retinal detachment are directly related to the amount of vitreous hemorrhage and presence of incarcerated vitreous in the wound.[17,18,28,39,43] Additional histopathologic studies have incriminated cellular proliferation and fibroglial ingrowth from the wound, injury to the lens and ciliary body, and vitreous hemorrhage in the formation of cyclitic membranes, which often progress to cause traction and ultimately retinal detachment.[15,17,26,51] Therefore removal of the components that stimulate fibrous proliferation (that is, vitreous condensations and blood clot) by vitrectomy may preclude the sequelae of penetrating injuries to the eye.[15,32,51] However, although initial results of vitrectomy in treatment of such injuries are encouraging,[4,16,27,35,40,45] the time at which such surgery should be performed remains a subject of controversy.[4,14,18,27,31] A previous review of 100 patients who underwent vitrectomy for penetrating eye injury seems to indicate that vitrectomy is most effective when performed from 4 to 14 days after injury.[47] Such studies are difficult to evaluate, however, because of the many variables that cannot be controlled in the clinical situation. To control more precisely the variables involved in penetrating ocular injury, we devel-

---

*F.R.C.S., Visiting Assistant Professor, Department of Ophthalmology, University of Southern California School of Medicine, Estelle Doheny Eye Foundation, Los Angeles, California.

oped an experimental animal model (adult rhesus monkeys) of posterior penetrating ocular injury.

ANIMAL MODEL

The goal of the initial aspect of the present study was to create reproducibly an injury that led to traction retinal detachment. This animal model was characterized histopathologically and found to undergo sequential development of cellular proliferation with the formation of cyclitic, transvitreal, epiretinal, and retroretinal membranes, which ultimately led to traction retinal detachment. These monkey eyes were studied at the ultrastructural level by electron microscopy and also by radiography in an effort to identify the origin of the proliferating cells.[9] In addition to the above studies, a controlled trial of pars plana vitrectomy was done in these animals.[13] Monkeys were assigned to groups that were to have vitrectomy performed at 1, 14, or 70 days after penetrating injury. Results of this study supported the hypothesis that vitrectomy after penetrating posterior segment eye injury is more effective than no surgery in prevention of the complication of retinal detachment.[13]

MECHANISM OF TRACTION RETINAL DETACHMENT

By use of a standard penetrating injury, we were able to produce traction retinal detachment in the rhesus monkey while avoiding direct damage to the retina, thereby excluding rhegmatogenous retinal detachment as a variable. In this animal mode, posterior vitreous detachment was first seen 1 to 2 weeks after injury and coincided with resorption of the blood clot. When retinal detachment subsequently occurred, the peripheral retina was pulled forward toward the pars plana. We interpreted this as evidence of traction on the peripheral retina. Similar findings were observed in human eyes after posterior penetrating injury[51] and in rabbits after experimental injury.[12] In our rhesus model, retinal detachment most commonly occurred between 7 and 11 weeks after injury. As in the human eye, it is believed that this detachment is caused by two mechanisms. First, incarcerated vitreous forms a scaffold upon which fibrous ingrowth can progress from the wound to form cyclitic membranes; second, the combination of traction on the peripheral retina to which the vitreous is attached and contraction of epiretinal fibrous tissue on the surface of the periphral and equatorial retina causes shortening of the retina, which may ultimately result in traction retinal detachment (Fig. 10-1). This sequence of events was very similar to that noted in our review of clinical cases.[46] Natural history and histopathologic studies in our experimental model thus support evidence from previous clinical studies that presence of blood in the vitreous is important in the development of vitreous traction and traction retinal detachment.[17,18,28,39]

To further define the precise mechanisms responsible for traction retinal detachment, we undertook an ultrastructural study of changes occurring after posterior penetrating injury. It was considered that changes in the collagen linkage in the vitreous or in the newly formed cyclitic membranes may produce a shrinkage that results in traction on the retina.[2,25,43] In our model, the wound-healing response, which shared many features with the normal systemic processes of wound healing, consisted of an inflammatory reaction that was followed by cellular proliferation with fibroplasia and collagen production; these are the processes that lead to scar formation and contraction. Although normal wound healing may be controlled by chemical factors, it appears to be aided by

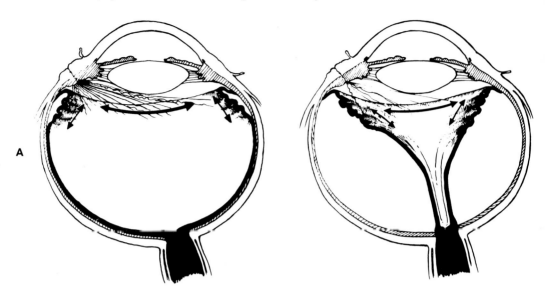

A

Fig. 10-1. The development of traction retinal detachment can be related to two mechanisms. **A,** Vitreous is incarcerated in the wound and fibrous ingrowth from the wound along the vitreous scaffold may result in traction on the peripheral retina over the vitreous base. **B,** Contraction of epiretinal fibrous tissue on the surface of the peripheral and equatorial retina may result in shortening of the retina. Either of these mechanisms, but usually the combination of both, results in traction retinal detachment. (From Cleary, P.E., and Ryan, S.J.: Am. J. Ophthalmol. **88:**212, 1979, published with permission from the American Journal of Opthalmology, copyright 1979 by the Ophthalmic Publishing Co., Chicago.)

the presence of a fibrin matrix that acts as a scaffold for proliferating fibroblasts, which in turn lay down collagen.[39] It is well documented that bonding between collagen fibers or collagen synthesis is not necessary for wound healing.[1,38] Recently, multipurpose cells that have electron microscopic features of both fibroblasts and smooth muscle cells, termed "myofibroblasts,"[24] have been described; they have created renewed interest in the mechanisms of wound contraction. These cells, which contain intracytoplasmic filaments of actinomyosin, which provides a mechanism for cell contraction,[26] are considered responsible for the contraction component observed in wound healing.[24] In addition, these cells have also been detected in human tissues from various fibrocontractive disorders.[5,19,23,33]

In our rhesus monkey model, classic myofibroblasts were seen in the intravitreous fibrous tissue and within epiretinal membranes. The precise origin of these myofibroblasts was difficult to determine, but it is known that, in both monkey and human eyes, retinal pigment epithelial cells can undergo metaplasia into fibroblast-like cells[28] and, in tissue culture, chick retinal pigment epithelial cells can express themselves as fibroblasts.[51]

Examination of the epiretinal membranes by electron microscopy also revealed cells that were obviously glial in origin; these were identical to glial cells seen in human and monkey eyes after rhegmatogenous retinal detachment[31,49] and in epiretinal membranes of human eyes.[3,8,20,21,30,43,45]

Considering the many layers and types of tissues involved in our experimental pen-

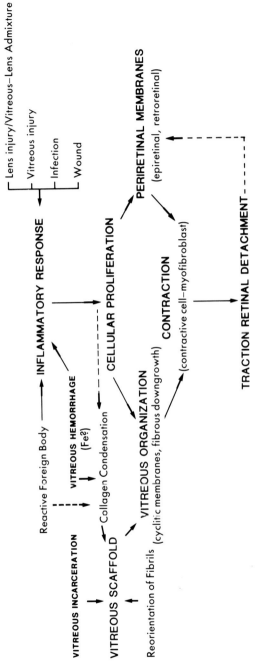

Fig. 10-2. Schematic diagram of the probable mechanisms of traction retinal detachment after a penetrating eye injury. (From Cleary, P.E., Minckler, D.S., and Ryan, S.J.: Am. J. Ophthalmol. **90:**829, 1980, published with permission from the American Journal of Ophthalmology, copyright 1980 by The Ophthalmic Publishing Co., Chicago.)

etrating eye injury, the variability of cellular elements within the fibrous ingrowth was not surprising. We found many typical myofibroblasts in the vitreous and in epiretinal membranes, and their presence may be directly responsible for contraction of epiretinal membranes, which results in traction retinal detachment of the monkey eye. These findings in the monkey eye are consistent with those in the human and form the basis for an understanding of the mechanisms responsible for traction retinal detachment after penetrating eye injury (Fig. 10-2).

Detailed knowledge of vitreoretinal anatomy is essential to an understanding of the mechanisms involved in the production of retinal traction and detachment. In the monkey eye, the vitreous readily separates from the posterior retina.[10,11] and complete detachment of the posterior hyaloid precudes anteroposterior vitreous traction. However, as the vitreous remains adherent to the retina at the vitreous base, a penetrating scleral wound with vitreous incarceration causes traction on the peripheral retina.

The intraocular cellular proliferation produces transvitreal, cyclitic, retroretinal, and epiretinal membranes that contain the recently described myofibroblasts, which are known to cause contraction. It is possible that in the future the contractile action of these cells may be altered by pharmacologic agents.[22,34] In the meantime, however, vitrectomy is the treatment of choice after penetrating ocular injury.

EFFECT OF TIMING OF VITRECTOMY ON OUTCOME

Although preliminary reports of results of open-sky and pars plana vitrectomy in the treatment of posterior penetrating injury are encouraging,[4,16,18,27,35,46] controversy remains as to when such procedures should be performed. Delayed vitrectomy may allow formation of cellular proliferation, membrane formation, and retinal detachment.[4,27] On the other hand, vitrectomy immediately after injury may result in uncontrolled hemorrhage.[18,31] Using our rhesus monkey model, we investigated the role of timing in the ultimate outcome of vitrectomy for posterior penetrating eye injury.

Pars plana vitrectomies were performed at 1, 14, and 70 days after standardized injury, a control group received no therapy. If performed at 1 to 14 days, vitrectomy prevented formation of epiretinal and cyclitic membranes and traction retinal detachment. It should also be noted that there was no statistically significant difference in eyes operated at 1 to 14 days. By contrast, vitrectomy at 70 days proved no more beneficial than no surgery at all. Significant differences were noted at vitrectomy between eyes operated on at 1 and 14 days. Specifically, there was a noticeable change in the color and consistency of the vitreous, possibly related to effects of iron or lysozomal enzymes activated by the inflammatory process.[11] This facilitated cutting the vitreous at 14 days. In addition, vitreoretinal adhesions were no longer present over the posterior retina though vitreous did remain firmly adherent to the peripheral retina. This is significant because it is known that traction on the peripheral retina is one of the contributing factors in the development of retinal detachments.[10]

In addition, epiretinal membranes, which were not encountered at 14 days, were prominent at 70 days.

Results of this controlled laboratory trial of vitrectomy in monkey eyes support the hypothesis that vitrectomy is an effective management of penetrating ocular injuries. Although there were no major differences in results of vitrectomy performed at 1 to 14 days, the procedure was less difficult technically when performed at 14 days. In the monkey eye there was no suprachoroidal or subretinal hemorrhage and no engorgement of choroidal vessels, thus, even at 1 day we did not encounter the problem of expulsive hemorrhage, which can occur in the clinical situation.

By 70 days, vitrectomy was successful in only 2 of 10 monkey eyes; the remainder were inoperable.

Results of this study further support the belief that there is a rationale for prophylactic vitrectomy in the treatment of posterior penetrating eye injury, with the use of an encircling scleral buckle; others have recommended this in all vitrectomy procedures,[6,34] but this may be particularly efficacious in the treatment of ocular trauma. Removal of the stimulus to inflammation plus the vitreous scaffold are the goals that may be achieved by vitrectomy. Thus we can now salvage eyes that were previously lost.

REFERENCES

1. Abercrombie, M., Flint, M.H., and James, D.W.: Wound contraction in relation to collagen formation in scorbutic guinea pigs, J. Embryol. Exp. Morphol. **4:**167, 1956.
2. Balazs, E.A.: The molecular biology of the vitreous. In McPherson, A., editor: New and controversial aspects of retinal detachment, New York, 1968, Harper & Row, Publishers.
3. Bellhorn, M.B., Friedman, A.H., Wise, G.N., and Henkind, P.: Ultrastructure and clinicopathologic correlation of idiopathic preretinal macular fibrosis, Am. J. Ophthalmol. **79:**366, 1975.
4. Benson, W.E., and Machemer, R.: Severe perforating injuries treated with pars plana vitrectomy, Am. J. Ophthalmol. **81:**728, 1976.
5. Bhathal, P.S.: Presence of modified fibroblasts in cirrhotic livers in man, Pathology **4:**139, 1972.
6. Charles, S.: Fluid-gas exchange in the vitreous cavity, Outcome Newsletter **2:**1, 1977.
7. Cinotti, A.A., and Maltzman, B.A.: Prognosis and treatment of perforating ocular injuries, Ophthalmic Surg. **6:**54, 1975.
8. Clarkson, J.G., Green, W.R., and Massof, D.: A histopathologic review of 168 cases of preretinal membrane, Am. J. Ophthalmol. **84:**1, 1977.
9. Cleary, P.E., Minckler, D.S., and Ryan, S.J.: Ultrastructure of traction retinal detachment in rhesus monkey eyes after a posterior penetrating ocular injury, Am. J. Ophthalmol. **90:**829, 1980.
10. Cleary, P.E., and Ryan, S.J.: Method of production and natural history of experimental posterior penetrating eye injury in the rhesus monkey, Am. J. Ophthalmol. **88:**212, 1979.
11. Cleary, P.E., and Ryan, S.J.: Histology of wound, vitreous, and retina in experimental posterior penetrating eye injury in the rhesus monkey, Am. J. Ophthalmol. **88:**221, 1979.
12. Cleary, P.E., and Ryan, S.J.: Experimental posterior penetrating eye injury in the rabbit. I. Method of production and natural history, Br. J. Ophthalmol. **63:**306, 1979.
13. Cleary, P.E., and Ryan, S.J.: Vitrectomy in penetrating eye injury: results of a controlled trial of vitrectomy in experimental posterior penetrating eye injury in the rhesus monkey, Arch. Ophthalmol. **99:**287, 1981.
14. Coleman, D.J.: Current concepts of vitreous including vitrectomy, St. Louis, 1976, The C.V. Mosby Co.
15. Coles, W.H., and Haik, G.M.: Vitrectomy in intraocular trauma, Arch. Ophthalmol. **87:**621, 1972.
16. Conway, B.P., and Michels, R.G.: Vitrectomy techniques in the management of selected penetrating ocular injuries, Ophthalmology **85:**560, Jan.-Dec. 1978.
17. Eagling, E.M.: Perforating injuries involving the posterior segment, Trans. Ophthalmol. Soc. U.K. **95:**335, 1975.
18. Faulborn, J., Atkins, J., and Olivier, D.: Primary vitrectomy as a preventive surgical procedure in the treatment of severely injured eyes, Br. J. Ophthalmol. **61:**202, 1977.
19. Feiner, H., and Kaye, G.I.: Ultrastructural evidence of myofibroblasts in circumscribed fibromatosis, Arch. Pathol. Lab. Med. **100:**265, 1976.
20. Foos, R.Y.: Vitreoretinal juncture: simple epiretinal membranes, Albrecht von Graefes Arch. Klin. Exp. Ophthalmol. **189:**231, 1974.
21. Foos, R.Y.: Vitreoretinal juncture: epiretinal membranes and vitreous, Invest. Ophthalmol. Vis. Sci. **16:**416, 1977.

22. Gabbiani, G., Hirschel, B.J., Ryan, G.B., Statkov, P.R., and Majno, G.: Granulation tissue as a contractile organ: a study of structure and function, J. Exp. Med. **135:**719, 1972.
23. Gabbiani, G., and Majno, G.: Dupuytren's contracture: fibroblastic contraction—an ultrastructural study, Am. J. Pathol. **66:**131, 1972.
24. Gabbiani, G., Ryan, G.B., and Majno, G.: Presence of modified fibroblasts in granulation tissue and possible role in wound contraction, Experientia **27:**549, 1971.
25. Havener, W.H.: Massive vitreous retraction, J. Ophthalmol. Surg. **4:**22, 1973.
26. Hirschel, B.J., Gabbiani, G., Ryan, G.B., and Majno, G.: Fibroblasts of granulation tissue: immunofluorescent staining with anti–smooth muscle serum, Proc. Soc. Biol. Med. **138:**466, 1971.
27. Hogan, M.J., and Zimmerman, L.E.: Ophthalmic pathology: an atlas and textbook, Philadelphia, 1964, W.B. Saunders Co., pp. 645 and 646.
28. Hutton, W.L., Snyder, W.B., and Vaiser, A.: Vitrectomy in the treatment of ocular perforating injuries, Am. J. Ophthalmol. **81:**733, 1976.
29. Johnson, S.: Perforating injuries: a five year study, Trans. Ophthalmol. Soc. U.K. **91:**895, 1971.
30. Kenyon, K.R., and Michels, R.G.: Ultrastructure of epiretinal membranes removed by pars plana vitreoretinal surgery, Am. J. Ophthalmol. **83:**815, 1977.
31. Laqua, H., and Machemer, R.: Glial cell proliferation in retinal detachment (massive periretinal proliferation), Am. J. Ophthalmol. **80:**602, 1975.
32. Machemer, R., and Norton, E.W.D.: A new concept for vitreous surgery. III. Indications and results, Am. J. Ophthalmol. **74:**1034, 1972.
33. Madden, J.W., Carlson, E.Z., and Hines, J.: Presence of modified fibroblasts in ischemic contracture of the intrinsic musculature of the hand, Surg. Gynecol. Obstet. **140:**509, 1975.
34. Madden, J.W., Morton, D., Jr., and Peacock, E.E., Jr.: Contraction of experimental wounds. I. Inhibiting wound contraction by using a topical smooth muscle antagonist, Surgery **76:**8, 1974.
35. Michels, R.G.: Vitrectomy for complications of diabetic retinopathy, Arch. Ophthalmol. **96:**237, 1978.
36. Michels, R.G., and Ryan, S.J.: Results and complications of 100 consecutive cases of pars plana vitrectomy, Am. J. Ophthalmol. **80:**24, 1975.
37. Moncreiff, W.F., and Scheribel, K.J.: Penetrating injuries of the eye: a statistical survey, Am. J. Ophthalmol. **28:**1212, 1945.
38. Newcombe, J.D.W.: Granulation tissue resorption during free and limited contraction of skin wounds, J. Anat. **95:**247, 1961.
39. Peacock, E.E., and Van Winkle, W., Jr.: Surgery and biology of wound repair, Philadelphia, 1971, W.B. Saunders Co.
40. Percival, A.P.B.: Late complications from posterior segment intraocular foreign bodies, Br. J. Ophthalmol. **56:**462, 1972.
41. Peyman, G.A., Huamonte, F.U., and Rose, M.: Management of traumatic retinal detachment with pars plana vitrectomy, scleral buckling, and gas injection, Acta Ophthalmol. (Kbh.) **53:**731, 1975.
42. Remky, H., Kobor, J., and Pfeiffer, H.: Traumatologie chirurgicale du segment antérieur, Ann. Inst. Barraquer **7:**487, 1967.
43. Rentsch, F.J.: The ultrastructure of preretinal macular fibrosis, Albrecht von Graefes Arch. Klin. Exp. Ophthalmol. **203:**321, 1977.
44. Roper-Hall, M.J.: The treatment of ocular injuries, Trans. Ophthalmol. Soc. U.K. **79:**57, 1959.
45. Roth, A.M., and Foos, R.Y.: Surface structure of the optic nervehead. I. Epipapillary membranes, Am. J. Ophthalmol. **74:**977, 1972.
46. Ryan, S.J.: Results in pars plana vitrectomy in penetrating ocular trauma, Int. Ophthalmol. **1:**5, 1978.
47. Ryan, S.J., and Allen, A.W., Jr.: Pars plana vitrectomy in ocular trauma: results in a consecutive series, Am. J. Ophthalmol. **88:**483, 1979.
48. Snell, A.C.: Perforating ocular injuries, Am. J. Ophthalmol. **28:**263, 1977.
49. van Horn, D.L., Aaberg, T.M., Machemer, R., and Fenzl, R.: Glial cell proliferation in human retinal detachment with massive periretinal proliferation, Am. J. Ophthalmol. **84:**383, 1977.
50. Watz, H., and Reim, N.: Statistics of injuries referred to provincial eye clinic, Klin. Monatsbl. Augenheilkd. **162:**648, 1973.
51. Wiggert, B., Masterson, E., Israel, P., and Chader, G.J.: Differential retinoid binding in chick pigment epithelium and choroid, Invest. Ophthalmol. Vis. Sci. **18:**306, 1979.
52. Winthrop, S.R., Cleary, P.E., Minckler, D.S., and Ryan, S.J.: Penetrating eye injuries: a histopathological review, Br. J. Ophthalmol. **64:**809, 1980.

11

Penetrating ocular trauma and pars plana vitrectomy

Stephen J. Ryan

Visual outcome after anterior segment injury has improved greatly in recent years, primarily because of technologic advances such as the operating microscope and newly developed and refined surgical techniques. As a result of these advances, normal ocular anatomy can be more readily approximated after such injury.[16,31,34-36,40,41,44,46] Unfortunately similar advances have not been made in repair of posterior segment injury.[15,24] In this type of injury, if the eye is not lost as a result of the injury itself, severe complications often result. These complications often result from an acute inflammatory response to the injured or infected tissue or to a foreign body. Cyclitic membranes can form, and they lead to hypotony or phthisis; similarly, transvitreal membranes may form, and they frequently result in retinal breaks or traction retinal detachments. If the retina becomes detached, it often becomes virtually encased in a massive periretinal proliferation, which makes reattachment much more difficult.[3,25,30]

Because ocular trauma is an important cause of blindness[2] (in some hospitals accounting for the majority of enucleations[11]), we believed that it was important to characterize changes occurring immediately after injury in an attempt to determine how they might stimulate the mechanisms responsible for the acute inflammatory response and eventual retinal detachment. By determining the sequence of histopathologic changes that result from severe penetrating injury, one may identify the optimal time at which pars plana vitrectomy should be performed.

Unfortunately one of the major problems encountered in such a study is the tremendous number of variables that cannot be controlled. These variables include the nature and severity of the wound, the types of tissues involved, the length of time between injury and initial repair, and the type of surgery that is feasible; in addition, the individual patient's response to the injury is important, as well as the patient's age. Ocular injury accounts for a tremendous economic loss because it most commonly occurs in young males who are otherwise healthy and productive.[13] This same age group is also more prone to severe fibrovascular ingrowth, which further complicates repair.

ROLE OF VITRECTOMY IN TRAUMA

Most ophthalmic surgeons now believe that pars plana vitrectomy has potential in the management of severe ocular trauma,* but the role of proper timing of such surgery remains controversial. In an animal model, we previously showed that vitrectomy, as opposed to no surgery, is beneficial in the treatment of severe posterior penetrating ocular injuries[9]; however, we found no difference in eventual outcome if vitrectomy were performed one day after trauma or if surgery were delayed for up to 14 days.

HISTOPATHOLOGIC STUDIES

To determine if results in our experimental model were relevant to the clinical situation, we reviewed our histologic findings in patients who had been treated for severe penetrating ocular injury between 1970 and 1977.[47] Tissues or histopathologic slides were available on 34 such cases that had undergone enucleation from 1 day to 3 years after trauma. All of these eyes were characterized by severe intraocular cellular proliferation that led to the formation of cyclitic, epiretinal, and retroretinal membranes, some of which ultimately resulted in retinal breaks and retinal detachment. Our results thus support previous clinical studies in which the primary cause of loss of vision after posterior penetrating injury was reported to be traction retinal detachment.[15,24,38,40]

Immediately after injury an expulsive hemorrhage frequently occurs with massive bleeding into the choroid beneath the retina and into the vitreous; if this hemorrhage results in prolapse of the ocular contents, vision can rarely be salvaged.[15] After this hemorrhage, an inflammatory reaction usually ensues; the extent of this inflammation is influenced by many variables, including extent of vitreous hemorrhage and vitreous-lens admixture and presence or absence of a foreign body. As this inflammation gradually subsides, intravitreal cellular proliferation occurs. These proliferating cells, in turn, give rise to cyclitic, transretinal, epiretinal, and retroretinal membranes. When these cells coalesce, traction is placed on the retina. Thus it is this cycle of trauma, inflammation, proliferation, and traction that results in traction retinal detachment, which is the main cause of visual loss after trauma.[4]

In our study, the inflammation had subsided, and cellular proliferation had begun within 1 week of injury; in most cases, a cyclitic membrane was identifiable by 6 weeks after injury though in several cases in which there was incarceration of lens material, vitreous, or blood, membranes were seen as early as 2 weeks after injury. Other factors that appeared to have an influence on the rapidity of membrane formation include the site of penetrating wound, adequacy of wound closure, extent of involvement of iris, lens, and vitreous, and presence of massive vitreous hemorrhage.

The cellular proliferation within the vitreous appears to arise from several sources, more specifically from the episclera and uvea in the case of perforating scleral or limbal wounds. Nonpigmented ciliary epithelium also proliferated in several cases; these cells, which were abnormally elongated, extended along vitreous fibrils into the vitreous cavity, and they were a contributing factor to the formation of cyclitic membranes. Similar hyperplasia of nonpigmented ciliary epithelium after trauma and inflammation has been reported by others.[11,21] The intravitreal fibroblastic response may also have been derived, at least in part, from macrophages and monocytes originating in the systemic

---

*See references 1, 10, 12, 17, 22, 29, 31-33, 42, 43.

circulation; however, experimental evidence indicates that fibroblasts involved in wound healing are derived locally.[20,37]

The intraocular cellular proliferation progressed to formation of epiretinal and retroretinal membranes by 1 to 2 weeks after injury. Membranes over the peripheral retina and, in eyes with double penetrating wounds (that is, entrance and exit wounds), membranes over the posterior retina appeared to be derived from fibroblastic ingrowth immediately adjacent to the wound. Again, this finding supports evidence reported in an experimental animal model of posterior eye injury.[6,7,45] In the case of epiretinal membranes, there appeared to be a connection to the retinal surface by bridges of tissue suggestive of glia, a feature that has also been described in animal models.[4,7] Retroretinal membranes also appeared to have a glial component and probably arose from retinal glial cells or retinal pigment epithelial cells. In addition, in the presence of choroidal and subretinal hemorrhage, fibroblasts were seen to proliferate from the choroid into the subretinal space through breaks in Bruch's membranes.

The hypothesis that damaged vitreous forms a scaffold, which in turn supports cellular proliferation, was supported by our findings of condensation of anterior vitreous fibrils. When there was incarceration of vitreous within the penetrating wound, vitreous strands formed between the wound and peripheral retina. Ingrowth of fibroblasts along these connecting strands is consistent with information derived from growth of fibroblasts in tissue culture, which demonstrated that cells use linear structures for directed proliferation.[37]

In 27 of the 34 eyes we studied, evidence of retinal traction was noted.[47] Although retinal breaks were observed in only two eyes, a rhegmatogenous component could not be excluded in the remainder. Of course, a severe penetrating injury can result in a retinal tear as a direct result of the contusion. In our study, however, the configuration of the detached retina, which was typically pulled anteriorly over the pars plana, along with the presence of retinal folds, which were related to epiretinal or retroretinal membranes, suggested that traction is a most important component in the formation of eventual total retinal detachment.

COMPARISON WITH EXPERIMENTAL MODEL

We have previously noted a similar appearance in an experimental animal model; in the model, we proposed that traction retinal detachment after a posterior penetrating injury resulted from vitreous traction on the peripheral retina and traction on the peripheral and equatorial retina by epiretinal and retroretinal membranes.[4,7,8] In double perforating injuries, in this study and in experimental animals,[5,6] anteroposterior vitreous traction may also be present.

Only in cases where there was incarceration of tissue in the wound or when wound closure was poor fibrous ingrowth from the corneal wound seen. In limbal or scleral wounds, on the other hand, particularly in the presence of lens damage or vitreous hemorrhage and despite good wound closure, fibrous ingrowth was common. This is in agreement with findings in animal models that suggested the importance of vitreous hemorrhage and damage to intraocular structures in the subsequent development of fibrous ingrowth.[6,7]

Our results indicate that significant cellular proliferation is present within the vitreous and along the surfaces of the retina as early as 2 weeks after posterior penetrating eye injury. Results also indicate that damage to the lens, with admixture of lens material and vitreous, and presence of vitreous hemorrhage contribute significantly to the degree of cellular proliferation. Unfortunately it has not been possible to study the effects of these various factors, individually, on the phenomenon of fibrous proliferation.[18]

From this study it is apparent that vitreous surgery may well be an important method for treatment of posterior penetrating ocular injury. Such surgical repair must, however, include careful exploration and débridement with close reapproximation of the wound edges. To remove the stimulus and scaffold for intravitreal fibroblastic proliferation, prolapsed or incarcerated tissue must be excised or repositioned anatomically. Since massive cellular proliferation and fibrous ingrowth may be well established as early as 2 weeks after injury, from our series it appears that vitrectomy is best performed within 2 weeks of injury. Pars plana vitrectomy performed at the optimal time can thus be successful in cases in which retinal detachment would previously have resulted in blindness.[14,19,23,26-29,32,33,39] On the other hand, in cases with extrusion of intraocular contents, extensive suprachoroidal and ciliary body hemorrhage, disruption or infarction of the retina, and surgery, including pars plana vitrectomy, has not proved to be beneficial. The presence of vitreous incarceration, in combination with vitreous hemorrhage, leads to vitreous condensation and organization, vitreoretinal traction, and, ultimately, retinal detachment.[5,7,15,24,40]

RESULTS WITH VITRECTOMY IN TRAUMA

Pars plana vitrectomy for repair of posterior segment injuries clearly has several attributes. The vitreous and blood clot scaffold upon which a fibrous ingrowth can build is removed; this reduces chances of vitreoretinal traction, which can progress to retinal detachment. Most importantly, vitrectomy also allows removal of damaged tissue, hemorrhage, and foreign bodies, which can stimulate fibrous proliferation and cellular response. In addition, by clearing the ocular media, vitrectomy allows visualization and repair of retinal breaks and detachments.

Although results of anterior segment injury are good, results of this series indicate that with posterior penetrating injury, only 49% of surgery will be successful. As reported previously,[3,15] results are even worse in cases of combined posterior and anterior segment injury. Removal of foreign bodies resulted in visual improvement with clearing of the vitreous and decreased inflammation in 61% of our cases.

Although the overall success rate (62%) for repair of anterior and posterior penetrating injuries may not seem high, as recently as 10 years ago surgery would not have even been attempted in most of these cases. Thus, in terms of the nature of the condition, pars-plana vitrectomy is a rational approach to treatment with an acceptable success rate.[12]

MANAGEMENT OF PATIENTS WITH OCULAR TRAUMA

In light of our clinical and experimental studies of ocular trauma, we have formulated the following suggestions:

1. A thorough preoperative evaluation should be made and primary repair made promptly. Primary repair should include exploration and careful débridement with excision or repositing of uveal tissue. Vitreous incarceration should be avoided though in posterior scleral wounds incarceration probably cannot be avoided.

Microscopic reapproximation of the cornea and sclera should be performed, and if a cataract is developing, lensectomy may be necessary.

2. Vitreoretinal evaluation, including electroretinography and ultrasonography, should be performed in the early postoperative period.
3. Retinal surgery may be necessary in individual cases.
4. In cases with endophthalmitis or chalcosis, vitrectomy should be performed immediately.
5. Vitrectomy should be performed within 4 to 14 days after injury in the presence of retinal detachment with an opaque vitreous, reactive nonmagnetic foreign body, double perforating injuries, significant admixture of lens and vitreous, and scleral rupture with extensive vitreous hemorrhage or vitreous loss.
6. Criteria for delayed vitrectomy (more than 14 days of injury) include persistent inflammation, glaucoma or corneal decompensation, long-standing vitreous hemorrhage, development of retinal detachment, and formation of membranous cataracts.

Although the principles of vitrectomy for trauma are similar to those for vitrectomy in other situations,[22] with surgical control being the key to success, in these procedures the surgeon must be even more ready to manage complications, including infusionand retinal detachment. Even though electroretinography and ultrasonography are performed preoperatively, the surgeon at all times must be concerned with the possibility of retinal detachment, ciliary body effusion, and cyclitic membranes. Complete rehabilitation of the eye is, of course, the ultimate goal of surgery; accordingly, one should perform as complete a vitrectomy as is needed to preclude subsequent transivtreal traction. Based on previous evidence,[13] we recommend removal of all accessible vitreous to within 1 to 2 mm of the internal limiting membrane in the area of the vitreous base; we further recommend encirclement of the globe to support the posterior vitreous base.

Retinal detachments should be dealt with at the time of surgery. Vitrectomy is technically more difficult in the presence of a freely mobile or bullous detachment. The use of gas or air, combined with cryotherapy and standard buckling techniques, usually makes the detachment easier to manage.

TIMING OF VITRECTOMY

In regard to recommended timing of vitrectomy, immediate intervention is mandated in certain instances. Because of the potentially devastating effects of endophthalmitis, as soon as such a diagnosis is made vitrectomy should be performed. Similarly, if retinal detachment is demonstrated, repair should be immediately undertaken before massive periretinal proliferation develops. In cases in which the patient has evidence of penetrating injury with dense vitreous hemorrhage and vitreous condensation and organization and yet has no evidence of retinal detachment (as determined by ultrasound), the physician is confronted with a dilemma. Should he observe the patient or perform surgery? Our recommendation in such cases is that the patient be evaluated within the first week after injury by a skilled vitreoretinal surgeon.

Controversy as to the appropriate timing of vitrectomy centers on the relative merits of early surgery (within 48 hours) versus late surgery (at approximately 14 days). Early vitrectomy has the advantage of removing vitreous scaffolds and inflammatory elements, which may stimulate fibrous proliferation; it has been demonstrated that prominent preretinal and retroretinal cellular membranes may be present very soon after injury. Removal of these scaffolds and stimulating factors may preclude or reduce formation of vitreous condensation, cyclitic membranes, and retinal traction. On the other hand, a major disadvantage of early surgical intervention is the possibility of uncontrolled hemorrhage. When surgical intervention is delayed 10 to 14 days after injury, the patient's condition can be followed and vitrectomy may, in fact, not prove necessary. Furthermore, as inflammation abates and the eye becomes quiescent, vitrectomy is technically easier and thus a more safe procedure. However, the progression of membrane formation and retinal detachment can occur during the waiting period.

It is our belief that the patient should have prompt repair performed by the primary ophthalmologist; this would include excising or repositioning uveal tissue and reapproximation of the wound. The patient can then be referred to a surgeon who has expertise in vitreous procedures, and he can then make the final decision as to whether surgery is indicated and, if so, the optimal time for such intervention.

In the series reported by Ryan and Allen[43] of 100 patients with ocular trauma treated with pars-plana vitrectomy, 62% had improvement in visual acuity; anterior segment injuries responded better than posterior segment injuries and retinal detachment was a poor prognostic sign. Improvement was greater in patients undergoing vitrectomy during the first 2 weeks after injury than those who had vitrectomy at a later date.

We believe 4 to 10 days after injury to be the optimal time for surgical intervention of ocular trauma. Vitrectomy performed during this time avoids the hazards of immediate vitrectomy and allows removal of damaged tissue and debris before serious or irreversible ocular changes occur.

REFERENCES

1. Benson, W.E., and Machemer, R.: Severe perforating injuries treated with pars plana vitrectomy, Am. J. Ophthalmol. **81:**728, 1976.
2. Blindness: facts on the major killing and crippling diseases in the United States today, New York, 1971, National Health Education Committee, Inc.
3. Cinotti, A.A., and Maltzman, B.A.: Prognosis and treatment of perforating ocular injuries, Ophthalmic Surg. **6:**54, 1975.
4. Cleary, P.E., Minckler, D.S., and Ryan, S.J.: Ultrastructure of traction retinal detachment in rhesus monkey eyes after a posterior penetrating eye injury, Am. J. Ophthalmol. **90:**829, 1980.
5. Cleary, P.E., and Ryan, S.J.: Experimental posterior penetrating eye injury in the rabbit. I. Method of production and natural history, Br. J. Ophthalmol. **63:**306, 1979.
6. Cleary, P.E., and Ryan, S.J.: Experimental posterior penetrating eye injury in the rabbit. II. Histology of wound, vitreous, and retina, Br. J. Ophthalmol. **63:**312, 1979.
7. Cleary, P.E., and Ryan, S.J.: Method of production and natural history of experimental posterior penetrating eye injury in the rhesus monkey, Am. J. Ophthalmol. **88:**212, 1979.
8. Cleary, P.E., and Ryan, S.J.: Histology of wound, vitreous, and retina in experimental posterior penetrating eye injury in the rhesus monkey, Am. J. Ophthalmol. **88:**221, 1979.
9. Cleary, P.E., and Ryan, S.J.: Vitrectomy in penetrating injury: the results of a controlled trial of vitrectomy in experimental posterior penetrating eye injury in the rhesus monkey, Arch. Ophthalmol. **99:**287, 1981.
10. Coleman, D.J.: Role of vitrectomy in trauma, In Gitter, K.A., editor: Current concepts of the vitreous, including vitrectomy, St. Louis, 1976, The C.V. Mosby Co.
11. Coles, W.H., and Haik, G.M.: Vitrectomy in intraocular trauma: its rationale and its indications and limitations, Arch. Ophthalmol. **87:**621, 1972.
12. Conway, B.P., and Michels, R.G.: Vitrectomy techniques in the management of selected penetrating ocular injuries, Ophthalmology **85:**560, Jan.-Dec. 1978.

13. Cox, M.S., and Freeman, H.M.: Retinal detachment due to penetration. I. Clinical characteristics and surgical results, Arch. Ophthalmol. **95:**1354, 1978.
14. Douvas, N.G.: Microsurgical pars plana vitrectomy, Trans. Am. Acad. Ophthalmol. Otolaryngol. **81:**371, 1976.
15. Eagling, E.M.: Perforating injuries involving the posterior segment, Trans. Ophthalmol. Soc. U.K. **95:**335, 1975.
16. Eagling, E.M.: Perforating injuries of the eye, Br. J. Ophthalmol. **60:**723, 1976.
17. Faulborn, J., Atkinson, J., and Olivier, D.: Primary vitrectomy as a preventive surgical procedure in the treatment of severely injured eyes, Br. J. Ophthalmol. **61:**202, 1977.
18. Faulborn, J., and Topping, T.M.: Proliferation in the vitreous cavity after perforating injuries: a histopathologic study, Albrecht von Graefes Klin. Exp. Ophthalmol. **205:**157, 1978.
19. Gitter, K.A.: Current concepts of the vitreous, including vitrectomy, St. Louis, 1976, The C.V. Mosby Co.
20. Grillo, H.C.: Derivation of fibroblasts in the healing wound, Arch. Surg. **88:**82, 1964.
21. Hogan, M.J., and Zimmerman, L.E.: Ophthalmic pathology: an atlas and textbook, Philadelphia, 1964, W. B. Saunders Co.
22. Hutton, W.C., Snyder, M.D., and Vaiser, A.: Vitrectomy in the treatment of ocular perforating injuries, Am. J. Ophthalmol. **81:**733, 1976.
23. Irvine, A.R., and Stone, R.D.: Indications for the newer vitrectomy techniques in ocular trauma, Trans. Pac. Coast Otoophthalmol. Soc. **55:**117, 1974.
24. Johnson, S.: Perforating injuries: a five year study, Trans. Ophthalmol. Soc. U.K. **91:**895, 1971.
25. Laqua, H., and Machemer, R.: Glial cell proliferation in retinal detachment (massive periretinal proliferation), Am. J. Ophthalmol. **80:**602, 1975.
26. Machemer, R.: Vitrectomy: a pars plana approach, New York, 1975, Grune & Stratton, Inc.
27. Machemer, R.: Surgical management of non-magnetic intraocular foreign bodies, Arch. Ophthalmol. **93:**1003, 1975.
28. Machemer, R., Buettner, H., and Norton, E.W.D.: Vitrectomy: a pars plana approach, Trans. Am. Acad. Ophthalmol. Otolaryngol. **75:**813, 1971.
29. Machemer, R., and Norton, E.W.D.: A new concept for vitrous surgery. 3. Indications and results, Am. J. Ophthalmol. **74:**1034, 1972.
30. Machemer, R., van Horn, D., and Aaberg, T.M.: Pigment epithelial proliferation in human retinal detachment with massive periretinal proliferation, Am. J. Ophthalmol. **85:**81, 1978.
31. Michels, R.G.: Early surgical management of penetrating ocular injuries involving the posterior segment, South. Med. J. **69:**1175, 1976.
32. Michels, R.G., Machemer, R., and Muller-Jensen, K.: Vitreous surgery: past, present, and future, Adv. Ophthalmol. **29:**22, 1974.
33. Michels, R.G., and Ryan, S.J.: Results and complications of 100 consecutive cases of pars plana vitrectomy, Am. J. Ophthalmol. **80:**24, 1975.
34. Moncreiff, W.F., and Scheribel, K.J.: Penetrating injuries, Am. J. Ophthalmol. **28:**1212, 1945.
35. Neubauer, H.: Microsurgery in ocular trauma, Adv. Ophthalmol. **22:**246, 1970.
36. Neubauer, H.: Treatment of perforating injuries with intraocular foreign bodies, Presented at the Retina and Vitreous Symposium, Bascom Palmer Eye Institute Dedication meeting, Miami, Florida, Jan. 11-15, 1976.
37. Peacock, E.E., and Van Winkle, W.: Surgery and biology of wound repair, Philadelphia, 1970, W.B. Saunders Co.
38. Percival, S.P.B.: Late complications from posterior segment intraocular foreign bodies with particular reference to retinal detachment, Br. J. Ophthalmol. **56:**462, 1972.
39. Peyman, G.A., and Diamond, J.G.: The vitreophage in ocular reconstruction following trauma, Can. J. Ophthalmol. **10:**419, 1975.
40. Roper-Hall, M.J.: The treatment of ocular injuries, Trans. Ophthalmol. Soc. U.K. **79:**57, 1959.
41. Remky, H., Kobor, J., and Pfeiffer, H.: Traumatologie chirurgicale du segment antérieur, Ann. Inst. Barraquer **7:**487, 1967.
42. Ryan, S.J.: Results of pars plana vitrectomy in penetrating ocular trauma, Int. Ophthalmol. **1:**1, 1978.
43. Ryan, S.J., and Allen, W.A.: Pars plana vitrectomy in ocular trauma, Am. J. Ophthalmol. **88:**483, 1979.

44. Snell, A.C.: Perforating ocular injuries, Am. J. Ophthalmol. **28:**263, 1945.
45. Topping, T.N., Abrams, G.W., and Machemer, R.: Experimental double-perforating injury of the posterior segment in rabbit eyes: the natural history of intraocular proliferation, Arch. Ophthalmol. **97:**735, 1979.
46. Waltz, H., and Rein, N.: Statistics of injuries referred to provincial eye clinics, Klin. Monatsbl. Augenheilkd. **162:**648, 1973.
47. Winthrop, S.R., Cleary, P.E., Minckler, D.S., and Ryan, S.J.: Penetrating eye injuries: a histopathological review, Br. J. Ophthalmol. **64:**809, 1980.

12

Treatment of rhegmatogenous detachment in massive preretinal retraction

J. Wallace McMeel
Sheldon M. Buzney*

Successful surgical repair of rhegmatogenous retinal detachment is now achieved in over 90% of cases, with massive preretinal retraction being the most common cause for failure. Massive preretinal retraction represents the most severe stage of development of intravitreous tissues exerting traction on the retina. Abnormalities within the vitreous tissue, as a result of aging or chronic inflammation, may produce a thickening and contraction of collagen components within the vitreous. This vitreoretinal traction may be either tangential to the surface of the retina, or centripetal. The centripetal vectors are most frequently associated with a shrinkage across the coronal plane at the level of the insertion of the anterior vitreous base.

The manifestation of tangential traction of a minor degree may show up as a fine rippling of the surface of the detached retina, termed "shagreen." More severe manifestion of the tangential traction is the appearance of scroll-like eversion of the posterior edge of a retinal tear, the "rolled edge." Several fixed folds emanating from one area, the "star fold," is another sign of significant tangential preretinal traction.

Centripetal traction produces a horseshoe type of tear, with the flap being directed anteriorly. Close observation frequently shows a faint vitreoretinal wisp that is the shrinking, adhering portion of the vitreous that has produced the tear. Equatorial folds in the region of the posterior edge of the anterior vitreous base are indicative of extensive, continuous centripetal traction on the retina in this portion of the eye.

The nomenclature relating to this phenomenon and the classification of its severity are in a state of flux. In addition to the term "massive preretinal retraction" (MPR), other terms used are "massive vitreous retraction," "massive periretinal proliferation," and "vitreoretinal membranes." Some authors include the term "massive" when ophthalmoscopically visible fixed folds are visible in only one or two quadrants of de-

---

*Acknowledgment: The review of the 34 cases of massive preretinal retraction was by Sheldon M. Buzney, M.D., Assistant Clinical Scientist, Eye Research, Institute of Retina Foundation, Harvard Medical School, Boston; Clinical Assistant in Ophthalmology, Retina Associates, Inc., Boston, Massachusetts.

137

tached retina. Others reserve the term "massive" until all quadrants are so involved. Among the last type, the detachments are usually total.

Among cases with fixed radiating folds in all four quadrants, the prime criteria for classification relate to the funnel form by the detached retina as it has been drawn forward from the optic nerve. three categories are wide funnel, narrow funnel, and closed funnel. In the last, the vitreous fibrotic tissues have pulled the circumference of the retina so tightly together that the disc is no longer visible.

In long-standing cases of massive preretinal retraction involving all four quadrants, one may occasionally see a rather sharp border between greatly thinned retina in the far periphery and a significantly thicker, much more convoluted retina within a circular border zone, which gives the appearance of the posterior zone being under traction by vitreoretinal adhesion and the more peripheral zone being retina that has been stretched to a considerable degree by this traction.

Examination of the vitreous gel by the slitlamp usually reveals a pronounced decrease in the mobility of the vitreous fibrils following a rapid movement of the eye upward and quick return to the primary position. Normally, the excursions show a reasonably wide sweep and take approximately 2 seconds to run their course. In eyes with massive preretinal retraction, the vitreous gel has much smaller excursions than those in the eye without massive preretinal retraction and the time duration of the excursions is much shorter, usually 1 second or less.

To see vitreous changes farther posteriorly, either indirect ophthalmoscopy or slit-lamp plus contact lens must be used. Certain entities that are associated with vitreous changes may mimic massive preretinal retraction, but the cause of the vitreous change may be different. These include cases of rhegmatogenous detachment with Wagner-Stickler syndrome, sickle cell retinopathy, or trauma.

Preretinal membrane with demonstrable cells have been seen in specimens of massive preretinal retraction for many years. Specific cell types have been demonstrated by Machemer, who showed growth on the retinal surfaces of pigment-containing cells.[1] Clarkson et al., obtaining material in closed vitrectomies, found other cell types as well.[3]

ETIOLOGY

Although most eyes developing massive preretinal retraction have had previous surgery, some eyes may reach this state in the absence of prior surgery. A low-grade uveitis is frequently seen in these latter instances. One cannot be certain whether this is a factor that enhanced the development of the massive preretinal retraction or was present merely in association with the long-standing retinal detachment. Most eyes having massive preretinal retraction have had prior surgery. A scleral buckle is the most common procedure. Cataract extraction is also a common precursor type of surgery. Aphakic detachments therefore probably have a slightly higher risk of developing massive preretinal retraction than eyes that are phakic.

In eyes that develop massive preretinal retraction after scleral buckling surgery, the period of the highest risk for its occurrence is approximately 4 to 8 weeks after operation. It may occur quite abruptly. Vision that may have been quite good (approximately 20/100 to 20/200) may start to develop a "shimmer." Within 12 hours after this premonitory symptom, the vision may have deteriorated to a level of hand motions. In retrospect, some of these eyes have had a continuing postoperative turbidity of the media. Preoperatively, immobility and haziness of the vitreous gel may have been noted. Extensive diathermy or cryopexy may have been applied at the time of the scleral buckling surgery, though massive preretinal retraction has been noted to occur in the athermal buckle technique.

MANAGEMENT

Treatment of rhegmatogenous retinal detachments with massive preretinal retraction requires the fulfillment of the same criteria necessary for the success of any retinal operation. This includes the permanent closure of all retinal breaks. To do this, one must expend a greater effort than that in cases not having massive preretinal retraction. Before the availability of vitrectomy surgery, one had to achieve this closure by creating a very high buckle that extended throughout the circumference of the eye. If there were multiple holes and posterior extensions from the 360-degree buckle might be necessary, meridional implants might be fitted beneath the circumferential implant. It was imperative that all retinal breaks be closed at the time or surgery because the central traction would not allow the retina to settle, as it so frequently does when a sponge is applied beneath a break in an area of localized detachment. Furthermore, a very careful preoperative fundus examination was necessary to be as certain as possible that no undiscovered holes would remain in radial folds or beneath preretinal bridges of tissue. If such a hole were not tightly closed, it could leak and result in a surgical failure. The surgical procedure I prefer was that of a 360-degree buckle with an implant having a width of approximately 8 to 10 mm. A thermal reaction, using discrete diathermy applications approximately 1.5 mm apart, was believed to inflict less thermal trauma upon the eye than cryopexy does. Transillumination at the 3 and 9 o'clock meridians was used to identify the long ciliary structures so that they might be avoided by the diathermy applications. This was to minimize the instance of anterior segment ischemia.

Because the retina was usually highly elevated throughout the eye, drainage of subretinal fluid could be performed at any desired point. The temporal region just above or below the long ciliary artery and nerve usually represented the best place to drain for subretinal fluid. The sclerotomy was usually made posterior to the buckle so that the buckle could be indented in its entirety when the mattress sutures were tightened and still with no compromise of the drainage process through the sclerotomy. After drainage, the fundus would be examined. If the retina were well in place on the high buckle, there was a reasonable chance for success. Sometimes injection of saline solution into the vitreous cavity through the pars plana with a 30-gauge needle could push the retina more firmly on the buckle if the tension in the eye were low. In many unfortunate instances, however, injected saline solution merely ran from the intravitreous compartment to the subretinal compartment, a result not enhancing the chances for success of the operation.

Injection of intravitreous silicone and cutting of transvitreous membranes were the first steps in intravitreous manipulation to solve the problems associated with massive preretinal retraction. With the advent of the closed vitrectomy operation, a dynamic additional dimension, was added to the treatment armamentarium. Current treatment, as I (J.W.M.) practice it, consists of the classic scleral buckle procedure as just described. This may be sufficient in eyes that have not reached the more severe degrees of massive preretinal retraction. However, any eye that has a narrow funnel and total detachment probably could not be successfully treated in this manner. A total detachment with a broad funnel, in most instances, is still a candidate for the full range of maneuvers now at our disposal.

In addition to a scleral buckling, the ancillary techniques consist of closed vitrectomy to remove transvitreous and preretinal membranes and to fill the vitreous cavity with a substance that can exert a constant outward pressure against the retina, holding it in contact with the buckle.

Indications for scleral buckle versus closed vitrectomy

Variations in sequence depend on various factors. In one sequence the scleral buckling operation is performed first, and in the other the closed vitrectomy is the initial part of the operation. The indications for doing the closed vitrectomy first are the possibility that the cornea may become hazy during the time the scleral buckling procedure is being performed, the risk that the pupil may become small while the scleral buckle is being done, a need to have a clearer medium within the vitreous cavity, and an uncertainity about the potential awareness that all the retinal holes have been found on prior preretinal examination. The instances in which the scleral buckling is performed first relate primarily to concerns about a leaking sclerotomy site and the associated soft, partially collapsed globe that would ensue. The conditions that are more likely to create this problem include an eye with thin sclera over the pars plana, holes lying far posteriorly particularly in the nasal quadrants, a lens already with haziness in which the preoperative examination had been performed with marginal capabilities, an eye in which an intraocular lens is in place, an eye with a lens with a poorly dilating pupil, or an eye in an elderly person in whom repetitive hypotony might have a higher chance of triggering a massive choroidal effusion postoperatively. When one uses an exoplant and cryopexy technique to produce a scleral buckle, most of the indications for doing the buckle before closed vitrectomy are less pertinent.

Localization of retinal holes

In all but the most unusual case, localization of the retinal holes is done before either closed vitrectomy or scleral buckling. If the retina is highly elevated, consideration must be given to where the hole will settle after drainage of subretinal fluid and indentation of the ocular wall by the buckle. Because a 360-degree buckle is probably being made, the prime consideration relates to its sagittal not its circumferential location. Because multiple holes are frequently present, those representing the most anterior and posterior limits are the most important to localize.

Closed vitrectomy

The closed vitrectomy surgery may require a single instrument with integrated function (suction cutting, illumination, infusion). A single instrument can often remove all the transvitreous membranes to the site of their junction with the retina. Keeping the cutting port on the inner side, away from the retina, reduces the chances of producing a iatrogenic hole. The blunt tip of the instrument can frequently be used successfully to tease tissue from the retina as it bridges from one radial fold to another. Once the wisps of tissue are floating freely, they can be removed by the nibbler. A single integrated instrument frequently cannot be as effective in removing preretinal membranes as when a second instrument is used also. A second instrument may be a pick, scissors, forceps, or endocoagulating device. The selection depends on the need. A forceps may be the optimal second instrument in situations in which membranes traverse crevices between radial folds. The forceps can grasp the bridging membrane while the nibbler gently dissects the retina away from the membrane. This is similar to the maneuver when the single integrated instrument is used, but it can be effective when the adhesions are stronger and not responsive to the single-instrument approach. Also the forceps as a second instrument can be used to protect the retina from the nibbler port when the forceps on a membrane are interposed between the retina and the nibbler port. On other occasions, the forceps can be used as a prehensile device to grasp the preretinal membranes and peel them. If the tissues are too tough for this maneuver or the retina appears particularly thin and subject to tearing, intravitreous scissors may be introduced as the second instrument and membranes may be cut, to be subsequently consumed by the suction cutter. An endocoagulating device can be inserted to produce a reaction about any posterior holes, either those noted preoperatively or iatrogenic in nature. A single probe with bipolarity at its tip is the most precise method of producing discrete, localized reactions to the retina.[2] Reactions to the retina alone may be sufficient to allow the holes to stay closed postoperatively.

I have found that constant low-volume automated removal of vitreous contents is the safest and most satisfactory way to remove membranes in a technically trying situation, as exists in these cases. The constancy of an automated aspiration device allows the surgeon to become familiar with the characteristics of flow at the suction port. The variable then becomes the position of the suction port in relation to the retina and membranous structures, giving the surgeon himself total control. The use of a paristaltic pump permits abrupt cessation of flow that an air-suction type of aspiration does not.

Scleral buckle

To make a buckle, I create a scleral bed by cutting approximately three fourths the distance through the thickness of the sclera and dissecting flaps anteriorly and posteriorly, which are wide enough to accommodate an intrascleral silicone rubber implant and an encircling band to hold it in place. The bed is incised so that it extends at least 3 mm beyond the edge of each retinal tear. Diathermy is performed with a conical electrode as noted above placed at 1.5 to 2 mm intervals, with avoidance of the long ciliary structures. Two 4-0 Dacron mattress sutures are placed in each quadrant. Once the implant, encircling band, and sutures are in place, the next step depends on the sequence of the operation. In some instances, the closed vitrectomy is done at this point. In cases in which the closed vitrectomy was the first portion of the sequence in the operation, the perforation for subretinal fluid is made by a sclerotomy. This procedure has been previously described.

Gas-fluid exchange

In eyes in which an extensive closed vitrectomy and removal of intravitreous contents has been performed, one has an opportunity to inject larger amounts of material to replace the fluid within the intravitreous cavity. This is usually done after the subretinal fluid has been drained and the scleral buckle has been indented by appropriate tightening of the mattress sutures. A gas-fluid exchange can be done in one of two ways. In one, the head is turned to one side and the sclerotomy site at the pars plana that is most dependent is loosened slightly to allow seepage of intravitreous fluid. Because these vitrectomies usually remove virtually all the intravitreous contents, the problems of blockage at the sclerotomy site by vitreous gel are minimal. The site for injection of the intravitreous gas is then selected at the opposite meridian in the pars plana. The head is turned so that the site for injection is the highest within the eye. A sudden bolus of approximately a half milliliter is injected. This should form a single bubble. The subsequent injection proceeds slowly into this bubble. The intravitreous contents should then flow slowly from the slightly open sclerotomy site. Pressure may be exerted on the inferior portion of the globe to increase the amount of intravitreous contents expressed through the sclerotomy site. The endpoint is when a small bubble of air starts to come out of the sclerotomy site. The sclerotomy site is then sutured, and the tension within the eye is taken. One continues to inject air through the pars plana site until the tension lies in range of 20 to 30 mm Hg. With this method, one can introduce a gas bubble that fills 75% or more of the vitreous cavity.

By another way, a 30-gauge needle on a 5 cc gas-filled syringe is inserted through the sutured sclerotomy site, with the sclerotomy being placed as dependent as possible. Gas is injected into the eye and clear watery fluid is removed from the vitreous cavity. This is repeated stepwise until the cavity lying above the sclerotomy site has had its fluid evacuated and replaced by air.

A third way of producing an extensive air-fluid exchange is to reinsert the integrated nibbler and, while one has good visualization, place it just anterior to the optic nerve. The site for injection for the gas to fill the vitreous cavity is made through the pars plana with a 30-gauge needle with a syringe of an appropriate size. The aspiration of contents is then begun with the inflow closed off. Air gradually supplants the contents of the vitreous cavity. An initial bolus of 0.5 ml should be injected to attempt to maintain a good view through a single bubble. This cannot always be done. One can usually have a reasonable idea of the amount of fluid by the air, even though multiple bubbles may be present. Optimally, virtually all the fluid within the eye may be replaced by gas. Over 75% air-fluid exchange can usually be obtained. In the systems with a special infusion part, gas is injected through this part as the nibbler removes the liquid.

Using air, I have never yet had a problem associated with undue increase in intraocular pressure using this procedure. A clinically valuable air bubble usually persists for approximately 5 days postoperatively. This is a sufficient time for tamponade in most cases. I have avoided sulfur hexafluoride (SF_6) because of the infrequent ephemeral reports of postoperative hypertension and closure of the retinal arterioles and because of the FDA restrictions on its use with the attendant medicolegal exposure this entails.

Other substances being injected into the vitreous cavity include hyaluronic acid and silicone oil. New gases under investigation have the potential advantage of maintaining their volume for longer periods of time.

In aphakic eyes and eyes with intraocular lenses, compromises may have to be made with regard to intravitreous injection material. A gas bubble might either displace the intraocular lens, forcing it against the endothelium of the cornea, or else push the iris diaphram forward and close the angle of the anterior chamber. A large air bubble is usually most effective when the patient is prone or lying to the right or left side. In the supine position, one has the least effect in pushing the retina against the buckle. Specific head positioning should take into account the retinal tears and the opportunities to press these areas of the retina against the buckle by positioning the head appropriately.

RESULTS

Results of surgery for massive preretinal retraction must be viewed critically. There is a broad spectrum of rhegmatogenous retinal detachment problems that are called massive preretinal retraction by various authors. One must have an idea of the problems being treated when one examines the results of surgery. This is exemplified by the efforts now being made to grade and classify the varying degrees of massive preretinal retraction and the various names associated with the entity. The results of a small series of cases personally treated and having adequate follow-up study are reviewed.

Of the 34 cases, the majority had had prior surgery. Twenty-three had had cataract extraction, 16 a previous primary buckle, and 7 multiple buckles. Their average age was 56 years with a range from 38 to 82 years. Approximately three fourths of the eyes had moderate to severe massive preretinal retraction with fixed folds in two to four quadrants or total detachment with a central funnel configuration. Visual acuity was maintained or improved in 19 of 34 (56%) and worsened in 15 of 34 (44%). Of those that maintained or improved their acuity, five had a vision of 20/400 or better (26%) and nine could count fingers or see hand motions (48%). These 14 eyes represented a visual salvage rate of 41%. The visual results in many instances of anatomic reattachment were impaired because of significant preretinal membrane formation in the region of the macula.

Of the 24 eyes with severe massive preretinal retraction, nine were fully attached, giving an anatomic success rate of 38%. If one includes those that maintained a partial reattachment, the anatomic success increases to 12 out of 24 (50%).

SUMMARY

The treatment of massive preretinal retraction is significantly more successful now than a decade ago. The development of new forms of intravitreous surgical techniques has been responsible for much of this. The availability of techniques that offer this potentially higher success rate make it more imperative than ever that the patient having this problem be carefully studied so that the proper techniques given in a optimal manner be made available to the patient. It is not unreasonable to expect that new surgical techniques, intravitreous expanders, and possibly intravitreous fibrolytic enzymes may play a part in the treatment of this entity within the next decade.

REFERENCES

1. Clarkson, J.G., Green, W.R., and Massof, D.: A histopathologic review of 168 cases of preretinal membrane, Am. J. Ophthalmol. **84:**1-17, 1977.
2. Grignolo, F.M., Delori, F.C., and Pomerantzeff, O.: Evaluation of retinal adhesion in vivo. In Pruett, R.C., and Regan, C.D.J., editors: Retina congress, New York, 1974, Appleton-Century-Crofts.
3. Lagua, H., and Machemer, R.: Clinical-pathological correlation in massive periretinal proliferation, Am. J. Ophthalmol. **80:**913, 1929, 1975.

13

Neovascular and anastomotic vascular connections between the uveal tract, retina, and vitreous

Morton F. Goldberg
Lee M. Jampol*

The anatomic separation between the choroidal and retinal vasculatures is usually absolute and is manifested by an intact Bruch's membrane and retinal pigment epithelium. In at least the five following clinical circumstances, this barrier is broken: (1) as variants of normal, (2) in association with elevated pressure in the central retinal vein, (3) at the site of inflammatory and cicatrizing foci involving both retina and choroid, (4) in scar tissue related to both blunt and perforating trauma, and (5) after fundus photocoagulation.[17] In some rare circumstances, either naturally occurring or iatrogenic, blood vessels originating from the anterior uveal tract[20,30] may also enter the vitreous cavity, which, of course, is completely avascular in the normal postnatal human eye.

Abnormal vascular connections between the uveal tract, retina, and vitreous may involve anastomoses of vessels of the adult type or may be frankly neovascular. The visual prognosis is rarely compromised by anastomoses though the pathologic process underlying formation of these vascular connections may interfere with normal vision. Neovascularization, however, can unfavorably influence vision from hemorrhage or transudation, but these events do not invariably cause visual symptoms.

EMBRYOLOGY AND NORMAL VARIATIONS

At about 4 weeks of gestation some hyaloid vessels leave the developing retinal cup, indenting its peripheral edge, and anastomose with the primitive choroidal vasculatures.[32] Under normal conditions of maturation, these connecting vessels atrophy as the edge of the cup extends anteriorly to develop into the epithelium of the ciliary body and iris. With failure to atrophy, so-called atypical colobomas of the ciliary body may develop. If the atrophy is less extensive, it has been proposed that the lip of the optic cup

---

*M.D., Professor of Ophthalmology, Department of Ophthalmology, University of Illinois College of Medicine and University of Illinois Eye and Ear Infirmary, Chicago, Illinois.

might grow around these vessels, entrapping them, and thereby permitting an embryonic mesenchymal connection to run from the vitreous through the sensory retina and pigment epithelium to the choroid,[32] even in the absence of a full-blown ciliary body coloboma. Because these connecting vessels occur before the development of the periphral blood vessels of the adult retina, they can create mesenchymal channels, which peripheral retinal vessels might follow later in development. Thus, even if the original hyaloid vessels completely disappear during gestational development, as is normally the case, an occasional adult might be expected to show uveoretinal vascular anastomoses in the region of the ora serrata. In fact, Daicker has demonstrated that such vessels do occur in some meridional folds of the normal ora serrata.[32] Histologic study has shown vessels with venous characteristics passing from the retina through Bruch's membrane to the choroid.[32] Such connections are rarely appreciated clinically however.[28]

The vasculatures of the retina and choroid develop quite independently and are separated by Bruch's membrane and the retinal pigment epithelium. Thus, for the broad expanse of the fundus posterior to the ora serrata, vascular connections between the retina and choroid do not normally occur except at the peripapillary region. In this location a variable vascular pattern is achieved. Both arterial and venous connections normally exist between retinal and posterior ciliary or uveal blood vessels at the optic nerve head.[17,47] Also a substantial percentage of normal individuals have cilioretinal arterioles supplying the macula and other portions of the central retina. Retinociliary veins also occur normally but are less common.

At the anterior edge of the developing optic cup, the embryonic vasculature has innumerable connections among the iris, both the anterior and the posterior portions of the tunica vasculosa lentis, and the retrolental hyaloid vascular system. Incomplete atrophy during pregestational maturation may give rise to the commonly observed and usually inconsequential persistent pupillary membranes.[22] At the other extreme, persistence of the hyaloid vasculature may cause a wide range of posterior segment pathologic conditions, including the full-blown persistent hyperplastic primary vitreous (PHPV) syndrome.[30] In the presence of an opaque lens or a large opaque retrolental mass, the diagnosis of PHPV may be difficult. The diagnosis is facilitated, however, if one can visualize a radial iris (iridohyaloid or capsulopupillary) vessel running prominently in the iris stroma to pass posteriorly around the pupillary sphincter (Fig. 13-1). From there, this embryonic vascular remnant passes into the posterior chamber, where it curves further posteriorly around the equator of the lens to anastomose with the retrolental hyaloid remnants. The anastomotic portion of the abnormal vessel may not be visible on physical examination. When the prominent iris vessel passes into the pupil, it lies within a very small but telltale notch (or atypical coloboma) in the pupillary sphincter. This notch may be so small that it can be seen only with 10 to 16 magnification, as with the operating microscope employed at the time of an examination of a patient under anesthesia. The presence of this notch (more than one may be present) and its accompanying vessel is rather good evidence for the presence of PHPV, even when the retrolental space and vitreous chamber cannot be visualized.[30]

Remnants of the embryonic hyaloid vascular system may also persist at the disc, forming the well-known Bergmeister's papilla.

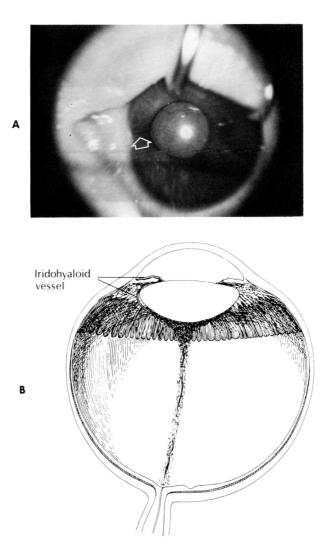

Fig. 13-1. A, Persistent hyperplastic primary vitreous syndrome with iridohyaloid vascular anastomosis, *arrow*. **B,** Schematic interpretation of **A.** (**A,** From Meisels, H.I., and Goldberg, M.F.: Am. J. Ophthalmol. **88:**179-185, 1979, published with permission from The American Journal of Ophthalmology, copyright by The Ophthalmic Publishing Co., Chicago.)

PATHOLOGIC ANASTOMOSES BETWEEN RETINAL AND CHOROIDAL VASCULATURES

Histologic confirmation of abnormal vascular anastomoses between the retina and choroid is limited to very few cases, but a substantial volume of clinical reports has demonstrated these connections either ophthalmoscopically or angiographically.

With respect to histologic documentation, Kennedy and Wise[25] confirmed a venous retinochoroidal vascular anastomosis after *Toxoplasma* retinochoroiditis, and Green and Gass[13] showed an arterial retinochoroidal anastomosis after presumed *Toxocara* chorioretinitis. Yanoff and Fine described similar, though less advanced, vascular connections between retina and choroid in the ringschwiele (ring-shaped wheal) associated with chronic retinal detachment.[48] In this clinical setting, tugging on the retinal pigment epithelium can cause it to break as well as proliferate. The break apparently allows choroidal vessels to anastomose with those of the sensory retina. In an experimental primate model, Wolf and Goldberg showed histologic documentation of large-caliber chorioretinal anastomoses after intense photocoagulation of the fundus.[46]

Clinical evidence of these types of anastomoses has been amassed in a wide variety of disease states, including mechanical resistance to venous outflow in the optic nerve; inflammatory diseases, such as toxoplasmosis, toxocariasis, and syphilis; senile disciform degeneration of the macula; myopic degeneration; organization of fundus hematomas; and conditions after either blunt or perforating ocular trauma and after intense fundus diathermy, cryotherapy, or photocoagulation.[17] Poletti has collected 44 such cases from the literature and has added nine of his own.[33] In most of these clinical circumstances, Bruch's membrane and the retinal pigment epithelium were damaged by inflammatory, neoplastic, or traumatic insults. This damage appears to be a necessary precondition for almost all pathologic retinochoroidal anastomoses but, by itself, is insufficient for their production. Anatomic contact of the two adjacent vasculatures (retinal and choroidal) is also required. Their interconnections can be achieved either directly through large-caliber mature vessels or by intermediary capillary connections. As healing proceeds, the capillary channels often become remodeled or involuted, leaving large-caliber vascular anastomoses. Even when both conditions are met (anatomic approximation of the retinal and choroidal vasculatures plus damage to Bruch's membrane and the retinal pigment epithelium), neovascularization and anastomoses do not necessarily occur, as the following case attests.

Case report

A 24-year-old Oriental male physicist was referred for evaluation immediately after he sustained an inadvertent laser lesion in his right foveola. In performing an unfamiliar alignment procedure on an experimental dye laser, he was exposed to a 10-nanosecond pulsed beam of 589-nanometer light. The estimated retinal irradiance, as calculated by Rockefeller Young, Ph.D., was 1.2 billion watts per square centimeter (about 10 times the threshold for a laser of this type having a 10 nsec pulse).

Central vision was reduced to counting fingers at 3 feet. There was a dense central scotoma of about 5 degrees. The fundus examination showed an intravitreal plume of blood emanating from the choroid in the center of the macular region. The retinal tissue in the center of the macula was missing, and appeared as if a sharp, tiny trephine had excised it from the foveolar region.

Within 5 days, vision improved to 20/100 (6/30) and remained at that level for the

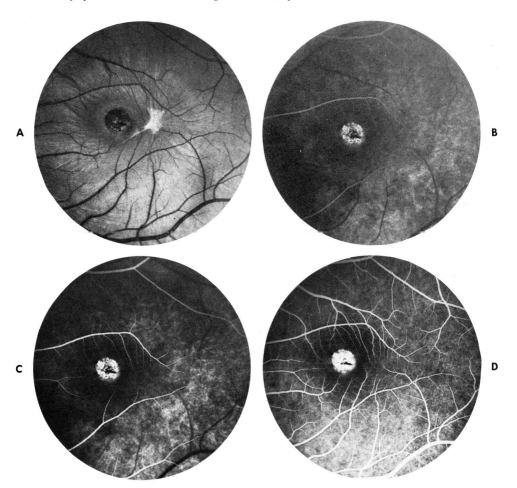

Fig. 13-2. Macular hole 4 months after inadvertent burn from an experimental laser. **A,** Fundus photograph. **B,** Early arterial phase of angiogram. Choriocapillaris is seen as a hyperfluorescent zone in the center of the macula. **C,** Later arterial phase of angiogram. **D,** Late venous phase of angiogram.

ensuing 4 months. Fundus angiography revealed the characteristic findings of a full-thickness macular hole, with early hyperfluorescence that remained confined to the involved area. The choriocapillaris in the center of the foveolar region appeared largely intact (Fig. 13-2). No chorioretinal anastomoses or neovascularization occurred.

Comment

Despite obvious rupturing of the choroid, retinal pigment epithelium, Bruch's membrane, and sensory retina and despite anatomic approximation of these damaged tissues in the center of a highly vascular zone (the central choroid), healing occurred without formation of subretinal, chorioretinal, or choriovitreal neovascularization. Chorioretinal anastomoses also failed to develop. Other factors, as yet unknown, including perhaps the size of the traumatized arterioles or venules in the contiguous choroid and retina, must play a role in the formation of such vascular anomalies.

MECHANICAL RESISTANCE TO VENOUS OUTFLOW

Increased hydrostatic pressure within the central retinal vein may, if sufficiently chronic, lead to opticociliary shunt vessel formation. Retinal venous blood bypasses the laminar portion of the central retinal vein and enters the uveal or posterior ciliary venous circulation at the border of the optic disc through enlarged capillary connections resembling red knuckles or curlicues. That these opticociliary collaterals do not represent epipapillary and peripapillary neovascularization can be angiographically demonstrated by the absence of fluorescein leakage.

Opticociliary shunts occur at the margin of the optic nerve where Bruch's membrane terminates. Thus they do not have to penetrate Bruch's membrane. These anastomotic vessels may occur when there is obstruction or mechanical resistance to venous outflow in the optic nerve. Such conditions have been described in the following diseases: thrombosis of the central retinal vein; hyaline bodies of the optic nerve head; arachnoid cysts of the intraorbital optic nerve; and spheno-orbital meningioma, where their presence, along with disc pallor and visual loss, constitutes a diagnostic triad.[10]

INFLAMMATORY DISEASES

Toxoplasma retinochoroiditis has been the most frequently described inflammatory cause of acquired retinochoroidal vascular anastomoses, probably because of the intense necrosis that can involve all layers of the eyewall. Owens, Goldberg, and Busse were able to document the formation of these anastomoses with prospective angiographic observations.[31] They showed that the direction of arteriolar anastomotic flow was from choroid to retina in one portion of the macula, whereas the direction of venular anastomotic flow was from retina to choroid in an adjacent area (Fig. 13-3). This suggested that the gradient of blood pressure or of vascular resistance was as follows: choroidal artery → retinal artery → retinal vein → choroidal vein.

A somewhat similar fundus appearance has been observed in other cases of *Toxoplasma* retinochoroiditis by Gass[13] and by Saari and colleagues.[37] In the case of Saari et al., angiography again revealed retinal venous input to large choroidal vessels. These authors postulated that extension of perivascular cuffs of inflammation contributed to venous thrombosis and necrosis and subsequent formation of a retinochoroidal venous anastomosis.

Wessing also showed a somewhat similar fundus appearance in a case of inactive disseminated chorioretinitis. Angiography demonstrated the anastomosis to be between a retinal artery and a large choroidal vessel, but the direction of flow was from the retina to the choroid.[44]

After studying presumed nematode infestation of the retina and choroid, Green and Gass showed clinical evidence of a retinal artery connected to a subretinal disciform mass. The direction of flow appeared to be from retina to choroid. Older ophthalmoscopic reports of macular toxocariasis have also shown dilated retinal vessels passing deeply through the outer retina into the choroidal mass.[2,45] The direction of blood flow was not determined in these cases because they antedated the availability of fundus angiography.

Retinochoroidal anastomoses in an area of chorioretinal scarring are highly characteristic of but not pathognomonic for toxoplasmosis or toxocariasis. They also have been observed in disciform types of senile macular degeneration.[21] Rossazza et al.[35] also

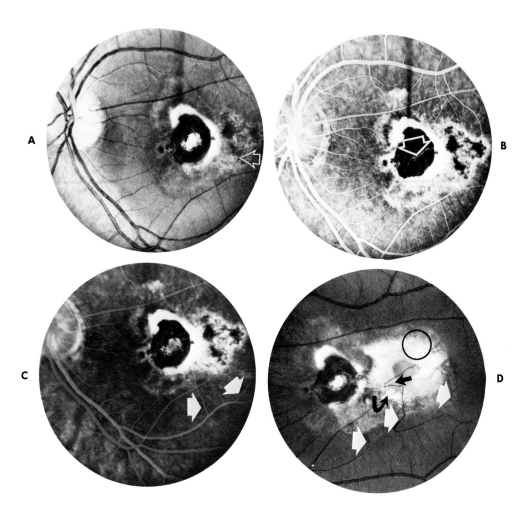

Fig. 13-3. Prospective observations of vascular anastomoses between choroid and retina in recurrent toxoplasmosis. **A,** Left macula in 1971. Ophthalmoscopic appearance of inactive fundus scar. *Arrow,* Site of future development of retinochoroidal venous anastomoses. **B,** Midvenous phase of angiogram shows capillary collateral, *arrow,* crossing the normally avascular foveola. No evidence for anastomoses between the retina and choroid is present. **C,** Late venous phase of angiogram shows some of the retinal venules, *arrows,* that subsequently became displaced and incorporated into anastomotic channels. **D,** Left macula in 1975. Ophthalmoscopic appearance of scar that now has inactive satellite lesion on its temporal border (see **A**). *White arrows,* Venules pulled into chorioretinal scar (see **C**); *curved black arrow,* choroidal vein; *straight black arrow,* confluence of retinal venular anastomoses as they drain into choroidal vein; *circle,* area of choroidal perfusion of retinal arterioles (not seen ophthalmoscopically). (**A** to **G,** From Owens, P., Goldberg, M.F., and Busse, B.J.: Am. J. Ophthalmol. **88:**402, 1979, published with permission from The American Journal of Ophthalmology, copyright by The Ophthalmic Publishing Co., Chicago.)

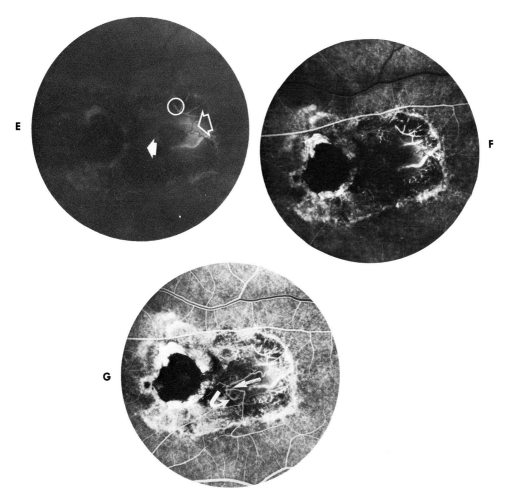

Fig. 13-3, cont'd. E, Arterial phase of choroidal perfusion. *Circle,* Area of choroidal perfusion of retinal arterioles; *solid arrow,* site of venous anastomoses; *open arrow,* anastomotic retinal venules that have not yet become perfused. **F,** Early venous phase of angiogram still shows nonfilling of both retinal and choroidal components of venous anastomoses. **G,** Midvenous phase of angiogram shows that anastomotic retinal venules, *straight arrow,* now drain into choroidal vein, *curved arrow* (see **D**).

reported a somewhat similar case of idiopathic submacular neovascularization and claimed that blood from the choroidal (subretinal) neovascular network drained into a retinal vein.

Careful angiography is necessary to confirm that actual anastomosis between retinal and choroidal vasculatures has been established by these enlarged macular vessels. Goldberg, for example, has described a case of presumed macular tuberculosis,[19] where highly resolved, magnified macular angiography was employed. The angiogram revealed that the dilated retinal vessel simply drained through enlarged capillary channels

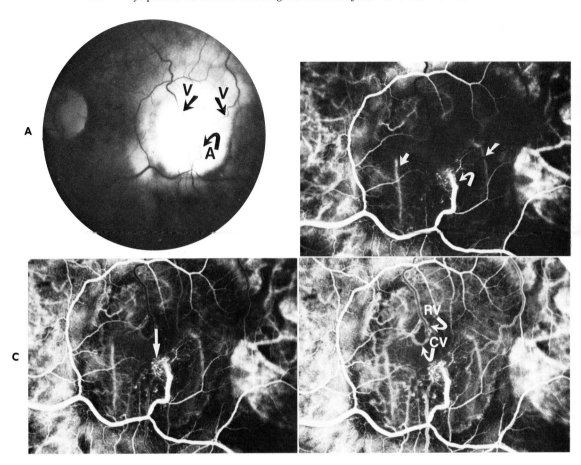

Fig. 13-4. Presumed tuberculous maculopathy with ophthalmoscopic appearance of enlarged vessels suggesting retinochoroidal anastomoses. Angiographic evidence, however, shows only that the enlarged retinal arteriole drains into adjacent retinal capillaries and venules. **A,** Ophthalmoscopic view of left macula. Note prominent retinal arteriole, *A,* at 6 o'clock region of white lesion and retinal venules, *V,* at the 10 and 2 o'clock regions that apparently dive into the substance of the mass. (See **E** and **F** for the angiographic appearance at same magnification.) **B,** Arterial phase of magnified angiogram of the left macular mass. Note early filling of inferior retinal arteriole, *curved arrow,* and of vessels within the lesion itself, *straight arrows.* **C,** Early venous phase of magnified angiogram. Note retinal capillary connections between adjacent arteriole and venule, *arrow.* No choroidal connections are seen. **D,** Later venous phase of magnified angiogram. Loop-shaped choroidal vessel, *CV,* at the 12 o'clock border of the foveola is in the choroidal mass and has no connection to the overlying retinal venule, *RV.* (**A** to **F,** From Goldberg, M.F.: Retina **2**:47, 1982.)

in the retina, and no connection to underlying choroidal vessels could be seen (Fig. 13-4), despite the suggestive ophthalmoscopic appearance.

A definitive explanation for retinochoroidal vascular connections after inflammatory and necrotic foci is lacking, but it is likely that histologic organization of the developing scar involves the growth of granulation tissue with proliferation of capillary buds and fibroblasts.[21] Newly formed capillary channels are presumably derived from both the retina and choroid and link up across defects in Bruch's membrane and the retinal

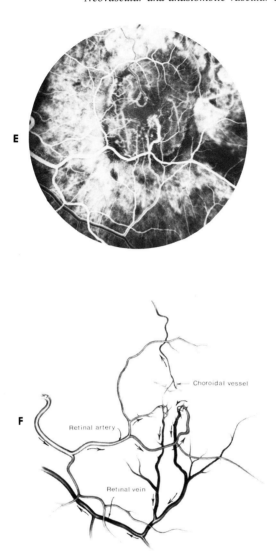

Fig. 13-4, cont'd. E, Venous phase of angiogram of left macula at normal magnification (compare **A**). **F,** Schematic interpretation of the blood flow pattern.

pigment epithelium. With progressive remodeling and maturation of these small vessels, gradients of blood flow ostensibly occur, enabling enlargement of some channels to develop. Preferential routes of flow develop, and the enlarged anastomosis may assume the angiographic appearance of a mature fundus artery or vein; for example, leakage of dye does not occur, possibly because of the loss of cytoplasmic fenestrations in maturing endothelial cells and the acquisition of tight intercellular junctions. Until electron microscopic inspection of a suitable human specimen or animal model occurs, this explanation must remain conjectural.

OCULAR TRAUMA

Ocular trauma may rather frequently result in vascular connections between the retina and choroid. Several types can develop: (1) discrete connections between mature arteries and veins of the retina and choroid, such as those occurring after choroidal and retinal rupture or after small chorioretinal perforations; (2) neovascular capillary connections, such as those developing after choroidal rupture and as a complication of angioid streaks or of high myopia, especially when such eyes are bluntly traumatized[38]; (3) diffuse fibrovascular adhesions among the retina, choroid, and sclera, as in chorioretinitis sclopetaria; and (4) anastomoses of mature vessels and of neovascular capillaries after intense fundus thermal injury, as in laser or xenon arc photocoagulation and in diathermy and cryopexy.

Choroidal rupture alone is unlikely to cause anastomoses of large, mature retinal and choroidal vessels because, although there has been a break in Bruch's membrane and retinal pigment epithelium, damaged vessels from both retina and choroid are not necessarily brought into anatomic proximity. Localized ruptures of contiguous portions of both choroid and retina, however, are capable of inducing such anatomoses in human eyes after as short a period as 6 weeks.[16] In one such patient the direction of arterial flow was from choroid to retina, and that of venous flow was from retina to choroid.[16] No neovascularization, fluorescein leakage, transudation, or hemorrhage occurred (Fig. 13-5).

In a similar patient (reported by Dr. J. Sebag, Department of Ophthalmology, Harvard Medical School), a virtually identical chorioretinal arteriolar anastomosis was seen 1 year after blunt ocular trauma. In this patient, however, the venous anastomosis also filled from choroid to retina. In addition, a small patch of neovascularization developed (Fig. 13-6). Vision was 20/40 (6/12).

In other cases, the healing of choroidal ruptures may be complicated by neovascularization, which results in transudative or hemorrhagic phenomena. Detachment of or hemorrhage within the macula can thus occur[11,24,40] with substantial visual disability, even when the rupture site is not located immediately in the center of the macula. Some of these cases may be aided by photocoagulation of the leaking neovascular tissue.

Small chorioretinal perforations may also be associated with anastomoses of large, mature retinal and choroidal vessels. In one such instance, a metallic foreign body lacerated both retinal and choroidal blood vessels.[18] As in the case of blunt rupture of both retina and choroid cited above, vascular connections between the retina and choroid were permitted by the breaching of Bruch's membrane and the retinal pigment epithelium and by the simultaneous juxtaposition of lacerated retinal and choroidal vessels. The anastomoses occurred within 10 months (Fig. 13-7). The direction of arterial flow was from choroid to retina, and that of venous flow was from retina to choroid. The clinical course was benign, apparently because no substantial amounts of neovascular tissue developed or persisted. Accordingly, there was no propensity for hemorrhagic or transudative activity.

Chorioretinitis sclopetaria is caused by a severe concussion to the sclera, retina, and choroid, usually because of a high-velocity missile, such as a bullet, transversing the orbit next to the globe. Extensive rupture of the choroid and retina occurs, often with cons derable intraocular hemorrhage. The sclera is not perforated in this disorder but participates in a dense fibrovascular reparative process involving all three tunics of the

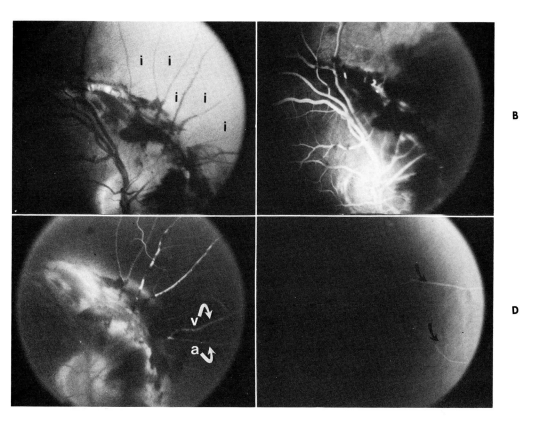

Fig. 13-5. Prospective observations of vascular anastomoses between choroid and retina after blunt ocular trauma with rupture of both retina and choroid. **A,** Five days after blunt trauma to the right eye, rupture of the choroid and retina is seen superonasal to the optic disc. Superonasal branch vessels are transected, and their blood columns are segmented and stationary. The corresponding quadrant of the retina is opaque because of ischemic infarction, *i*. The other retinal quadrants had normal coloration and markings. **B,** During the early arteriovenous phase of fluorescein angiography, there is no perfusion of superonasal vessels or retina. **C,** During the late venous phase of angiography, the superonasal venules carry dye from the retinal periphery up to but not across the rupture site. The superonasal arterioles are perfused in the retrograde direction up to but not across the rupture site. *a,* Arteriole; *v,* venule. **D,** Six weeks after trauma, distal segments of transected arterioles, *arrows,* are perfused during the early arterial phase of angiography (unlike that in **B**). (**A** to **F,** From Goldberg, M.F.: Am. J. Ophthalmol. **82:**892, 1976, published with permission from The American Journal of Ophthalmology, copyright by The Ophthalmic Publishing Co., Chicago.)

Continued.

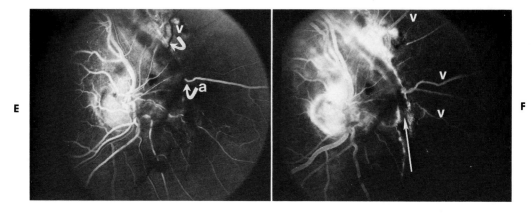

Fig. 13-5, cont'd. E, Early arteriovenous phase. Note large-caliber distal segment of arteriole at 2:45 position, *a,* and lack of connection with proximal segment. The proximal segment is less well perfused than distal segment. Also note 1:30 position nonperfused venule, *v,* and its lack of connection with proximal segment. **F,** Late arteriovenous phase. Connections between proximal and distal segments of venule, *v,* at 1:30 position and arteriole and venule at 2:45 position are not seen. One small venule, *arrow,* at 3 o'clock bridges the defect.

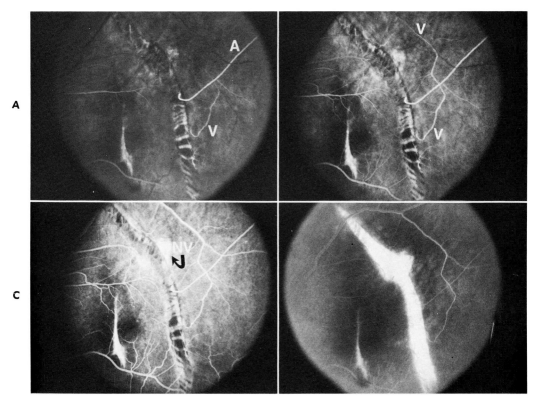

Fig. 13-6. Angiograms of vascular anastomoses between the retina and choroid after blunt trauma to the eye. **A,** Arterial phase showing choroidal origin of both retinal arteriole, *A,* and retinal venule, *V.* **B,** Early venous phase. Retinal venule, *V,* is fully perfused. **C,** Late venous phase shows leakage from neovascular tissue, *NV.* **D,** Very late venous phase. (Courtesy of Dr. J. Sebag, Harvard Medical School, Boston.)

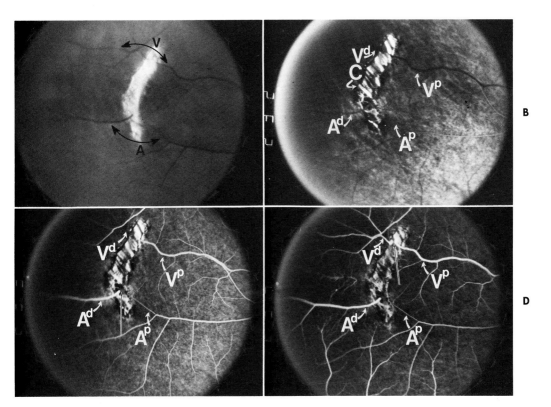

Fig. 13-7. Vascular anastomoses between the choroid and retina after perforating ocular trauma. **A,** Chorioretinal scar 10 months after perforating injury. Note deviated retinal arteriole, *A,* at lower pole of scar and retinal venule, *V,* at upper pole of scar. **B,** Early arterial phase of angiogram. Note choroidal perfusion, *C,* early filling of distal segment of interrupted retinal arteriole, A^d, but absence of filling of its proximal segment, A^p. Neither the distal nor the proximal segment of the retinal venule is perfused yet, V^d and V^p. **C,** Early venous phase of angiogram. Note discontinuous retinal arteriole, A^d and A^p, and choroidal origin of distal segment of retinal arteriole, *long arrow.* The proximal portion of the retinal venule, V^p, is perfused, but the distal segment, V^d, is not. **D,** Late venous phase of angiogram. Note apparent discontinuity in retinal venule, *long arrow.* (**A** to **D,** From Goldberg, M.F.: Am. J. Ophthalmol. **85:**171, 1978, published with permission from The American Journal of Ophthalmology, copyright by The Ophthalmic Publishing Co., Chicago.)

eyewall. The result is a tightly adherent adhesion of sclera to choroid and retina. Extensive histopathologic organization of connective tissue occurs, with proliferation of vessels from both the retina and choroid.[34] This condition has been called chorioretinitis proliferans. Enmeshed in the chorioretinal scar are large numbers of capillaries connecting the retina and choroid. Despite the severity of the trauma, retinal detachment rarely occurs because the scar tissue is tightly adherent to the sclera.

PHOTOCOAGULATION

Fundus photocoagulation has been responsible for creating neovascular and mature vascular connections between retina and choroid in both experimental and therapeutic settings. Using a primate experimental model of argon laser photocoagulation, Wolf and Goldberg exposed large retinal arteries to extremely high energy densities. The energy was sufficiently intense to close the arteries and also induce hemorrhage or visible disruption at the level of Bruch's membrane and retinal pigment epithelium. Ophthalmoscopically visible chorioretinal anastomoses developed at nine of 19 fundus sites so treated (Fig. 13-8). The shortest period after photocoagulation at which an anastomosis was detected was 7 weeks, and the majority occurred within 10 weeks.

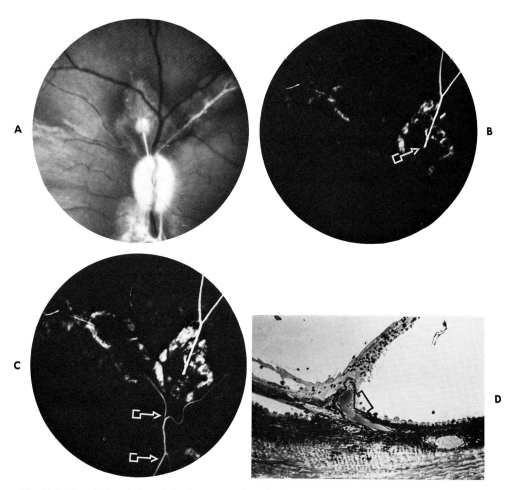

Fig. 13-8. Choroidal perfusion of distal segments of monkey's retinal arterioles after laser-induced proximal occlusion. **A,** Ophthalmoscopic appearance after laser burns. Note obstructed arterioles. **B,** Early arterial phase of angiogram 10 weeks after laser photocoagulation of retinal arteriole adjacent to disc (case similar to that seen in **A**). Note that retinal arteriole, *arrow,* becomes perfused during choroidal phase of angiogram (that is, before the central retinal artery). **C,** Later arterial phase of angiogram. The central retinal artery and its branches are now perfused, *arrows.* **D,** Histology of chorioretinal vascular anastomosis, *arrow.* Retinal detachment is artifactual. (**A** to **D,** From Wolf, E.D., and Goldberg, M.F.: Ophthalmic Surg. **11:**30, 1980.)

In this experimental model, the direction of arterial anastomotic flow was choroid to retina, and that of venous anastomotic flow was retina to choroid. The clinical course was not complicated by late onset of transudation, hemorrhage, or retinal detachment, apparently because neovascular tissue did not occur to any appreciable extent. In fact, there was no ophthalmoscopic, angiographic, or histologic evidence of neovascularization over a follow-up period that extended for up to 24 months. Because the anastomoses were not created immediately at the time of laser burns to the retinal arteries, organizing granulation tissue with capillary budding must have occurred and must have facilitated the development of the large-vessel anastomoses that developed. These neovascular capillaries were ostensibly small and transient because no evidence for their presence could be detected subsequently.

An interesting human case of arteriolar chorioretinal anastomosis occurring after laser photocoagulation was reported by Poletti[33] and another similar case was reported by Douenne and LeRebeller.[7] The direction of flow in these arterial anastomoses was choroid to retina, as in the primate model of Wolf and Goldberg. Similarly, neovascular tissue was not present. Archer and Gardiner also showed mature anastomoses in their monkey model[1] but additionally demonstrated ample evidence of laser-induced neovascularization (p. 164).

It would appear from these clinical and experimental studies that intense photocoagulation burns overlying major retinal arteries can give rise to large-vessel chorioretinal anastomoses, whereas somewhat less intense burns not involving major retinal arteries, but possibly involving retinal veins,[1] may be more likely to induce neovascularization. The creation of anastomoses involving large arterial vessels in the retina may have permitted the development of a hemodynamic "steal" that allowed or induced rapid shunting of blood past incipient neovascular capillary buds.[46] The neovascular tissue might thus have been deprived of a blood supply suitable for sustaining or enhancing its growth.

From the burgeoning case material being published on the subject of acquired chorioretinal anastomoses, certain clinical conclusions can be drawn.[33] The anastomoses may be arterial or venous. Arterial flow is usually in the direction of choroid to retina. Angiograms purporting to show the opposite direction for arterial flow[21,33] have not been very convincing up to now. Venous flow is usually in the direction of retina to choroid though the opposite direction can occur (Fig. 13-6); again, most published angiograms have not been convincing primarily because of the absence of early-phase angiographic photographs and incomplete labeling of surrounding blood vessels.[33] The development of chorioretinal anastomoses may occur within weeks or months of the inciting pathologic fundus condition. The ophthalmoscopic appearance of a large-caliber retinal vessel plunging into the subretinal space is highly characteristic though not truly diagnostic (Fig. 13-4) without proper angiograms. Many of these anastomoses appear to become permanent, with little or no tendency to break or bleed. Clinically detectable neovascular tissue is often absent. Symptoms rarely, if ever, can be attributed to the anastomoses by themselves, and treatment is not indicated, unless neovascularization supervenes and threatens the macula.

CHOROIDAL NEOVASCULARIZATION

Neovascularization arising from the choroid can be distinguished from chorioretinal anastomosis by its incompetence to sodium fluorescein. The absence of intercellular tight junctions or the presence of cytoplasmic fenestrations in the endothelia of these vessels (in comparison to normal retinal vessels, which ordinarily have tight junctions and no fenestrations) is easily recognized by profuse leakage during the fluorescein angiogram. Three types of choroidal neovascularization can be recognized: (1) subretinal neovascularization, (2) chorioretinal neovascularization (occurring in the plane of the retina), and (3) choriovitreal neovascularization (with growth of the blood vessels into the vitreous cavity). Subretinal neovascularization is a common entity, whereas chorioretinal neovascularization and choriovitreal neovascularization are rarer and are usually seen as complications of intense photocoagulation. Each of these three types of choroidal neovascularization are now discussed.

Subretinal and choroidal neovascularization. Although there is considerable evidence that many normal adult eyes have sub–pigment epithelial neovascularization in the peripheral fundus,[9,41] these new vessels are not usually recognized clinically and do not appear to cause significant morbidity. On the other hand, subretinal neovascularization in the posterior pole, particularly in the macular and peripapillary areas, may frequently cause loss of vision. Subretinal neovascularization[23] can develop in patients with senile macular degeneration, angioid streaks, high myopia, or macular dystrophies (such as Best's dystrophy) or in association with tumors (such as choroidal melanoma), trauma (choroidal rupture), inflammatory diseases (presumed ocular histoplasmosis and serpiginous choroiditis), and other clinical entities. Subretinal neovascularization may also occur after photocoagulation of the macular area[8] (as for central serous choroidopathy). It may be difficult to determine if the neovascularization is secondary to the photocoagulation or is part of the natural course of the underlying disease. The occurrence of subretinal neovascularization in the macula can result in disciform degeneration with destruction of macular function.

Many entities causing subretinal neovascularization are associated with degenerative changes in Bruch's membrane, which apparently predispose to the ingrowth of choroidal vessels into the sub–pigment epithelial space. Since some patients with degeneration or disruption of Bruch's membrane do not develop subretinal neovascularization, other factors must also be important. It has been suggested that, for example, the detachment of the photoreceptors can be associated with retinal hypoxia, which might provide an angiogenic stimulus for ingrowth of choroidal neovascularization.[39] Similarly, inflammatory cells in the outer retina might also stimulate choroidal neovascular growth. A tumor-angiogenic factor might account for the appearance of subretinal neovascularization in association with neoplasms. Experimental models for the production of subretinal choroidal neovascularization have been developed in the hope of determining the mechanisms of growth of these new vessels (p. 164).

Chorioretinal and choriovitreal neovascularization (Figs. 13-9 and 13-10). The development of choroidal neovascularization with growth into the retina (chorioretinal neovascularization) or into the vitreous (choriovitreal neovascularization) can be seen as a complication of intense photocoagulation in the fundus. This entity was probably first noted by Theodossiadis and Velissaropoulos in 1973.[43] These authors described four patients with Eales' disease who developed choriovitreal neovascularization after intense fundus photocoagulation.

Subsequently, the development of choriovitreal neovascularization was reported from our clinic in two patients with sickle cell disease and one patient with sarcoidosis who

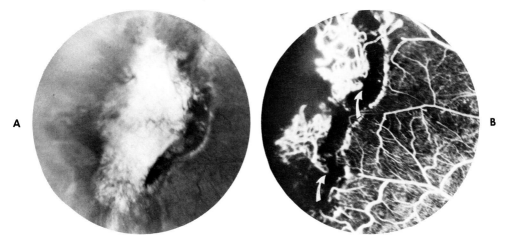

Fig. 13-9. Chorioretinal neovascularization after argon laser photocoagulation of sickle-cell sea fans. **A,** Ophthalmoscopic view. **B,** Angiographic view of neovascularization emanating from choroid, *arrows,* but lying in plane of retina.

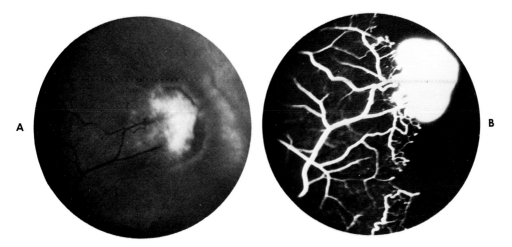

Fig. 13-10. Development of choriovitreal neovascularization after overly intense laser treatment of sickle-cell sea fan. **A,** Ophthalmoscopic view of preretinal neovascular sea fan before photocoagulation. **B,** Angiographic appearance of sea fan before photocoagulation.   *Continued.*

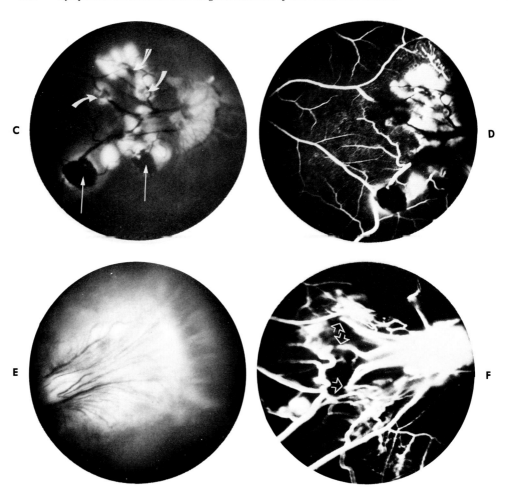

Fig. 13-10, cont'd. C, Ophthalmoscopic view of sea fan immediately after intense laser treatment. Note ruptures in Bruch's membrane and retinal pigment epithelium, *curved arrows,* as well as hemorrhage from choroid, *straight arrows.* **D,** Angiographic appearance of **C.** Note that feeder vessels and neovascular sea fan are no longer perfused. **E,** Ophthalmoscopic appearance of enormous choriovitreal fibrovascular frond originating from area of previously ruptured Bruch's membrane and retinal pigment epithelium. **F,** Angiographic appearance of **E.** Note choroidal origin of many of the nutrient vessels, *arrows.*

had also received intense fundus photocoagulation.[12] We noted at that time that very small burn diameters of high intensity could disrupt Bruch's membrane with the secondary development of choroidal neovascularization. In a short-term follow-up study of a group of 53 eyes that had received xenon arc or argon laser photocoagulation for proliferative sickle cell retinopathy, choriovitreal neovascularization was noted in 5.7% of the cases.[15] With longer follow-up study of the same 53 photocoagulated eyes,[6] we have subsequently reported choroidally fed neovascularization in at least 21 of the 53 eyes (40%). Fortunately, visual loss has been infrequent. Choroidal neovascularization has been noted in both argon laser– and xenon arc–treated eyes. In 11 of these 21 eyes, the neovascularization was chorioretinal, and in 10 it was choriovitreal.

Re-treatment of flat chorioretinal neovascularization with photocoagulation was noted, on occasion, to stimulate its growth and sometimes converted it to choriovitreal neovascularization.[6] In this series of eyes, we found that patients with chorioretinal neovascularization usually did well, with only the rare occurrence of local vitreous hemorrhaging. The choroidal neovascularization in these eyes usually remained within the photocoagulation scar and appeared to stabilize after an initial period of growth. The occurrence of choriovitreal neovascularization, on the other hand, was much more ominous. Recurrent vitreous hemorrhaging and, in some patients, retinal detachments were noted. The destruction of choriovitreal neovascularization proved to be extremely difficult. Very intense photocoagulation temporarily halted perfusion of the new vessels in some cases. However, in most cases the new vessels reperfused, and in many instances treatment with intense photocoagulation, diathermy, or cryotherapy appeared either to stimulate or to have no inhibitory effect on further growth of the vessels.

Iatrogenic choroidal vascularization after photocoagulation has also been described by several other authors in patients with both sickle cell and diabetic retinopathy.[3-5] Again, very intense focal photocoagulation resulted in disruption of Bruch's membrane with the development of subretinal, chorioretinal, or choriovitreal neovascularization. Similar choriovitreal neovascularization has also been described in several eyes that received intense cryopexy for lattice degeneration with retinal detachment.[42] One case of spontaneous chorioretinal neovascularization in a patient with sickle cell disease has also been detected.[29]

Based on our experience in patients with diabetes and with sickle cell disease, we currently recommend that no treatment be given for iatrogenic chorioretinal neovascularization. We have also not treated most patients with choriovitreal neovascularization unless the growth of the vessels is threatening the eye. Even in these cases, however, we have not had much success in closing these vessels with partially penetrating diathermy, cryotherapy, or repeat photocoagulation. Based upon animal and human studies, we presently recommend that intense photocoagulation using small spot sizes (such as 50 or 100 μm) be avoided, unless special precautions are taken (see Chapter 5) in the hope of preventing disruption of Bruch's membrane and therefore minimizing the occurrence of choroidal neovascularization. The larger and much less intense photocoagulation burns employed with scatter (panretinal) photocoagulation are unlikely to disrupt Bruch's membrane and cause choroidal neovascularization. With the great decrease in the use of focal treatment in patients with diabetes and other proliferative retinopathies, choroidal neovascularization appears to be occurring less frequently. On the other hand, since feeder vessel photocoagulation is very effective in patients with sickle cell disease, choroidal neovascularization still remains a potential problem for these patients. The use of a two-stage technique for the photocoagulation of retinal neovascularization in sickle cell disease (see Chapter 5) minimizes the chances of development of choroidal neovascularization.

The precise pathogenesis of chorioretinal and choriovitreal neovascularization occurring after photocoagulation remains uncertain. Mechanical disruption of Bruch's membrane undoubtedly facilitates the ingrowth of these choroidal vessels. It is possible that the inner retinal ischemia present in patients with diabetes and sickle cell disease might stimulate the growth of choroidal vessels. In addition, the intense photocoagulation probably causes considerable inflammation. Inflammatory cells are well known to produce angiogenic factors that might stimulate ingrowth of choroidal vessels. Another factor that might be responsible for the ingrowth of choroidal vessels is the occurrence of choroidal ischemia after intense photocoagulation.[14] Closure of the choroidal capillaries may set the stage for the development of choroidal neovascularization. Histopathologic studies of an eye treated with xenon arc photocoagulation for proliferative diabetic retinopathy showed breaks in Bruch's membrane, destruction of choriocapillaries, and the growth of fibrovascular tissue from the choroid into the subretinal space and the damaged retina.[27] These findings appear to correspond to subretinal and chorioretinal neovascularization as described on p. 160.

EXPERIMENTAL MODELS OF SUBRETINAL, CHORIORETINAL, AND CHORIOVITREAL NEOVASCULARIZATION IN PRIMATE EYE

Wolf and Goldberg[46] attempted to produce choroidal neovascularization in cynomolgus monkeys by using very intense argon laser photocoagulation. They were successful in producing chorioretinal vascular anastomoses in monkey eyes when the photocoagulation was intense enough to occlude a major retinal arteriole and disrupt both choroidal and retinal vasculatures. However, as noted above, long-term follow-up study showed no subretinal, chorioretinal, or choriovitreal neovascularization. In this study, argon laser burns over branch retinal arteries were created with a power of 200 to 500 milliwatts (mW), a 0.5-second duration, and burn diameters of 50 to 500 μm.

Subsequently, Ryan[36] was successful in producing subretinal neovascularization using very intense argon laser photocoagulation in rhesus monkeys. Initially, he utilized moderately intense photocoagulation (50 to 100 μm spot size and powers of less than 500 mW) in combination with attempts to close retinal veins. In some eyes, subretinal neovascularization did develop. However, with utilization of much more intense photocoagulation burns (750 to 950 mW), again using small spot sizes, Ryan was frequently able to produce subretinal neovascularization, even when no attempt was made to disrupt the retinal vasculature. He demonstrated that the subretinal neovascularization in these photocoagulated monkey eyes was easily produced in the posterior pole, but rarely occurred in the nasal retina or in the fundus periphery. He also noted that spontaneous involution occurred in 71 of the 90 photocoagulation burns that developed subretinal neovascularization. Of the 90 loci with subretinal neovascularization, 27 demonstrated at least one episode of spontaneous hemorrhaging. Ryan did not describe growth of the vessels into the sensory retina or the vitreous cavity in this study.

Archer and Gardiner[1] reported a related technique to produce choroidal neovascularization in rhesus monkey eyes. In this study 28 rhesus monkeys received very intense retinal photocoagulation. In all these eyes, attempts were made to close retinal veins. The exact details of photocoagulation are not specified, but the authors utilized small, high-intensity burns. Vitreous hemorrhaging was seen in many of the eyes at the time of treatment. Subsequently, the occurrence of choroidal neovascularization was noted in many instances.

Archer and Gardiner noticed the growth of choroidal neovascularization into the subretinal space in some eyes. In five eyes, however, the neovascularization grew from the choroid through the necrotic retina into the vitreous cavity. This would appear to be an excellent model of iatrogenic choriovitreal neovascularization. In addition, mature chorioretinal anastomoses, similar to those reported in monkeys by Wolf and Goldberg[46] and in the patient by Poletti,[33] were also seen.

A review of the studies by Wolf and Goldberg,[46] Ryan,[36] and Archer and Gardiner[1] enables us to reach the following conclusions: Very intense photocoagulation is obviously capable of disrupting Bruch's membrane. In some eyes the occurrence of chorioretinal vascular anastomoses is noted. In others, subretinal, chorioretinal, and choriovitreal neovascularization can occur, and spontaneous hemorrhaging may develop. In many of these eyes, choroidally fed neovascularization will show spontaneous involution. The reasons are unknown. Why some eyes develop anastomoses and others develop neovascularization is also unknown. Differences in size or number of photocoagulated retinal arteries or veins may play a role, as may the size and number of underlying choroidal vessels. It is unclear, as yet, whether the stimulus for the ingrowth of the new vessels is related to inflammation from intense photocoagulation, retinal or choroidal ischemia from vascular closure, or simply mechanical factors such as disruption of Bruch's membrane (and the retinal pigment epithelium). Other, unidentified factors may also contribute to the pathogenesis.

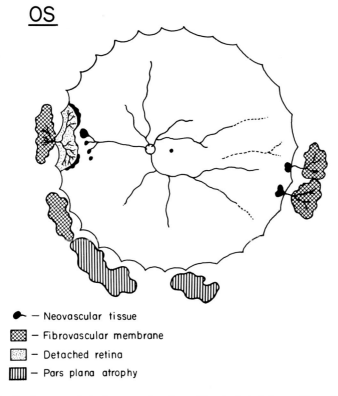

OS

- Neovascular tissue
- Fibrovascular membrane
- Detached retina
- Pars plana atrophy

Fig. 13-11. Intravitreal neovascularization emanating from ciliary body in left eye. (From Goldberg, M.F., and Ericson, E.S.: Ophthalmic Surg. **8:**62, 1977.)

CILIARY BODY NEOVASCULARIZATION

Intravitreal neovascularization emanating from the ciliary body is a rare event, but it can cause visually disabling intraocular hemorrhages.[20] Preexisting severe ocular disease appears to be a prerequisite and often has included thermal damage to the ciliary body in an attempt to control severe glaucoma (Fig. 13-11). Thermal, inflammatory, or hypoxic breakdown of the basement membranes and epithelia separating ciliary body vessels from the vitreous space may have contributed (in analogy to damage to Bruch's membrane and the retinal pigment epithelium described earlier in this chapter) to passage of neovascular tissue through the normally avascular membranes and epithelia into the vitreous chamber.[20]

Ciliary body neovascularization may also occur as a result of fibrovascular organization of granulomatous tissue, such as occurs in toxocariasis or pars-planitis.[26]

REFERENCES

1. Archer, D.B., and Gardiner, T.A.: Morphologic, fluorescein angiographic, and light microscopic features of experimental choroidal vascularization, Am. J. Ophthalmol. **91**:297, 1981.
2. Ashton, N.: Larval granulomatosis of the retina due to *Toxocara,* Br. J. Ophthalmol. **44**:129, 1960.
3. Benson, W.E., Townsend, R.E., and Pheasant, T.R.: Choriovitreal and subretinal proliferations: complications of photocoagulation, Trans. Am. Acad. Ophthalmol. Otolaryngol. **86**:283, 1979.
4. Chandra, S.R., Bresnick, G.H., Davis, M.D., Miller, S.A., and Myers, F.: Choroidovitreal neovascular ingrowth after photocoagulation for proliferative diabetic retinopathy, Arch. Ophthalmol. **98**:1593, 1980.
5. Condon, P.I., Jampol, L.M., Ford, S.M., and Serjeant, G.R.: Choroidal neovascularization induced by photocoagulation in sickle cell disease, Br. J. Ophthalmol. **65**:192, 1981.
6. Dizon-Moore, R.V., Jampol, L.M., and Goldberg, M.F.: Chorioretinal and choriovitreal neovascularization, Arch. Ophthalmol. **99**:842, 1981.
7. Douenne, J.L., and LeRebeller, M.-J.: Anastomoses choriorétiniennes acquises: à propos de 3 cas, Bull. Soc. Ophtalmol. Fr. **80**:291, 1980.
8. François, J., de Laey, J.J., Cambie, E., Hanssens, M., and Victoria-Troncoso, V.: Neovascularization after argon laser photocoagulation of macular lesions, Am. J. Ophthalmol. **79**:206, 1975.
9. Friedman, E., Smith, T.R., and Kuwabara, T.: Senile choroidal vascular patterns and drusen, Arch. Ophthalmol. **69**:220, 1963.
10. Frisen, L., Hoyt, W.F., and Tengroth, B.M.: Optociliary veins, disc pallor, and visual loss: a triad of signs indicating spheno-orbital meningioma, Acta Ophthalmol. **51**:241, 1973.
11. Fuller, B., and Gitter, K.A.: Traumatic choroidal rupture with late serous detachment of macula: report of successful argon laser treatment, Arch. Ophthalmol. **89**:354, 1973.
12. Galinos, S.O., Asdourian, G.K., Woolf, M.B., Goldberg, M.F., and Busse, B.: Choroidovitreal neovascularization after argon laser photocoagulation, Arch. Ophthalmol. **93**:524, 1975.
13. Gass, J.D.M.: Stereoscopic atlas of macular disorders, St. Louis, 1970, The C.V. Mosby Co.
14. Goldbaum, M.H., Galinos, S.O., Apple, D., Asdourian, G.K., Nagpal, K., Jampol, L.M., Woolf, M.B., and Busse, B.: Acute choroidal ischemia as a complication of photocoagulation, Arch. Ophthalmol. **94**:1025, 1976.
15. Goldbaum, M.H., Goldberg, M.F., Nagpal, K., Asdourian, G.K., and Galinos, S.O.: Proliferative sickle cell retinopathy. In L'Esperance, F., editor: Current diagnosis and management of choriovitreal disease, St. Louis, 1976, The C. V. Mosby Co.
16. Goldberg, M.F.: Choroidoretinal vascular anastomoses after blunt trauma, Am. J. Ophthalmol. **82**:892, 1976.
17. Goldberg, M.F.: Bruch's membrane and vascular growth (Editorial), Invest. Ophthalmol. **15**:443, 1976.
18. Goldberg, M.F.: Chorioretinal vascular anastomoses after perforating trauma to the eye, Am. J. Ophthalmol. **85**:171, 1978.
19. Goldberg, M.F.: Presumed tuberculous maculopathy, Retina **2**:47, 1982.
20. Goldberg, M.F., and Ericson, E.S.: Intravitreal ciliary body neovascularization, Ophthalmic Surg. **8**:62, 1977.
21. Green, W.R., and Gass, J.D.M.: Senile disciform degeneration of the macula, Arch. Ophthalmol. **86**:487, 1971.

22. Gutman, E.D., and Goldberg, M.F.: Persistent pupillary membrane and other ocular anomalies: feature photo, Arch. Ophthalmol. **94:**156, 1976.

23. Henkind, P.: Ocular neovascularization, Am. J. Ophthalmol. **85:**287, 1978.

24. Hilton, G.F.: Late serosanguineous detachment of the macula after traumatic choroidal rupture, Am. J. Ophthalmol. **79:**997, 1975.

25. Kennedy, J.E., and Wise, G.N.: Retinochoroidal vascular anastomosis in uveitis, Am. J. Ophthalmol. **71:**1221, 1971.

26. Kenyon, K.R., Pederson, J.E., Green, W.R., and Maumenee, A.E.: Fibroglial proliferation in pars planitis, Trans. Ophthalmol. Soc. U.K. **95:**391, 1975.

27. Kodama, Y., Ishikawa, Y., Nomura, T., and Taniguchi, Y.: Choroidal neovascularization in the photo-coagulated retina with diabetic retinopathy: a light and electron microscopic study, Jpn. J. Ophthalmol. **24:**35, 1980.

28. Larsson, L., and Osterlin, S.: Retinal vessels in the ora region: possible role in the vitreo-retinal pathology in aphakia, Acta Ophthalmol. **59:**526, 1981.

29. Liang, J., and Jampol, L.M.: Spontaneous peripheral chorioretinal neovascularization in association with sickle cell anemia. (Submitted for publication.)

30. Meisels, H.I., and Goldberg, M.F.: Vascular anastomosis between the iris and persistent hyperplastic primary vitreous, Am. J. Ophthalmol. **88:**179, 1979.

31. Owens, P., Goldberg, M.F., and Busse, B.J.: Prospective observation of vascular anastomoses between the retina and choroid in recurrent toxoplasmosis, Am. J. Ophthalmol. **88:**402, 1979.

32. Ozanics, V., in discussion of Daicker, B.: Retino-choroidal venous anastomoses in the ora serrata, Surv. Ophthalmol. **14:**81, 1969.

33. Poletti, J.: Anastomose chorio-rétinienne acquise, J. Fr. Ophtalmol. **3:**737, 1980.

34. Richards, R.D., West, C.E., and Meisels, A.A.: Chorioretinitis sclopetaria, Am. J. Ophthalmol. **66:**852, 1968.

35. Rossazza, C., Poletti, J., and François, J.-H.: Anastomose choriorétinienne au cours d'une uvéite, Bull. Soc. Ophtalmol. Fr. **78:**901, 1978.

36. Ryan, S.J.: Subretinal neovascularization after argon laser photocoagulation, Albrecht von Graefes Arch. Klin. Exp. Ophthalmol. **215:**29, 1980.

37. Saari, M., Miettinen, R., Nieminen, H., and Raisanen, S.: Retinochoroidal vascular anastomosis in toxoplasmic chorioretinitis, Acta Ophthalmol. **53:**44, 1975.

38. Shilling, J.S., and Blach, R.K.: Prognosis and therapy of angioid streaks, Trans. Ophthalmol. Soc. U.K. **95:**301, 1975.

39. Smith, R.J.H.: Rubeotic glaucoma, Br. J. Ophthalmol. **65:**606, 1981.

40. Smith, R.E., Kelley, J.S., and Harbin, T.S.: Late macular complications of choroidal ruptures, Am. J. Ophthalmol. **77:**650, 1974.

41. Spitznas, M., and Bornfeld, N.: Development and ultrastructure of peripheral subretinal neovascularizations, Albrecht von Graefes Arch. Klin. Exp. Ophthalmol. **208:**125, 1978.

42. Theodossiadis, G.P.: Choroidal neovascularization after cryoapplication, Albrecht von Graefes Arch. Klin. Exp. Ophthalmol. **98:**1593, 1980.

43. Theodossiadis, G.P., and Velissaropoulos, P.: Choroidal vascular involvement in Eales' disease, Ophthalmologica **166:**1, 1973.

44. Wessing, A.: Fluorescein angiography of the retina: textbook and atlas, St. Louis, 1969, The C.V. Mosby Co.

45. Wilder, H.C.: Nematode endophthalmitis, Trans. Am. Acad. Ophthalmol. Otolaryngol. **55:**99, 1950.

46. Wolf, E.D., and Goldberg, M.F.: Chorioretinal vascular anastomoses resulting from photocoagulation in cynomolgus monkeys, Ophthalmic Surg. **11:**30, 1980.

47. Wybar, K.C.: Anastomoses between the uveal and retinal circulations, and their significance in vascular occlusion. In XVII Concilium Ophthalmologicum, Toronto, 1955, University of Toronto Press, vol. 1, p. 204.

48. Yanoff, M., and Fine, B.S.: Ocular pathology: a text and atlas, Hagerstown, Md., 1975, Harper & Row.

14

Related hereditary macular dystrophies

Robert C. Watzke

The cause of the yellow, opaque lesions so typically found in fundus flavimaculatus and Best's vitelliform macular dystrophy has been an enigma for generations. These lesions are certainly subretinal and probably at the level of the pigment epithelium. They are irregular in shape, often oval, yellowish in color, and quite opaque. They appear in a normal fundus and evolve into areas of atrophic pigment epithelial scars. They may occur as a large cyst in Best's disease or in irregular oval flecks in the posterior pole and midperiphery in fundus flavimaculatus or Stargardt's degeneration.

On fluorescein angiography they are typically hypofluorescent in the early stages of the angiogram, particularly when the yellow lesions are opaque and not surrounded by any areas of pigment epithelial degeneration. Occasionally there may be very faint staining. After evolution into atrophic scars, they become hyperfluorescent.

Recently these lesions have been characterized by pathologic study. Eagle found in studying eyes removed from a 24-year-old patient with fundus flavimaculatus that the yellow flecks corresponded to areas of enormously swollen pigment epithelial cells.[2] Within the cytoplasm of these cells was an abnormal PAS-positive material that had the staining characteristics of lipofuscin. Adjacent pigment epithelial cells appeared normal. In studying the eyes of a patient with Best's vitelliform degeneration Weingeist found a similar abnormal lipofuscin material within abnormally enlarged and degenerative pigment epithelial cells and also in cells that were liberated into the subretinal space.[9] Both investigators also found that pigment epithelial cells containing the lipofuscin material were often degenerative and had desquamated into surrounding tissues. The overlying photoreceptors were usually abnormal.

We have recently studied two families who show various lesions that clinically, morphologically, and angiographically appear identical to this material. Both families belong to the clinical entity known as "pattern dystrophy." The features of patients from these two pedigrees suggests to me that there is a similar basic defect in this group of hereditary macular dystrophies and that the pattern dystrophies may also represent a disorder of pigment epithelial metabolism with accumulation of abnormal lipofuscin material in the degenerative pigment epithelium.

PATTERN DYSTROPHIES

The pattern dystrophies are a group of hereditary macular dystrophies characterized by yellow-white lesions in the retinal pigment epithelium in varying degrees of size, opaqueness, atrophy, and pigmentation. Depending on their arrangement in linear, stellate, butterfly, or clustered patterns, they have been separately reported as reticular,[7] macro reticular,[6] butterfly dystrophy,[1] grouped pigmentary dystrophy,[3] fundus pulverulentus,[8] and foveomacular dystrophy.[4]

The transmission is autosomal dominant, the onset is usually after the second decade, and visual loss is usually minimal. The electro-oculogram (EOG) usually shows an abnormality. These dystrophies have an extremely variable appearance, but with experience one can recognize the characteristic lesions. I believe that this is an extremely common condition, probably the most common of the hereditary macular dystrophies. It is easy to diagnose this as "senile macular degeneration," but the pathogenesis and prognosis are much different.

Certain representative individuals from two families with pattern dystrophy will be briefly described to present the typical features of this hereditary macular dystrophy.

Family 1

Family 1 is a large pedigree of English extraction comprising 53 individuals. Forty-two of these individuals were examined (Fig. 14-1).

Two members of the first generation were examined. These persons were 90 and 81 years old. They had lost reading vision and had cataracts, and their fundi showed atrophy of the pigment epithelium and choriocapillaris in the posterior pole.

In the second generation six of 10 persons were definitely affected in varying degrees (two persons could not be examined).

Patient II-1 was 67 and had lost vision in her late forties. Vision was light perception and projection in both eyes. Both fundi showed striking loss of the entire pigment epithelium and choriocapillaris so that only the large vessels of the choroid were visible. There was secondary atrophy of the discs and slight attenuation of the vessels. The electroretinogram (ERG) was nonrecordable. This patient showed the most severe affection in this entire pedigree.

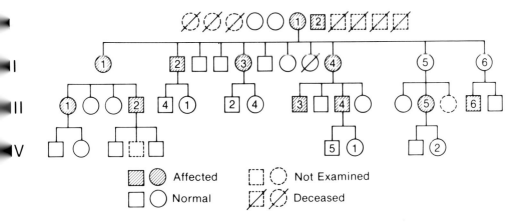

Fig. 14-1. Pedigree of family I with pattern dystrophy.

In contrast to patient II-1 was her brother (II-2) who was 57 years old with a vision of 20/20 OD and 20/25 OS. There were several subtle, pigmented spots grouped in a linear and branching pattern in both foveas. These spots consisted of faint yellow subretinal material with gray-pigmented centers in a dot-and-halo pattern (Fig. 14-2). There were also some yellow lesions near the temporal arcade in the left eye.

A 53-year-old sister (II-3) had 20/50 vision OD and 20/25 OS. Both fundi showed a striking stellate pattern of yellow, slightly atrophic pigment epithelial lesions centered in the foveas. Color vision was normal by AO pseudoisochromatic testing, and the ERG was normal. On fluorescein angiography certain portions of the stellate figure where the

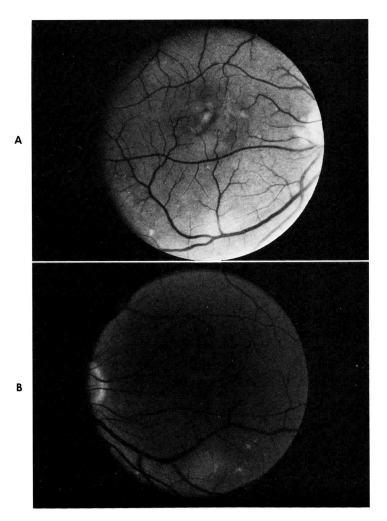

Fig. 14-2. Patient II-2. A 57-year-old man with subretinal grayish spots and surrounding pigment epithelial atrophy in both foveas. Note the yellow subretinal flecks in the left eye inferotemporally. **A,** Right eye (OD). **B,** Left eye (OS).

yellow subretinal lesions were most opaque were hypofluorescent. The atrophic areas were hyperfluorescent.

Another sister (II-4) was 63 years old and had experienced loss of central vision in the left eye at about age 60. Vision was 20/100 OD and 20/20 OS. Both fundi showed extensive atrophy of the retinal pigment epithelium and choriocapillaris, with only islands of intact pigment epithelium in both eyes. In the left eye and foveal pigment epithelium was intact (Fig. 14-3). The EOG showed an abnormality (1.40 OD and 1.38 OS).

A 55-year-old sister (II-5) had 20/25 vision OD and 20/70 OS. The pertinent findings were similar stellate patterns of linear yellow deposits centered on the fovea of both eyes. In addition, there were numerous pisciform, yellow, opaque, irregular deposits in the posterior pole and midperiphery. On fluorescein angiography these were hypofluorescent early and showed very faint late staining, except for the atrophic pigment epithelial lesions, which were hyperfluorescent throughout the angiogram. The EOG showed normal results for both eyes.

A 50-year-old sister (II-6) was the last in this generation of 10 persons to have subtle pigment epithelial lesions of the dot-and-halo type. Vision was normal.

There were 24 persons in the third generation, and all except one were examined. Six persons had fundi with pattern dystrophy.

Patient III-1 was a 45-year-old woman who had poor vision in her right eye since infancy. Vision was count-fingers at 2 feet OD and 20/20 OS. Both fundi showed striking and almost complete loss of the pigment epithelium and choriocapillaris, with only a few islands of intact pigment epithelium remaining. The patient refused further testing.

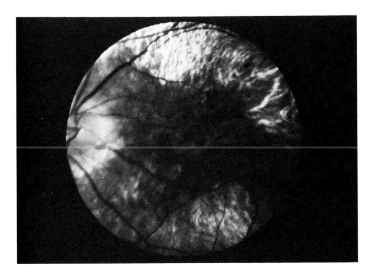

Fig. 14-3. Patient II-4. A 63-year-old woman with extensive atrophy of the pigment epithelium and choriocapillaris in both eyes (OU). Vision was 20/100 OD, 20/20 OS. A cataract precluded photographic presentation OD.

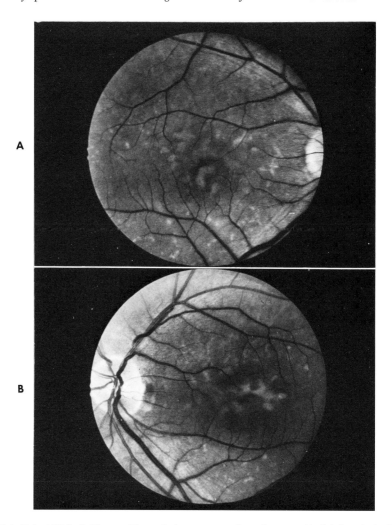

Fig. 14-4. Patient III-2. A 43-year-old man had numerous yellow-pigment epithelial deposits in the posterior poles OU. The foveal lesions were arranged in a linear pattern with some pigmentation. Vision was 20/20 OU. **A,** Right eye. **B,** Left eye.

A 43-year-old brother (III-2) had no visual complaints, and vision was 20/20 OU. Both fundi contained numerous atrophic, pale, yellow, irregular deposits in the retinal pigment epithelium, and they filled the entire posterior pole (Fig. 14-4). The foveal lesions had a branching pattern and were more atrophic with pigmented centers. The EOG showed an abnormality (1.3 OD and 1.4 OS). There was no significant color defect on Farnsworth-Munsell 100-hue testing. On angiography the deposits generally were hypofluorescent early and faintly hyperfluorescent in late stages (Fig. 14-5).

A 39-year-old brother (III-3) had no visual complaints, and vision was 20/15 OU.

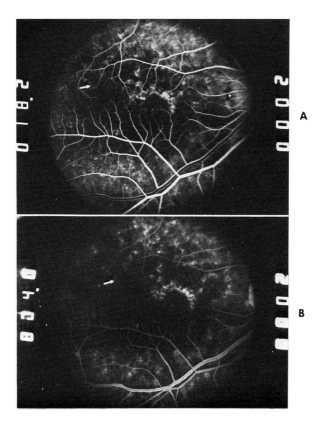

Fig. 14-5. Fluorescein angiogram of right eye of patient in Fig. 14-4. The atrophic foveal lesions are hyperfluorescent early, **A,** and stain late, **B.** Many parafoveal lesions are hypofluorescent early, **A,** *arrow,* and show faint late staining, **B,** *arrow.*

Both fundi contained small, opaque, irregular, yellow lesions with pigmented centers (dot-and-halo lesions) in the posterior pole and equator. On fluorescein angiography the lesions acted like window defects, with blocking corresponding to the central pigment.

A 45-year-old man (III-4) the fourth member of this generation also had 20/15 vision OD and 20/25 OS. Both fundi showed dot-and-halo lesions centered on the foveola of both eyes.

Two other members of this generation (patient III-5 and patient III-6) were 30 years old and 28 years old, respectively. Both had normal vision and similar irregularly opaque yellow deposits and atrophic dot-and-halo lesions in the posterior pole.

Nineteen of 28 members of the fourth generation were examined. All of these were younger than 17 years, and none had any evidence of a pathologic fundus.

Family 2

The second family was of German extraction and comprised four generations. There were 12 family members and all were examined (Fig. 14-6).

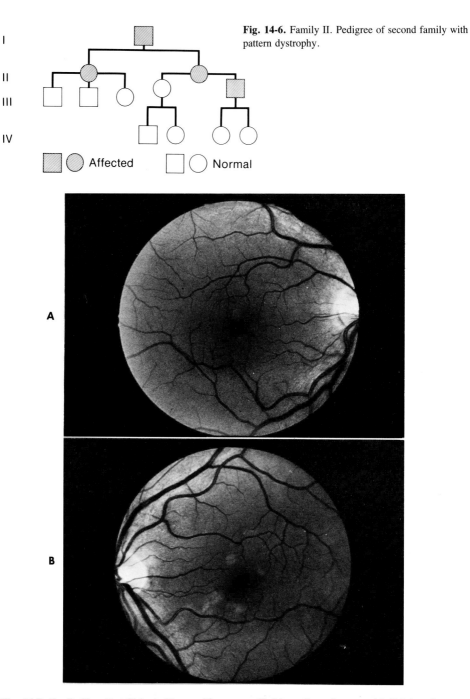

Fig. 14-7. Family II, patient II-1. A 46-year-old woman with faint yellow-pigment epithelial deposits parafoveally OU. **A,** Right eye. **B,** Left eye.

The first generation consisted of an 81-year-old man (I-1) who had had normal vision in his middle thirties. In his fifties he became unable to read. Vision was 20/750 OD and 20/500 OS. Both fundi had complete atrophy of the pigment epithelium and choriocapillaris in a symmetrically circular fashion centered on the fovea. The appearance was that of a central areolar choroidal dystrophy.

Both daughters were examined. One 46-year-old daughter (II-1) had no visual complaints and had 20/20 vision OU. Yet both fundi contained numerous linear, winged, and dotlike spots of increased pigmentation surrounded by halos of yellowish pigment epithelial atrophy (Fig. 14-7). The EOG showed normal results.

A 51-year-old woman (II-2) had vision of 20/30 OU. She was referred to Dr. Gass because of metamorphopsia. Both fundi showed striking stellate or butterfly-shaped lesions consisting of yellow subretinal masses arranged in a stellate fashion centered on the fovea. There were varying degrees of opaqueness, atrophy, and pigmentation. The material was subretinal.

There were five members of the third generation and only one was affected. This patient (III-1) was a 28-year-old man who had slight blurring of vision in his right eye. Vision was 20/20 OD and 20/15 OS. Both foveas contained dot-and-halo subretinal lesions at the level of the pigment epithelium. During an observation period of 1 year a new subretinal lesion appeared and enlarged just temporal to the right fovea. The EOG showed an abnormality (1.6 OD and 1.6 OS).

There were four members of the fourth generation, and none were older than 13 years. Vision and ocular examinations showed normal results.

DISCUSSION

These two families both broaden the spectrum of the pattern dystrophies and suggest a unified concept for the disease.

Patients with this condition have a basic lesion consisting of an opaque, yellow material situated at the level of the pigment epithelium. These lesions are 50 to 400 µm in diameter and irregularly oval in shape. They initially appear to be opaque but can show varying degrees of atrophy and pigmentation. They are frequently arranged in lines, and the lines may be arranged in a stellate, butterfly, winged, or reticulated configuration.

The opaque yellow lesions appear morphologically and angiographically identical with the flecks seen in fundus flavimaculatus and the subretinal yellow material in early stages of Best's disease. This similarity between fundus flavimaculatus, Best's disease, and the pattern dystrophies is reinforced by a recent report of a patient with a typical Best's vitelliform lesion in one eye and a butterfly pigment epithelial dystrophy of the fellow eye.[5]

I suggest as a working hypothesis that the pattern dystrophies, fundus flavimaculatus, and vitelliform dystrophy are caused by a basic metabolic defect in the pigment epithelial cells. This defect leads to an accumulation of an abnormal lipofuscin material within these enormously swollen cells. As groups of these cells enlarge and there is atrophy and loss of the pigment granules in such cells, this material becomes clinically evident as yellow, opaque lesions scattered about the posterior pole in various plaques, cysts, lines, and figures.

Angiographically this lipofuscin material blocks choroidal fluorescence, and the lesions are hypofluorescent. With progressive degeneration of the pigment epithelial cells, fluorescein stains these cells and they become hyperfluorescent.

In these two families there was a range of pigment epithelial changes from opaque yellow lesions to various degrees of pigment epithelial atrophy and loss of the choriocapillaris. If the process of accumulation of lipofuscin material, degeneration of the pigment epithelium, and secondary degeneration of overlying photoreceptors and choriocapillaris were to be progressive, we would expect some patients to lose vision in later life and to show the clinical findings of a retinal pigment epithelial atrophy and choriocapillaris atrophy. This was the case.

We do not know whether there is one or many enzyme deficiencies as the cause of the accumulation of this abnormal lipofuscin material in degenerating retinal pigment epithelial cells. Is the differentiation between the various forms of pattern dystrophy, fundus flavimaculatus, and vitelliform dystrophy only one of degree or is it attributable to specific enzyme defects? Many of these patients in later stages would be mistaken for senile macular degeneration, and only a family survey of this type could differentiate these lesions.

The causes of macular degeneration are so diverse that it is advantageous to separate out this group of macular dystrophies as a specific type characterized by lipofuscin accumulation within degenerative pigment epithelial cells and secondary loss of photoreceptors and choriocapillaris.

(Ocular findings from the examination of patient II-2 of family II were furnished by Dr. Gass.)

REFERENCES

1. Deutman, A.F., van Blommestein, J.D.A., Henkes, H.E., Waardenburg, P.J., and Solleveld van Driest, E.: Butterfly-shaped pigment dystrophy of the fovea Arch. Ophthalmol. **83:**558, 1970.
2. Eagle, R.C., Jr., Lucier, A.C., Bernardino, V.B., Jr., and Yanoff, M.: Retinal pigment epithelial abnormalities in fundus flavimaculatus: a light and electron microscopic study, Ophthalmology **87**(12):1189, 1980.
3. Forgacs, J., and Bozin, I.: Manifestation familiale de pigmentations groupées de la région maculaire, Ophthalmologica **152:**364, 1966.
4. Gass, J.D.M.: A clinicopathologic study of a peculiar foveomacular dystrophy, Trans. Am. Ophthalmol. Soc. **72:**150, 1974.
5. Gutman, I., Henkind, P., and Walsh, J.B.: Best's disease and butterfly-shaped dystrophy in an individual, Br. J. Ophthalmol. **66:**170-173, 1982.
6. Mesker, R.P., Oosterhuis, J.A., and Delleman, J.W.: A retinal lesion resembling Sjögren's dystrophia reticularis laminae pigmentosae retinae. In Winkelman, J.K., and Crone, R.A. editors: Perspectives in ophthalmology, Amsterdam, 1970, Excerpta Medica Foundation, vol. 2.
7. Sjögren, H.: Dystrophia reticularis laminae pigmentosae retinae, Acta Ophthalmol. **28:**279, 1950.
8. Slezak, H., and Hommer, K.: Fundus pulverulentus, Albrecht von Graefes Arch. Klin. Exp. Ophthalmol. **178:**177, 1969.
9. Weingeist, T.A., Kobrin, J.L., and Watzke, R.C.: Histopathology of Best's macular dystrophy, Arch. Ophthalmol. **100:**1108-1114, 1982.

15

Early treatment of trauma

D. Jackson Coleman

Because of the exquisite delicacy of ocular structures and the great variation in type and severity of ocular trauma and its sequelae, considerable variation in the approach to management is possible.

Roper-Hall[18] cogently summarized three critical areas in the salvage of eyes after trauma: (1) severity of trauma, (2) efficiency of early treatment, and (3) management of complications. We have no way of modifying the severity of the injury that presents to us, but we can modify treatment and reduce complications. The efficiency of early treatment is dependent on the techniques of surgery and the timing of intervention.

The techniques of intervention relate to two aspects: early and efficient diagnosis of the severity of the disease, and application of instrumentation and methodology that can be used to modify the effects of healing in ocular trauma.

DIAGNOSTIC TECHNIQUES

In the last decade we have seen the development of two imaging technologies that have resulted in significant improvement in diagnosis. These are ultrasonography to show soft tissue changes and computed tomography (CT scans) to show bone and orbital change as well as improved localization of intraocular foreign bodies. After any trauma, a plain x-ray film for the detection of the presence of foreign bodies is still recommended. Localization, once dependent on special techniques, such as Sweet's or Comberg-Pfeiffer localization, has now been largely supplanted by the use of computed tomography. CT views of the globe and orbit can allow quick identification of the presence of a foreign body and its location within or outside the globe and give a relatively precise estimate of its size (Fig. 15-1). Axial and special views can be included, and precise measurements from the foreign body to the cornea or the zygoma can be presented.[20] The presence of extraorbital damage is a major advantage offered by CT, since often unsuspected extraocular damage such as blow-out fracture or intracranial damage can be seen (Fig. 15-2).

Ultrasound offers a superb means of evaluating ocular soft-tissue changes.[6] Anterior segment disorders, such as hyphema, deepening of the angle, and suspected dialysis can be uniquely shown with ultrasound. Blood forming along the planes provided by the anterior hyaloid and zonules can outline these structures (Fig. 15-3) so that they are well appreciated, and defects can be noted. The presence of a dislocated lens (Fig. 15-4)

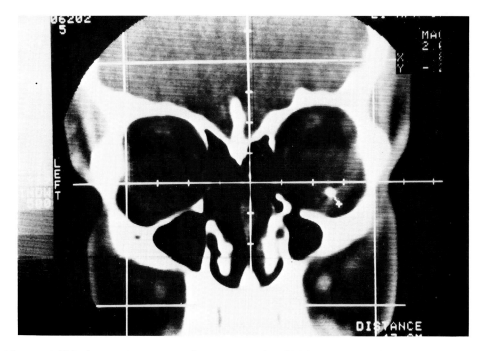

Fig. 15-1. Computed tomogram of a patient with a foreign body inferiorly in the left orbit. Different scan planes can be reconstructed for perspective advantages.

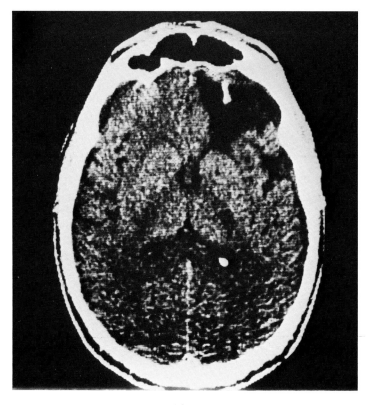

Fig. 15-2. Computed tomogram (CT) of a patient referred for a questionable ocular foreign body. CT scan showed atrophy of left frontal lobe. History revealed a penetration of periorbita with a wire coat hanger 20 years previously.

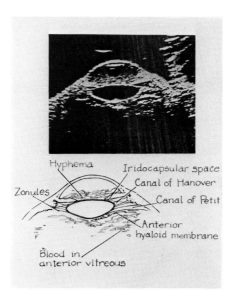

Fig. 15-3. Ultrasonogram of a traumatized eye showing hyphema and blood accentuation of lens-vitreous relationships. The deep anterior chamber and iris angles suggest iridodialysis, but none is seen in this section.

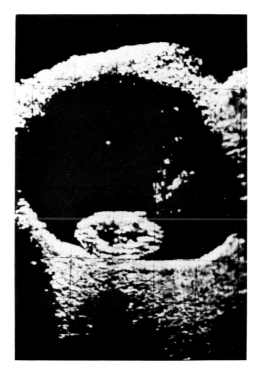

Fig. 15-4. Ultrasonogram of a traumatized eye with lens dislocated, appearing cataractous and resting on the posterior pole.

or of a posterior capsule rupture (Fig. 15-5) is often an indication for surgery and detection may thus determine or modify the surgical technique. The presence of retinal detachment is a most important contribution of ultrasonic diagnosis. Localized retinal disruption and traction forces are an important feature to evaluate and may be delineated with ultrasound (Fig. 15-6). Retinal detachment, combined with vitreous hemorrhage, is an indication for early vitreous surgery. Certainly, one of the most important contributions of ultrasound is the ability to determine the presence and position of foreign bodies relative to other ocular structures (Fig. 15-7). The magnetic properties of foreign bodies can be preoperatively determined when one observes their movement on A-, B-, or M-scan ultrasound in the presence of a magnetic field. Determining this will expedite preparation and procedures for foreign-body removal by alerting the surgeon for possible magnetic extraction.

Contusion injury that can produce severe vitreous hemorrhage usually does not produce structural damage of the type seen with laceration injuries or foreign-body perforations. Generally these cases have less immediacy for vitreous surgery. In addition, the presence of a thickened choroid (Fig. 15-8) identifiable by ultrasound may well be an indication for a further delay in surgery because of the greater possibility of hemorrhage during surgery. Even in cases where laceration or penetrating trauma has occurred and structural damage is seen, definitive vitreous surgery may well be deferred in the presence of choroidal thickening (Fig. 15-9). The concept of staged surgery can thus be related to evaluation of abnormal swelling or thickening of the choroid.

On the basis of a retrospective study of patients referred for ultrasonic diagnosis, prognostic values were extracted concerning eyes that would require vitreoretinal surgery for salvage.[5] The indications for surgical intervention are summarized in the following list. These criteria are the same as those proposed by Ryan[19] and form the basis of what would be regarded as severe ocular injury.

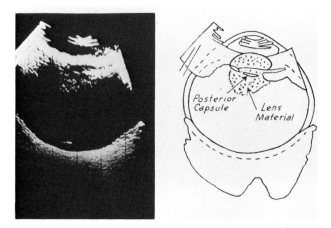

Fig. 15-5. Ultrasonogram of a traumatized eye with a rupture of the posterior lens capsule, which normally appears as a smooth, continuous line.

Indications for vitreous surgery after trauma
1. Vitreous incarceration in wound with either clear or opaque medium
2. Vitreous hemorrhage with retinal detachment
3. Severe vitreous hemorrhage with posterior lens rupture
4. Vitreous hemorrhage with retained reactive foreign body or retinal tear, or both
5. Vitreous hemorrhage with severe ciliary body laceration or posterior perforation, or both

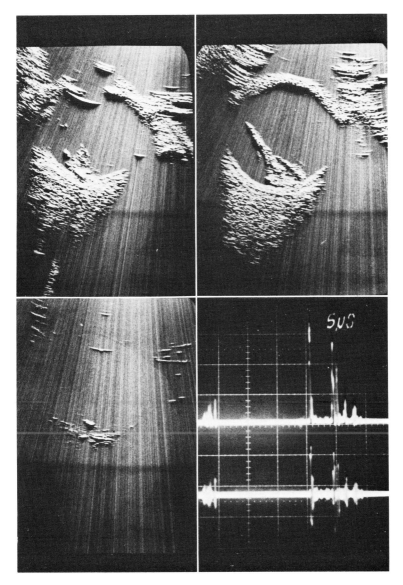

Fig. 15-6. Ultrasonogram of dense vitreous traction membranes surrounding an intraocular foreign body.

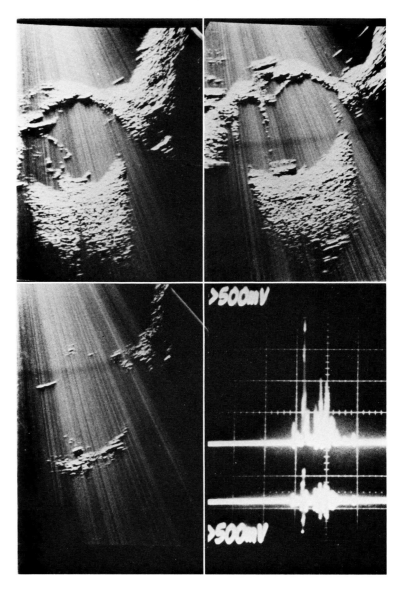

Fig. 15-7. Ultrasonogram of a penetrating injury with a foreign body that penetrated the lens and produced a posterior capsule rupture. The vitreous track is seen, and the relation of the foreign body to surrounding ocular structures is well seen.

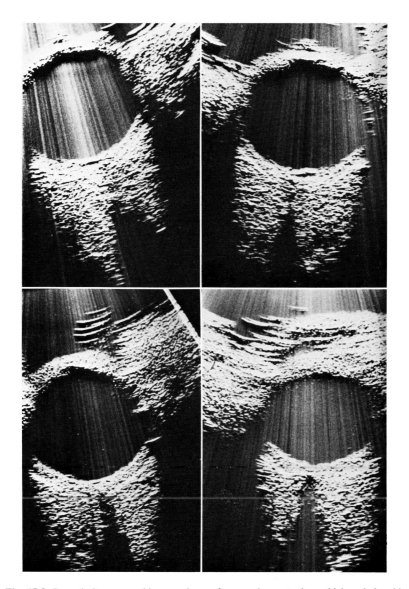

Fig. 15-8. Several ultrasonographic scan planes of an eye demonstrating a thickened choroid.

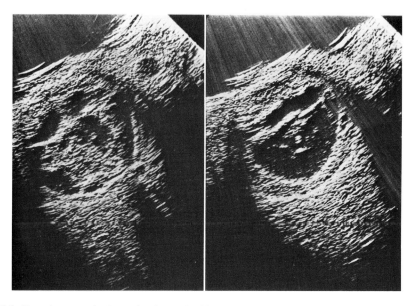

Fig. 15-9. Severely traumatized eye showing noticeable choroidal thickening, *right*. Accompanying vitreous hemorrhage and developing cyclitic membrane seen 1 week after injury, *left*.

TECHNIQUES OF SURGERY

Microsurgery and microsurgical instruments such as vitreous-suction cutting instruments have revolutionized our approach to surgical repair. The concept of closed, controlled vitreous removal based on the pioneering work of Kasner[11] and Machemer[14], has made major changes in our vitreous management techniques in the past decade. Cibis[1], Coles[9], Haik[10], Cleary[2], and Ryan et al.[3] have considered and demonstrated the mechanical traction and scaffolding effects of vitreous injury and proposed the need to disrupt traction membranes in order to preserve ciliary and epithelial function. At present, most surgical techniques stress closed surgical methods that are used within an intact globe. Thus immediate restoration of the integrity of the globe after trauma, always a prime consideration, remains of paramount importance in traumatic ocular emergencies.

Corneal wounds

The use of 10-0 nylon or Prolene sutures for closure of corneal wounds greatly reduces the chance of neovascularization of the cornea and allows us to proceed with vitreous surgery while maintaining corneal clarity immediately after injury. Healon can be used to reform the anterior chamber, facilitating corneal closure while maintaining intraocular volume and pressure and thus preventing ocular bleeding. Either Healon or air is also useful in bluntly removing lens material or lens capsule from the posterior corneal wound (Fig. 15-10). In the presence of lens rupture, Muga and Maul[16] have indicated the benefit of early removal of the ruptured lens, preferably at the time of initial repair. Ultrasound, if it indicates that the posterior lens capsule is intact, is useful

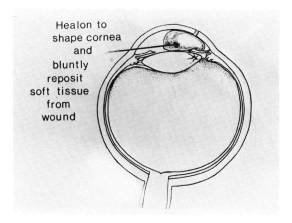

Fig. 15-10. Schematic drawing of injury similar to that in Fig. 15-7. The cornea is lacerated as well as the lens. Healon injection can reform the cornea, facilitating surgery, bluntly removing tissue traction from the posterior corneal injury, and reducing later adhesion and neovascularization.

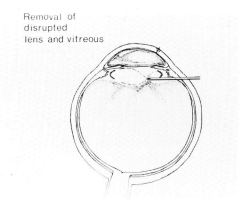

Fig. 15-11. Drawing of pars plana removal of cataract and anterior and posterior lens capsule.

when one is deciding whether a limbal or pars plana incision is of most value. When the posterior capsule is intact, we prefer a limbal incision with removal of the lens, using either a suction cutter or, in older individuals, a phakoemulsifier in order to preserve posterior capsule integrity. When the posterior capsule is ruptured and the vitreous compartment will need some degree of clearing, the pars plana incision is generally selected (Fig. 15-11). The use of a bimanual technique permits removal of the lens and capsule so that the vitreous compartment can be visualized. Transferring instruments can optimize cutter exposure to all areas of vitreous and optimize a variety of illumination techniques, such as direct, retro-, and "shadow" illumination to identify the ocular terrain.

Early surgical intervention allows clearing of vitreous blood clots while the remainder of the vitreous may still be clear and is easily cut and removed. It is important with intraocular foreign bodies to clear completely the vitreous compartment so that the site of a possible posterior retinal tear can be found and treated with endocryopexy, external cryopexy, or photocoagulation before the retina becomes detached.

Intraocular gas tamponade after vitrectomy can be of inestimable aid in repositioning or retaining the retina in the proper position and in helping to prevent choroidal engorgement during the postoperative period.

Foreign-body removal

Foreign bodies of reactive material such as iron and brass are generally regarded as toxic to the eye and therefore should usually be removed very quickly. Several routes of foreign-body removal are possible, including the limbal cornea, the pars plana, or direct sclera routes through the retina. The use of a pars plana incision in a closed technique with direct visualization of the foreign body offers many advantages, especially allowing the foreign body to be grasped with the appropriate instrument and removed under direct and controlled visualization. Magnetic foreign bodies, I believe, are best removed with the use of an intraocular magnet tip. Advantages of the intraocular magnet tip rest primarily in the fact that precise control of the foreign body can be exercised and there is less likelihood of incarceration of the choroid between foreign body and an externally applied magnet tip. Incarceration of the choroid may produce intraocular bleeding. In addition, since magnetic foreign bodies align themselves along their long axis in a magnetic field, the smallest diameter is thus presented to the wound and the least exit wound size and trauma can be afforded (Fig. 15-12). Nonmagnetic foreign bodies require manual removal and a slightly different surgical approach. Unusually shaped brass or wire fragments found in the eye are often difficult to remove while their smallest diameter is presented. When feasible, an attempt can often be made to reorient a foreign body once it is grasped while it is still in the vitreous, so that the smallest diameter is presented to the wound of exit. Regrettably, one may not always find this possible, and large exit wounds may result. Once a foreign body is removed from the eye, the exit wound should be quickly sutured closed so that reconstitution of globe pressure and a controlled intraocular pressure can be maintained. If further bleeding should become excessive at this point, intraocular evaluation can become difficult. We use intraocular gases to provide internal tamponade. A variety of gases have been made available to us for intraocular surgery, and they are of great value. In addition to air, Lincoff[12] has proposed the use of xenon and a number of perfluorocarbon gases, whereas Norton[17] and others have advocated the use of sulfur hexafluoride (SF_6) for maintaining intraocular volume. The advantage of these gases over air is that many of them expand postoperatively, thus aiding in internal tamponade. Lincoff[13] has described a series of gases that are absorbed at different rates, thus providing a menu for specific surgical needs.

Choroidal surgery

One of the more difficult problems facing trauma surgeons is the situation in which the choroid becomes massively engorged. Patients with expulsive choroidal hemorrhage during cataract extraction or with eyes that have progressed to hypotony after trauma are typical examples. In these situations, particularly if the retina becomes detached, routine methods of retinal repair are seriously impaired because of the inability to apply

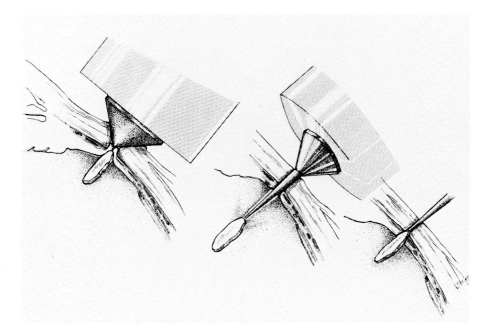

Fig. 15-12. An intraocular magnet tip has less pulling power, but this is compensated for by better control of foreign body removal. There is less chance of choroidal tearing from an incarcerated choroid between the foreign body and externally applied magnet. The foreign body aligns along its long axis for easy removal with the intraocular tip.

thermal injury to the pigment epithelium in order to provide appropriate scarring. In these situations, the use of staged chorioretinal surgery with controlled choroidal drainage is recommended. I advocate a technique of controlled drainage utilizing an intravitreal and a choroidal needle system. The advantage of this procedure over routine sclerotomy lies primarily in that an elevated intravitreal pressure provides a uniform pressure to the retina and tunica ruyschiana, thus reducing the chance of a sudden gush of fluid through an open sclerotomy, which in turn produces scleral apposition of the tunica ruyschiana and consequent failure to drain adequately the entire suprachoroidal space. With a controlled drain, a slow pressure reduces the chances of renewed choroidal bleeding and allows a maximized evacuation of the choroidal volume. A blood clot may not easily be removed with this method, but by the use of reverse flushing most of the hemorrhagic material can be removed.

Ultrasound evaluation during surgery is of great value in determining the progress and degree of choroidal drainage. The prevention of retina-to-retina apposition is the major surgical objective in these situations. After choroidal decompression, the vitreous volume can be augmented with expanding gas to put the globe in a ''holding'' situation while healing proceeds over several days and, one would hope, normal physiologic clearing of the vitreous continues. Normally, 1 to 2 weeks after initial choroidal drainage, a second procedure can be employed using conventional retinal surgical techniques.

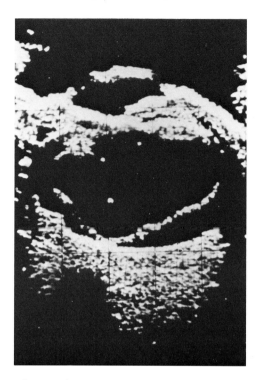

Fig. 15-13. Ultrasonogram of a severely traumatized eye showing prephthisic signs of shortened anteroposterior length, cyclitic membrane, and thickened choroid. Removal of the cyclitic membrane can allow retinal detachment surgery and improved visual recovery in a significant number of these patients.

Cyclitic membranes

After injury, many eyes are lost because of the development of cyclitic membranes that are formed in response to injury of the nonpigmented ciliary epithelium. In much the same manner that the retinal pigment epithelium can undergo transformation into migrating fibroblasts as outlined by Machemer[15], the nonpigmented ciliary epithelium also can be transformed. Interruption of the mechanical stress in these situations is essential to allow continued function of the ciliary body. Cyclitic membranes can develop relatively rapidly and are a major cause of the hypotonous state that we have described as prephthisic. The ultrasonic criteria of the prephthisic eye include (1) shortened anteroposterior length, (2) thickened choroid, and (3) presence of cyclitic membrane.[7] These three changes seen in eyes evaluated with ultrasound (Fig. 15-13) have invariably progressed to phthisis. Surgical interruption of cyclitic membranes allows many of these eyes to be salvaged.

TIMING OF SURGERY

The second major facet of the efficiency of early surgery relates to the time and extent of early surgical intervention. There are presently two prevailing views on the optimum time for vitreous intervention. The first view recommends vitreous surgery as part of the primary repair or secondarily within 72 hours, if possible, to reduce complications from inflammation.[4] The second view recommends such surgery after 72 hours to reduce complications of recurrent hemorrhage.[15a,19] Similar indications are ascribed in both views, and there is also general agreement recommending prompt primary closure of lacerated globes. Although aggressive surgical intervention of the vitreous is certainly not indicated in all trauma, I believe that cases of severe injury as outlined on p. 181 should be considered for early surgery. In evaluating a series of 112 consecutive patients of my own with severe trauma, I found that 23 eyes were operated on within the first 72 hours. When compared to globes with similar injuries operated on at later intervals, I found a better chance of good visual recovery (20/20 to 20/40) when early intervention was utilized, rather than when delayed repair was preferable or unavoidable.[4] The following list compares the advantages of early versus deferred surgery:

Reasons for immediate definitive surgery
1. Technically easier removal of damaged lens and vitreous
2. Good corneal transparency
3. Earlier detection of occult retinal damage
4. Less secondary inflammation
5. Not all vitreous requires removal
6. Better statistical prognosis

Reasons for deferred surgery
1. Thorough evaluation may not be possible
2. Surgical equipment may not be available
3. Surgical and operating room staff may not be optimal
4. Other injuries may take precedence
5. Bleeding may be better controlled
6. Vitreous retraction may make vitrectomy technically easier

Many other trauma surgeons recommend a delay between primary repair and definitive vitreoretinal surgery, believing that advantages of possible retraction of the vitreous from the posterior retina may be obtained and that the chance of recurrent hemorrhage will be reduced.[19] There is no question that recurrent hemorrhage can be a serious problem. Serious hemorrhage can be encountered at any time,[1a] and no one knows yet how to predetermine this eventuality. For now, my recommendation is for immediate lensectomy and vitrectomy when the lens has been ruptured. I also prefer an immediate vitrectomy when the retina is detached and there is a strong suspicion that a posterior retinal tear has been created by an intraocular foreign body. Should severe vitreous bleeding be encountered, I believe that the use of intraocular gas tamponade offers no greater risk than would have been obtained by delaying. In cases where posterior perforations are present, no foreign body remains in the eye, and the retina remains in place, there may be an advantage to treating the eye conservatively because there is often severe choroidal "contusion" injury. With an ultrasonically demonstrable thickening of the choroid, a delay may be preferable if the lens is intact and the retina is in place. I like to suture posterior perforations that are easily accessible, but those that occur directly at the posterior pole are not easily sutured and it is probably preferable to leave them for natural closure. A schematic representation of early versus delayed surgery in terms of time "windows" is shown in Fig. 15-14.

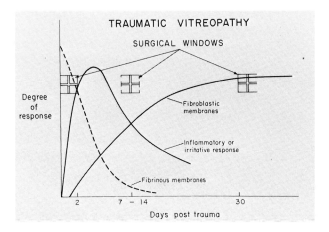

Fig. 15-14. Schematic drawing of traumatic vitreopathy after trauma, indicating the three significant "windows" for surgery after injury: immediate; 3 to 7 days after injury; delayed. (From Coleman, D.J.: Am. J. Ophthalmol. **93:**543, 1982.)

SUMMARY

Modern diagnostic techniques have allowed surgeons to evaluate the traumatized eye far more efficiently and knowledgeably than in the past. Thus we are able to make decisions as to the need for vitreous surgery very quickly after injury. Modern technology has kept pace with our diagnostic advances, providing us with instrumentation and techniques to remove vitreous hemorrhage and membranes, treat retinal tears, and remove foreign bodies in an efficient, controlled manner. The concept of controlled removal of vitreous scaffolds, controlled treatment of retinal injury, and controlled drainage of choroidal hemorrhage are the most recent advances in the management of ocular trauma. Intraocular gas and vitreous substitutes allow us to stabilize the retina and tunica ruyschiana so that later definitive retinal surgery can be performed. The concept of staged choriovitreoretinal surgery has thus evolved. In my opinion, in those cases of severe injury where vitrectomy is indicated, early intervention within the first 72 hours is preferable to a delay of 3 to 14 days. When there is ultrasonic and clinical evidence of choroidal thickening however, there is a greater likelihood for recurrent hemorrhage, and here it may be preferable to delay vitreous surgery to this second "window"—at 3 to 14 days.

REFERENCES

1a. Brinton, G.S., et al.: Surgical results in ocular trauma involving the posterior segment, Am. J. Ophthalmol. **93:**271-278, 1982.
1. Cibis, P.: Vitreoretinal pathology and surgery in retinal detachment, St. Louis, 1965, The C.V. Mosby Co.
2. Cleary, P., and Ryan, S.: Histology of wound, vitreous, and retina in experimental posterior penetrating eye injury in the rhesus monkey, Am. J. Ophthalmol. **88:**221, 1979.
3. Coleman, D.J.: The role of vitrectomy in traumatic vitreopathy, Trans. Am. Acad. Ophthalmol. Otolaryngol. **81:**406-413, 1976.
4. Coleman, D.J.: Early vitrectomy in the management of the severely traumatized eye, Am. J. Ophthalmol. **93:**543-551, 1982.

5. Coleman, D.J., and Franzen, L.A.: Vitreous surgery: preoperative evaluation and prognostic value of ultrasonic display of vitreous hemorrhage, Arch. Ophthalmol. **92:**375-379, 1974.

6. Coleman, D.J., Lizzi, F.L., and Jack, R.L.: Ultrasonography of the eye and orbit, Philadelphia 1977, Lea & Febiger.

7. Coleman, D.J.: Indications and techniques of surgery of the pre-phthisical eye, Presented at the Retina Society meeting, Houston, Texas, 1978.

8. Coleman, D.J., and Weininger, R.: Ultrasonic M-mode technique in ophthalmology, Arch. Ophthalmol. **82:**475, 1969.

9. Coles, W., and Haik, G.M.: Vitrectomy in intraocular trauma: its rationale and its indications and limitation, Arch. Ophthalmol. **87:**621, 1972.

10. Haik, G.M., and Coles, W.: Intraocular injuries: their immediate surgical management, Philadelphia, 1972, Lea & Febiger.

11. Kasner, D.: Vitrectomy: a new approach to the management of vitreous, Highlights Ophthalmol. **11:**304, 1968.

12. Lincoff, H., and Kressig, I.: Intravitreal behavior of perfluorocarbons. In Blankenship, G., Daicker, B., Gailloud, C., et al., editors: Current concepts in diagnosis and treatment of vitreoretinal diseases, vol. 2 of Straub, W., series editor: Developments in ophthalmology, Basel, 1981, S. Karger AG.

13. Lincoff, H., Mardirossian, J., Lincoff, A., Liggett, P., Iwamoto, T., and Jakobiec, F.: Intravitreal longevity of three perfluorocarbon gases, Arch. Ophthalmol. **98:**1610-1611, 1980.

14. Machemer, R.: (1) A new concept for vitreous surgery; (2) Surgical technique and complications, Am. J. Ophthalmol. **74:**1022, 1972.

15. Machemer, R.: Massive periretinal proliferation: a logical approach to therapy, Trans. Am. Ophthalmol. Soc. **75:**556, 1978.

15a. Michels, R.G.: Vitreous surgery, St. Louis, 1981, The C.V. Mosby Co.

16. Muga, R., and Maul, E.: The management of lens damage in perforating corneal lacerations, Br. J. Ophthalmol. **62:**784, 1978.

17. Norton, E.W.D.: Intraocular gas in the management of selected retinal detachments, Trans. Am. Acad. Ophthalmol. Otolaryngol. **77:**85-98, 1973.

18. Roper-Hall, M.J.: A retrospective study of eye injuries, Ophthalmologica **158:**12, 1969.

19. Ryan, S., and Allen, A.: Pars plana vitrectomy in ocular trauma, Am. J. Ophthalmol. **88:**483, 1979.

20. Trokel, S.L.: Radiologic evaluation of ophthalmologic trauma. In Freeman, H.M., editor: Ocular trauma, New York, 1979, Appleton-Century-Crofts.

16

Current concepts in retrolental fibroplasia

Arnall Patz

Retrolental fibroplasia (RLF) was first identified by Terry in 1942.[21] In recent years, many investigators have elected to use the term "retinopathy of prematurity" (ROP) for this disorder of the premature infant retina. After Terry's identification of retrolental fibroplasia in the early 1940s, isolated case reports of this disorder appeared in the medical literature. By the late 1940s, RLF had reached epidemic proportions and became the leading cause of child blindness in the United States. Many pediatricians who were involved in the care of the premature infant during the late 1940s and early 1950s have looked back to determine the reasons for the liberal use of oxygen that came into popular use during the late 1940s. Graham and co-workers[7] demonstrated that irregular, almost Cheyne-Stokes-like respirations are common in the samll premature infant shortly after birth. These investigators observed that increasing the oxygen concentration inhaled led to more regular breathing. It was naturally assumed that a more regular respiration was more healthy and physiologic, and it was also recognized that the small premature infant who had episodes of cyanosis might be protected from these episodes of cyanosis and periodic apnea known to occur in small infants. The closed incubator that was developed permitted the administration of a higher concentration of oxygen. The common practice of administering oxygen routinely to small premature infants purely because of prematurity became a standard practice in many nurseries. With the closed incubator systems, high concentrations of ambient oxygen in the range of 60 to 70 percent were readily achieved. It is of interest that when we initiated our controlled clinical trial of the role of oxygen on RLF[15] most nurseries rarely measured the actual concentration of oxygen in the incubator but simply recorded the number of liters of flow from the oxygen tank or wall source of oxygen. It was generally believed that ambient oxygen inhalation had little, if any, side effects. The recognition that oxygen can be lifesaving at times for the premature infant with severe cyanosis led to the widespread adoption of routine high oxygen concentrations throughout many major nurseries in this country.

EARLY STUDIES ON OXYGEN

Campbell[4] first suggested that the overuse of oxygen might be responsible for the development of RLF based on retrospective studies conducted in Melbourne, Australia. The first controlled clinical trial implicating the role of oxygen in RLF was reported in

1952,[15] and the experimental production of RLF was achieved in experimental animals in 1953.[2,15] The cooperative nursery study on oxygen involving 18 hospitals in the United States was reported in preliminary form in 1955.[11] The collaborative study gave final documentation to the etiologic role of oxygen in RLF.

The precise mechanism of oxygen damage to the premature retina is still not fully understood. Ashton and co-workers[2,3] have best elucidated this mechanism. Studies conducted on kittens indicated that the incomplete vascularization of the retina was fundamental to the RLF experimental lesion; the fully vascularized retina showed no injury. The response of the immature retinal vasculature was directly proportional to the duration of oxygen administration and to the concentration of oxygen used, and it was inversely proportional to the degree of maturity of the retina. Experimental production of RLF in mice, kittens, and puppies[16] demonstrated the common susceptibility of the immature retina to oxygen.

MECHANISM OF OXYGEN EFFECTS ON PREMATURE RETINA

From experimental observations, the oxygen response of the immature retina can be conveniently divided into two distinct stages: The *primary* stage, seen with prolonged inspiration of oxygen, involves closure of the most immature retinal vascular complexes, which are the most anterior; normal vascularization of the retina anteriorward toward the retinal periphery is then halted during oxygen exposure. The *secondary* stage, which occurs upon return to ambient air, involves those retinal vessels not totally destroyed; they undergo vasoproliferation with a classical picture of retinal neovascularization (Figs. 16-1 to 16-3). The new vessels erupt through the internal limiting membrane in a form of intravitreal neovascularization. Further progression of the retinopathy beyond this stage depends on the degree of hemorrhage and subsequent traction on the new vessels by the cortical vitreous (Fig. 16-4). The end stage of total detachment and disorganization of the retina with the retina adjacent to the posterior lens capsule prompted Terry's designation of the condition as "retrolental fibroplasia."

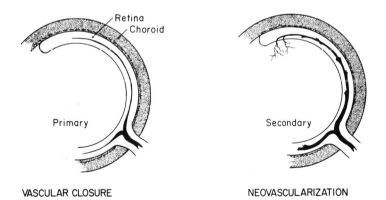

Fig. 16-1. Schematic diagram of the effect of oxygen on the incompletely vascularized retina in retrolental fibroplasia. *Left,* The most anterior or immature vascular complexes are closed after a moderate exposure to oxygen. *Right,* Retinal neovascularization immediately adjacent to the areas of vascular closure develops after removal to room air.

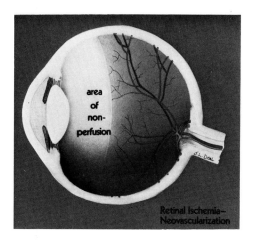

Fig. 16-2. The anterior temporal periphery containing the most immature vessels is selectively closed, resulting in nonperfusion.

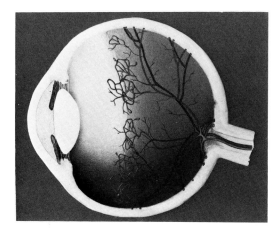

Fig. 16-3. Neovascularization results at the zone of vascularized retina and ischemic or nonperfusing retina.

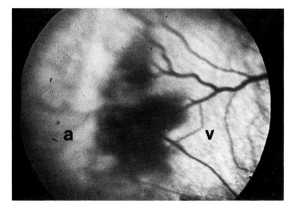

Fig. 16-4. Fundus photograph of infant with active proliferative retrolental fibroplasia involving the temporal periphery. Overlying hemorrhage has resulted from the retinal neovascularization. *v,* Vascularized retina; *a,* avascular anterior retina.

During the secondary stage of retinal neovascularization, fluorescein angiography shows dye leakage, and focal hemorrhages occur. We have demonstrated by fluorescein angiography in newborn kittens that the location and degree of vascular closure usually, but not invariably, determines the locus of the secondary neovascularization; for example, after 24 hours of oxygen at 50% to 60% oxygen inhalation, only anterior vessels are initially closed and the secondary neovascularization is in the anterior periphery, frequently temporally. With prolonged high concentrations of oxygen, such as 7 days at 80% concentration, parts of the entire retinal vascular bed were frequently closed, and this closure leads to disc neovascularization on removal to air. In these latter cases, the retina never revascularized normally after returning to room air, with multiple fine twigs of vessels in the posterior pole developing in the peripapillary area.

RECENT STUDIES

With the advent of fluorescein angiography and its wide usage during the past decade, retrolental fibroplasia has been studied along with the other major proliferative retinopathies. We have used fluorescein angiography extensively in the animal model, and Flynn and co-workers[6] have greatly improved our understanding of RLF pathogenesis by its use in human RLF.

Common to each of the proliferative retinopathies, such as diabetic retinopathy, retrolental fibroplasia, sickle cell retinopathy, and the neovascularization occurring after branch vein occlusion, the vascular closure generally precedes the development of retinal neovascularization. The vascular closure, demonstrated on fluorescein angiography, is believed to lead to retinal ischemia. Consistent with the earlier concept of Michaelson[12] and Ashton,[3] retinal ischemia is presumed to liberate a vasoproliferative or angiogenic substance, which stimulates the development of neovascularization. This hypothesis remains to be documented; however, the clinical and experimental findings are consistent with this working hypothesis.

In the experimental model of RLF, the initial vasoconstriction is believed to lead to ultimate vascular closure, particularly of the capillary bed. Recent studies by Flower et al.[5] suggest that retinal vasoconstriction may possibly be a physiologic mechanism to protect the immature retina from the damaging effects of increased oxygen concentrations. These investigators suggest that the vasoconstriction observed in the premature infant exposed to oxygen may be only an extreme of the normal physiologic response by which retinal blood flow is modulated during in utero development of the retinal vasculature. They suggest that it is conceivable that the susceptibility of the eye to oxygen associated retinopathy after birth depends on the extent to which the vasoconstrictive response is functional, taking into account that the immaturity of the retina is still fundamental to the response to oxygen. These investigators made these observations when they found that oxygen-treated young bealges had more significant final damage when vasoconstriction was inhibited by the combined breathing of a mixture of carbon dioxide and oxygen. Flower et al.[5] reasoned that retinal vasoconstriction may be more a protective response than a pathologic process in response to hyperoxia. They suggested that since more severe RLF was produced when oxygen-treated beagles also had carbon dioxide, which inhibited the vasoconstriction response, the retinal vascular damage may result primarily from cytotoxic effects of oxygen on endothelial cells, rather than secondarily to the vasoconstriction and diminished blood flow that was postulated as a possibility by Ashton and Pedler.[1] Thus, if the retinal vascular channels were dilated while the increased blood-oxygen levels were present, the endothelial vessel wall would be in contact with the presumed oxygen-toxic radicals, which are known to damage cell membranes.

CURRENT INCIDENCE OF RLF

In the past decade, a moderate increase in the incidence of RLF in the United States has occurred. This probably is attributable to modern neonatology practices, which have resulted in a striking reduction in small premature infant mortality. For example, Phelps[17] has indicated that the survival rate of infants weighing under 1 kg at birth has risen from 8% in 1950 to approximately 35% in 1980. The survival rate of these small premature infants with a birth weight under 1000 g in the Johns Hopkins Neonatology Unit is the in 40% to 50% range, a rate suggesting that Phelps' calculations are a conservative estimate. It is these extremely small infants that have the greatest susceptibility to RLF. A fourfold to fivefold increase in survival of these infants is significant, since during the epidemic years these extremely low birth weight infants would not have survived long enough to develop the disease. Furthermore, more cases of early active or proliferative RLF are being diagnosed currently, utilizing indirect ophthalmoscopy, which was not generally available during the epidemic of the early 1950s.

With the survival of the high-risk, low birth weight infants, RLF is occurring despite the most meticulous monitoring of oxygen therapy by precise blood-gas monitoring. It would seem that prematurity by itself may be responsible for most of the current cases of RLF, in contrast to the overuse of oxygen being the major cause 3 decades ago.

ANTIOXIDANTS IN RLF: ALPHA-TOCOPHEROL (VITAMIN E)

The use of vitamin E was first advocated in the prevention of RLF by Owens and Owens.[13] Although their initial controlled studies showed a protective effect in the prevention of RLF, these observations were not repeatable in the early 1950s because other investigators tested the prophylactic use of vitamin E for RLF. Its use was gradually discontinued once oxygen was incriminated in the early 1950s.

The rationale of therapy by Owens and Owens was based on the known deficiency in alpha-tocopherol in small premature infants and the experimental findings in animals of cerebral degeneration that developed in experimental vitamin E–deficient animals. At the time of the Owens' nursery studies, the role of *oxygen* in RLF was unknown and the possible "antioxidant" protective effect of vitamin E was not considered. Some 20 years later Johnson and co-workers initiated a nursery study utilizing alpha-tocopherol acetate by parenteral injection as a possible prophylactic agent in the prevention and also treatment of early active RLF.[10,20] Phelps and Rosenbaum,[18] utilizing the experimental RLF model in kittens, demonstrated an apparent protective effect of large doses of parenteral vitamin E on the experimental lesion. Johnson and her co-workers and Phelps and co-workers are at present conducting controlled clinical trials in the nursery to test the prophylactic role of vitamin E administration on RLF.

Recently, Puklin and co-workers[19] reported on a controlled clinical trial involving 100 neonates who received intramuscular vitamin E injection. These infants received vitamin E during the acute phase of therapy for the respiratory distress syndrome. Intramuscular doses were administered twice weekly to these infants as long as they remained in an oxygen-enriched environment and could not tolerate feedings and vitamin supplements by mouth. Control infants received intramuscular phacebo injections. There was no difference noted in the incidence of retrolental fibroplasia between the infants receiving vitamin E injections and their controls. The mean level of serum vitamin E in treated infants was significantly elevated over controls. For example, after 1 week the serum E level in those infants receiving intramuscular vitamin E was 3.9 mg/dl in contrast to the placebo group with 0.8 mg/dl.

Hittner and co-workers[9] reported the results of a controlled clinical trial on the efficacy of 100 mg/kg of vitamin E orally administered daily from birth on retrolental fibroplasia in infants who had the respiratory distress syndrome. Control infants received 5 mg/kg. Plasma vitamin E levels in those infants on high oral doses of vitamin E averaged approximately 1.2 mg/dl, whereas the control group averaged approximately 0.6 mg/dl.

Using multivariate analysis, Hittner and co-workers reported that the severity of RLF was found to be significantly reduced in those infants who received large doses of vitamin E. Hillis[8] raised questions on the data analysis in Hittner's report and suggested that more data would be required to make definitive recommendations on the use of large doses of vitamin E. Hillis cautioned that large doses of vitamin E, just as the high concentrations of oxygen administered in the 1950s, might have as yet unrecognized side effects. It would seem appropriate at this time to await the larger controlled clinical trials that are in progress by Johnson and co-workers and Phelps and co-workers, as well as further observations from Hittner and co-workers, before one draws final conclusions on the efficacy of large doses of vitamin E on either the prevention, reduction in severity, or therapy of active RLF.

Palmer[14] addressed the question of optimal time for examining the premature infant to detect active proliferative RLF. His nursery study data revealed that if only a single examination is to be made, the most productive time for that examination would be between 7 and 9 weeks of age. This would allow the detection of the majority of active proliferative RLF cases, and the likelihood that the disease would develop subsequently when the examination was found normal at this time was considered small.

SUMMARY

The role of oxygen in retrolental fibroplasia is summarized. Newer studies further elucidating the mechanism of oxygen action are briefly discussed. The current status of the potential role of the antioxidant vitamin E in prevention of retrolental fibroplasia is updated. The recent increase in RLF cases observed in recent years probably results from the improved survival of the extremely low birth weight infants made possible by modern neonatalogy practices.

REFERENCES

1. Ashton, N., and Pedler, C.: Studies on developing retinal vessels. IX. Reaction of endothelial cells to oxygen, Br. J. Ophthalmol. **46:**247, 1962.
2. Ashton, N., Ward, B., and Serpell, G.: Role of oxygen in the genesis of retrolental fibroplasia: preliminary report, Br. J. Ophthalmol. **37:**513, 1953.
3. Ashton, N., Ward, B., and Serpell, G.: Effect of oxygen on developing retinal vessels with particular reference to the problem of retrolental fibroplasia, Br. J. Ophthalmol. **38:**397, 1954.
4. Campbell, K.: Intensive oxygen therapy as a possible cause of retrolental fibroplasia: a clinical approach, Med. J. Aust. **2:**48-50, July 1951.
5. Flower, R.W., Hall, M.O., and Patz, A.: Oxygen. In Sears, M., editor: Handbook of experimental pharmacology: pharmacology of the eye, New York, 1982, Springer Publishing Co., Inc.

6. Flynn, J.T., O'Grady, G.E., Herrera, J., Kushner, B.J., et al.: Retrolental fibroplasia. I. Clinical observations, Arch. Ophthalmol. **95**(2):217-223, Feb. 1977.
7. Graham, B.D., Reardon, H.S., Wilson, J.L., Tsao, M., and Bauman, M.L.: Physiologic and chemical response of premature infants to oxygen-enriched atmosphere, Pediatrics **6**:55, 1950.
8. Hillis, A., Vitamin E in retrolental fibroplasia, N. Engl. J. Med. **306**:867, 1982 (Correspondence).
9. Hittner, H.M., Godio, L.B., Rudolph, A.J., et al.: Retrolental fibroplasia: efficacy of vitamin E in a double-blind clinical study of preterm infants, N. Engl. J. Med. **305**:1365-1371, 1981.
10. Johnson, L., Schaffer, D., and Boggs, T.R.: The premature infant, vitamin E deficiency and retrolental fibroplasia, Am. J. Clin. Nutr. **27**:1158-1173, 1974.
11. Kinsey, V.E., and Hemphill, F.M.: Etiology of retrolental fibroplasia and preliminary report of cooperative study of retrolental fibroplasia, Trans. Am. Acad. Ophthalmol. **59**:15, 1955.
12. Michaelson, I.C.: Retinal circulation in man and animals, Springfield, Ill., 1954, Charles C Thomas, Publisher.
13. Owens, W.C., and Owens, E.U.: Retrolental fibroplasia in premature infants: studies on prophylaxis of disease: use of alpha-tocopherol acetate, Am. J. Ophthalmol. **32**:1631-1637, Dec. 1949.
14. Palmer, E.A.: Optimal timing of examination for acute retrolental fibroplasia, Ophthalmology **88**:662-668, 1981.
15. Patz, A., Hoeck, L.E., and de la Cruz, E.: Studies on the effect of high oxygen administration in retrolental fibroplasia: nursery observations, Am. J. Ophthalmol. **35**:1248, 1952.
16. Patz, A., Eastham, A., Higgenbotham, D.H., and Kleh, T.: Oxygen studies in retrolental fibroplasia: production of the microscopic changes of retrolental fibroplasia in experimental animals, Am. J. Ophthalmol. **36**:1511, 1953.
17. Phelps, D.L.: Vision loss due to retinopathy of prematurity, Lancet **1**(8220):606, March 1981 (Letter to editor).
18. Phelps, D.L., and Rosenbaum, A.L.: Vitamin E in kitten oxygen-induced retinopathy. II. Blockage of vitreal neovascularization, Arch. Ophthalmol. **97**:1522-1526, 1979.
19. Puklin, J.E., Simon, R.M., and Ehrenkranz, R.A.: Influence on retrolental fibroplasia of intramuscular vitamin E administration during respiratory distress syndrome, Ophthalmology **89**:96-102, 1982.
20. Schaffer, D.B., and Johnson, L.: A classification of retrolental fibroplasia to evaluate vitamin E therapy, Ophthalmology **86**:1749-1760, 1979.
21. Terry, T.L.: Extreme prematurity and fibroblastic overgrowth of persistent vascular sheath behind each crystalline lens. I. Preliminary report, Am. J. Ophthalmol. **25**:203-204, Feb. 1942.

17

Behçet's disease

G. Richard O'Connor

The ocular form of Behçet's disease is fortunately a rare cause of uveitis among individuals seen in the United States and Canada. In the main, it affects individuals of Oriental or Mediterranean background. Behçet's disease represents no more than 0.2% of Schlaegel's large series[31] of uveitis cases surveyed in 1977 and no more than 0.4% of our own series of uveitis cases at the University of California.

Despite its rarity, the disease deserves additional attention because it has an almost uniformly bad prognosis. The acute anterior uveitis that ushers in the disease may respond well to corticosteroid medication, but the occlusive retinal vasculitis that almost invariably accompanies the later stages of the disease may be refractory to corticosteroid therapy. Eventually the occlusive disease of the retinal vessels may be complicated by hemorrhage, and massive vitreous opacity may result.

The material of this paper has been gleaned from (1) a study of our own 28 patients at the Uveitis Survey Clinic of the Proctor Foundation in whom a "definite" or "probable" diagnosis of Behçet's disease was made, (2) a review of recent world literature on this subject, and (3) a personal study of the histopathologic features of the ocular and cerebral manifestations of the disease.

Our criteria for diagnosis are essentially the same as those of Shimizu[34] and are based on the recommendations of the Behçet's Disease Research Committee of Japan.[3] The major signs of Behçet's disease are said to consist of recurrent aphthous ulcerations of the mouth (Fig. 17-1), skin lesions, eye lesions, and genital ulcerations. The minor signs consist of arthritic changes, gastrointestinal lesions, epididymitis, systemic vascular lesions, and central nervous system involvement. In the complete type of Behçet's disease, all four of the major lesions can be documented. In the incomplete type ("probable" diagnosis), three of the four major lesions can be documented, or the patient will be found to have eye disease plus one of the other major lesions. As stated above, the ophthalmic form of Behçet's disease is relatively rare in the United States. Furthermore, most of our cases represent the "incomplete" form of the disease ("probable" Behçet's disease).

One of the major questions to be answered is the following: "Is Behçet's disease an Oriental disease?" If one judges from the fact that over half of our group of patients with ophthalmic Behçet's disease are of white (principally northern European) origin, the answer is likely to be no. However, the answer must be modified by other consid-

199

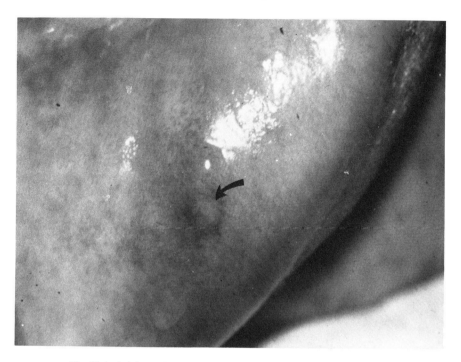

Fig. 17-1. Aphthous ulcer of the tongue in a patient with Behçet's disease.

erations. Approximately half of our white group of patients had the HLA antigen B5, and Lehner and Batchelor[18] reported the presence of HLA B5 in 8 out of 16 British (white) patients with the ocular form of the disease ($p = 0.0002$).

In virtually every study of Behçet's disease the importance of HLA B5 in the ocular form emerges. Is it an Oriental gene? Ohno et al.[27] showed that it was present in 72% of Japanese males with the complete type of Behçet's disease and in 62% of patients (of both sexes) with uveitis. These figures are to be contrasted with 55% incidence of B5 positivity among Japanese patients with the nonocular forms of Behçet's disease and with a 28% incidence of B5 among Japanese patients with eye disease unrelated to uveitis. It also emerges in Bloch-Michel's[4] and Rosselet's[29] studies of Behçet's disease among French patients and in Sanders'[30] study of ophthalmic Behçet's disease among British subjects. Of the latter, 11 of 15 patients were said to be B5 positive and, among these, six were definitely stated to be white.

If B5 is an oriental gene, it appears to have been liberally sprinkled throughout the Caucasoid populations of the world. Important trade routes between present-day Lebanon and the Orient were established by the Phoenicians (Semitic whites) in ancient times. The Phoenicians also made extensive forays throughout North Africa and the southern European countries bordering on the Mediterranean. Swedish vikings are known to have traveled through present-day Russia and Romania as far as the gates of Istanbul. Marco Polo established the silk route to China, and Genghis Khan is known to have invaded southern Europe in 1224. None of these peoples was distinguished by reputations of chastity, and the likelihood of miscegenation was great. It is thus possible that B5, an important genetic marker of the ophthalmic form of Behçet's disease, was established early among many populations of the Northern Hemisphere of the world through the adventures of various travelers and the extention of trade routes.

At the same time, it appears likely that factors other than those related to HLA may play an important role in the epidemiology of Behçet's disease. It cannot be denied that Behçet's disease in both its complete form and its ophthalmic form is much more highly concentrated in some parts of the world than in others. One must remember that Behçet's disease is well documented among patients who have none of the HLA types commonly associated with the disease (B5, B12, or B27). Thus it appears likely that the disease may be a response to environmental factors and that individuals with a certain immunogenetic background merely respond to the disease in a certain patterned way. Patients with HLA B5 are more likely to have eye disease; patients with HLA B12, mucocutaneous disease; and patients with HLA B27, joint disease.

PATHOGENESIS

It is tempting to think that Behçet's disease results from an immunogenetic predisposition *plus an infectious trigger*. Such combinations are well recognized in other diseases such as Reiter's syndrome where HLA B27 lays the genetic background for the disease, and an infectious trigger brings it on. Minor epidemics of Reiter's syndrome have been described among B27-positive populations exposed to *Yersinia* in Finland.[1] Reiter's syndrome has also been found to be associated with *Chlamydia* infection.[28] This illustrates that any one of a number of infectious triggers could bring on Reiter's syndrome, provided that the patient has the proper immunogenetic background. It would appear that damage resulting from the attack of a microorganism on normal tissue is necessary to provoke the autoimmune reaction that takes place in this disease, and it seems that the autoimmune reaction continues long after the infectious agent has been satisfactorily treated.

Numerous attempts have been made to isolate viruses from the ocular tissues of patients with Behçet's disease. The experiments of Sezer,[32] Ikui,[16] and Mortada[26] are most notable among these. An almost equal number of investigators[7,24] have failed to isolate infectious agents from the tissues of patients with Behçet's disease, but a virus has been isolated from the central nervous system by Evans et al.[10] These conflicting results pinpoint the need for a more concerted effort to isolate infectious agents from patients with Behçet's disease using recently developed techniques such as cocultivation. Technologic advances in virus isolation have proceeded at a rapid pace since Sezer's original isolation of a virus on chorioallantoic membranes.

One of the principal manifestations of Behçet's disease is an attack on the basement membranes of blood vessels. This is apparent in the retina, brain, lung, and kidney. In this connection Dilşen's[9] study on type C viruslike particles in the glomerular basement membrane of patients with Behçet's disease is most interesting. However, since electron microscopic studies are notoriously plagued by artifacts and no attempt was made to confirm the presence of virus by cultivation of the agent or by labeling it in the tissue with fluorescein- or peroxidase-tagged antibodies, such studies remain inconclusive. The same is true of the studies of Tawara et al.[38] showing aggregation of microtubules in the cytoplasm and nucleus of cells observed in the skin lesions. Such studies may suggest the presence of viruses, but do not prove it. Indirect evidence of a viral cause for Behçet's disease has been published by Denman et al.[8] These authors showed that the lymphocytes of untreated Behçet's disease patients could not be infected with herpes simplex virus; this is indirect evidence that these cells are infected with other viruses. The same authors also showed chromosome abnormalities, presumably caused by virus infection, in a large number of patients with Behçet's disease. The same acquired chromosomal defect was found in two members of the same family, indicating perhaps a common exposure to the same agent.

All these studies can be summarized by saying that it is likely that a viral agent either causes the disease or triggers an autoimmune reaction that is responsible for the disease. An endemic viral disease would account for the appearance of the disease in isolated, closely knit groups and for its relatively high concentration in certain geographic areas. If virus infection is persistent in such individuals, it is likely that it is of the slow-virus type. This makes detection and isolation of the virus difficult, and this difficulty in turn may account for the highly variable reports that have thus far been encountered in the literature.

Several other environmental stimuli could conceivably produce the disease. It is tempting to look for chemical agents in the air or drinking water of the affected individuals or to find other elements of environmental pollution as possible triggers of the disea e. Studies in Japan, where the incidence of the disease has increased enormously since the end of World War II, indicate a correlation between increased levels of copper both in the serum and in the ocular tissues of patients suffering from Behçet's disease.[35] The same appears to be true of organic chloride and organic phosphorus,[14] an indication that perhaps the use of organic pesticides containing these substances might play a role in the pathogenesis of the disease. It might equally well be argued that patients suffering from Behçet's disease have a metabolic defect that does not allow them to mobilize these elements from the tissues, as in Wilson's disease. Against this argument is the fact that serum copper level elevations seem to occur immediately before an attack of the disease.[35]

It has been speculated that the inflammatory lesions of Behçet's disease in both the eye and the brain take their origin from the deposition of immune complexes in the blood vessels of these organs. It is regrettable that there is so little immunohistopathologic data to substantiate the immune complex hypothesis. Unlike the lesions of the skin and mucous membranes, which have been extensively biopsied under conditions that would allow for the detection of immune complex components and complement in the tissue site, most specimens of the eye and brain have been fixed in formalin, embedded in paraffin, and subjected to staining by one of a number of histochemical stains useful for light microscopy alone.

A high percentage of patients with the ocular form of Behçet's disease have circulating, soluble immune complexes in their blood. Thus Levinsky and Lehner[20] were able to show that 72% of patients with the ocular form had circulating immune complexes, as compared with 67% of patients with the arthritic form and 40% of patients with the mucocutaneous form. Furthermore, Burton-Kee et al.[6] were able to show that the major components of the serum complexes in patients with the ocular form of the disease were IgG, IgM, and C1q. These are components that one would expect to find involved in the inflammatory process if the classic pathway of complement activation were followed. Indeed it seems likely that this is the case, for Shimada et al.[33] have shown a dramatic lowering of the level of all complement components in the sera of eye patients immediately before the onset of a uveitis attack. These are restored to normal or higher-than-normal levels 3 days after the beginning of such an attack. This would seem to indicate a massive binding of complement to immune complex deposits immediately before an attack of uveitis or retinal vasculitis.

Although both the ocular lesions and the neurologic lesions of Behçet's disease are characterized by an occlusive vasculitis with surrounding zones of acute and chronic inflammatory cells, the two diseases seem to be characterized by different sets of acute-phase products in the serum.[19] Both may show elevated levels of C9 and C-reactive protein, but patients with neurologic disease have large amounts of circulating factor B. Patients with the ocular form have large amounts of lysozyme and of alpha-1–acid glycoprotein in their serum. In the case of the former, the release of large amounts of lysozyme into the serum may result from the rapid destruction of granulocytes.[11] This is consistent with the rapid appearance and disappearance of polymorphonuclear leukocytes in the hypopyon so characteristic of the ocular form of Behçet's disease (Fig. 17-2). Hypopyon may take place very rapidly in the anterior chamber of an eye that does not otherwise look very inflamed. Although the nature of the increased leukotactic activity in Behçet's disease is not well understood, it has been well documented by objective methods of laboratory examination.[23] Presumably it is attributable to the

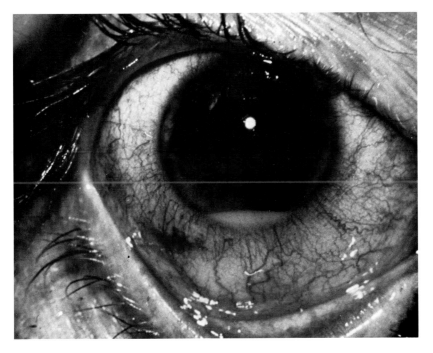

Fig. 17-2. Hypopyon iridocyclitis in a patient with Behçet's disease.

sudden accumulation of immune complexes and complement in the anterior uvea. Leukocytes entering the eye appear to be extremely short-lived effector cells. Thus a hypopyon filling one third or more of the anterior chamber may disappear within a few hours. If this breakdown and absorption of leukocytes is a generalized phenomenon affecting the whole body, it is easy to see why the serum lysozyme level might be elevated. Lehner et al.[17] have demonstrated the presence of damaged membrane fragments in the blood of patients with Behçet's syndrome. These membrane fragments contain holes, presumably caused by damage from complement. It is likely that this kind of damage is also taking place within the eye when a hypopyon is noted to disappear very rapidly.

The finding of elevated levels of alpha-1–acid glycoprotein in the sera of patients with the ocular form of Behçet's disease is of particular interest in view of the histopathologic findings in the retinas of such patients. By use of the periodic acid–Schiff stain and Masson trichrome stain it is easy to demonstrate a presumptive glycoprotein in the thickened basement membranes of retinal vessels affected by occlusive vasculitis (Fig. 17-3). It is tempting to think that this may represent a deposit of alpha-1–acid glycoprotein, though other possibilities must certainly be kept in mind. It is well known that the retinal blood vessels are abnormally permeable in Behçet's syndrome, possibly because of the release of lysosomal enzymes from cells with unstable lysosomal membranes.[22] It is entirely possible that the deposits seen in Fig. 17-3 represent pseudocol-

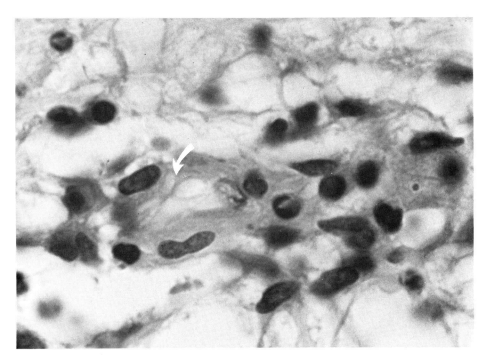

Fig. 17-3. Microscopic appearance of a diseased retinal blood vessel in a patient with Behçet's disease. Note thickened basement membrane, *arrow.* (PAS stain, 1200 × .)

lagen that has been formed in the wake of fibrin deposition, as described by Ashton[2] in diabetic retinopathy. This and other related matters await confirmation by electron microscopic studies.

Retinal vein involvement has been unduly emphasized in the past as an ocular manifestation of Behçet's disease. In my opinion, retinal arterioles and veins become equally involved, particularly in the later stages of the disease. Studies by Bonamour et al.[5] correctly describe the sequence of events in early inflammatory disease of the posterior segment of the eye: periphlebitis with venous dilation, capillary leakage, superficial hemorrhages, tributary vein thrombosis, and eventually central vein thrombosis. These changes are presumably caused by an immunologic attack on the endothelium of normal capillaries and postcapillary venules, followed by leakage of fibrinogen, other plasma proteins, and cells into the basement membranes and outer layers of the vessel wall. A defect in the fibrinolytic activity of plasma in patients with Behçet's disease has been documented, though Urgancioğlu et al.[39] could not correlate this with phlebitic activity in the retina. It is highly likely, however, that this defect in fibrinolysis contributes to the persistence and organization of blood clots once formed in the retina or elsewhere in the body.

By far the most serious damage occurs to both the retina and the brain when arterioles become involved by the inflammatory process. This may occur with frightening rapidity, leaving the retina or the periarteriolar brain tissue starved of nutrition. Fukuda et al.[12] have described the softening and necrosis of brain tissue in the immediate vicinity of such occluded vessels, and an identical picture can be seen in the retina. The ultimate fate of such vessel-deprived (Fig. 17-4) tissue is massive atrophy. This may be complicated by subretinal neovascular membrane formation in the macula, as described by Michelson et al.[25] or it may be accompanied by massive atrophy of the optic nerves, as described by Hyman and Sagar.[15] In the latter case, it is only fair to say that there was also considerable evidence of simultaneous central nervous system disease in the patient described by these authors.

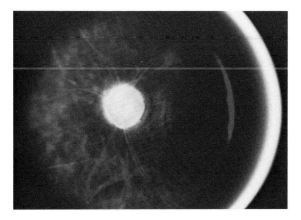

Fig. 17-4. Massive retinal vessel occlusion and optic atrophy in a patient with Behçet's disease.

DIAGNOSIS

The diagnosis of the ocular form of Behçet's disease is based on (1) the clinical appearance and course of the lesions, (2) the geographic and genetic background of the patients, and (3) selected laboratory tests. As mentioned above, many of the patients believed to have Behçet's disease failed to qualify as cases of ''complete'' Behçet's disease, as stipulated by Shimizu.[34] The clinical picture of hypopyon uveitis in a patient who has suffered from aphthous ulcers of the mouth or genitalia is highly suggestive of the disease. There is nothing diagnostic about the hypopyon, however. This may be seen in patients with Reiter's syndrome or in any acute uveitis such as that accompanying ankylosing spondylitis. One of the characteristics of the hypopyon of Behçet's disease is that it is often very short lived, and often it may appear in an eye that is not otherwise very inflamed.

The occlusive retinal vasculitis is generally a manifestation of the later stages of the disease. It may well affect veins exclusively in the early phase of the disease, but sooner or later both arterioles and veins are involved. In the wake of branch artery occlusions large areas of nonperfusion can be seen in the retina by fluorescein angiography. Neovascularization may occur in the areas of nonperfusion, and these newly formed vessels may bleed giving rise to hemorrhage in the overlying vitreous.

The extraocular manifestations of Behçet's disease may include arthropathy, particularly of weight-bearing joints, erythema nodosum, and other vasculitic lesions of the skin. The skin may sometimes reflect the excessive chemotactic activity that is seen elsewhere in the body. This can be demonstrated by microabcess formation at the site of a sterile needle injection on the forearm.

The ethnic and geographic background of the patient may be helpful. The majority of patients seen in our clinic come from eastern Mediterranean backgrounds, though this is not universal. HLA typing is useful, particularly in patients who do not come from an obvious Mediterranean background. The HLA antigen B5 is present in about 60% of all our patients with the ocular form of Behçet's disease, and among this group the subtype B51 carries a high correlation with the expression of ocular disease. HLA appears to be useful, particularly in those patients who lack other essential elements of the disease. It may also be useful in the identification of members of a given family who are at risk for the later development of the disease. It is of interest that although the ocular disease and the cerebral disease have many points of similarity as far as pathogenesis is concerned, the presence of HLA B5 does not correlate significantly with the cerebral form of Behçet's disease.

Serologic studies on patients with the ocular form of Behçet's disease may show elevated levels of C9. They may show a depression of C3 and C4 immediately before or during the early phases of an attack. Acute-phase reaction products such as alpha-1–acid glycoprotein may also be present at high levels in patients with the ocular form of Behçet's disease. Last, immune complex levels may be elevated in the serum of patients with Behçet's disease, and these show cross-reactivity with those of patients suffering from herpetiform ulcers of the mouth.

Fluorescein angiography may show important changes in the early phases of the retinal disease. Leakage of fluorescein from retinal veins may become apparent before there are obvious signs of occlusive vasculitis. In the later stages of the disease, when occlusive phenomena are more obvious, areas of nonperfusion of the retina can be identified, and zones of neovascularization can be located. Often there are focal infiltrates in the retina that appear to be independent of diseased retinal vessels. These show a pattern of blocked fluorescence during the early phase of the angiogram but may show staining in the later phases.

TREATMENT

In the early phases of the ocular form of Behçet's disease the lesions seem to be readily responsive to corticosteroid therapy. If the early manifestations of disease are confined to iridocyclitis, satisfactory therapeutic responses can be obtained with the frequent instillation of prednisolone acetate drops (1%). This is combined with atropine 1% applied as a single drop two or three times a day. As the pain and photophobia begin to subside, the long-acting cycloplegic should be abandoned in favor of a frequently applied short-acting dilator-like cyclopentolate 1%.

If a more diffuse uveitis is present, giving rise to extensive infiltration of the vitreous body, systemic corticosteroid therapy needs to be administered from the outset. Prednisone in doses ranging from 80 to 100 mg per day should be initiated early in the attack and should be administered initially in divided doses. After 7 days, the dosage regimen can be shifted to a single, early-morning dose. After a satisfactory anti-inflammatory effect has been obtained, alternate-day dosage, requiring the use of double the normal dosage every other day at breakfast time, may be instituted.

There is general agreement that the posterior lesions of Behçet's disease respond well to systemically administered corticosteroid therapy in the early phases of the disease. The vitreous opacities may resorb quickly, and the retinal infiltrates may melt away. Later in the disease, however, the posterior lesions seem to be resistant to corticosteroid therapy. This is particularly true of the retinal vasculitis that cannot be reversed by the use of systemic corticosteroids. Certainly corticosteroid therapy will do nothing to reverse the occlusion of a vessel once it has occurred. As a matter of fact, corticosteroid therapy may even predispose to vessel occlusion in the same way it appears to predispose to thrombosis of the leg veins in persons receiving long-term therapy. In the case of the diseased retinal vessels of Behçet's disease, the failure of the occluded vessels to recanalize may be directly related to a defect in fibrinolysis.

In general, Behçet's disease must be considered a malady of bad prognosis. Many patients reach a stage of irreversible inflammatory defects early in the course of their disease; others go for many years with easily reversible lesions. When corticosteroid therapy in moderate doses no longer reverses the inflammatory lesions of Behçet's disease, the ophthalmologist must consider other forms of therapy. These include but are not limited to immunosuppressive therapy. The most widely used immunosuppressive agent in the treatment of Behçet's disease is chlorambucil. The effectiveness of chlorambucil in treating the inflammatory lesions of Behçet's disease has been demonstrated by Mamo[21] and by Godfrey.[13] The patient is given a minimal dose of the agent at the beginning of therapy. Generally, 2 mg of chlorambucil are administered daily in the initial period to ascertain whether the patient will have an idiosyncratic reaction to the drug. Thereafter the dosage is increased to 4 mg per day in the second week, to 6 mg per day in the third week, and so on. The dosage is gradually increased in this manner until there is improvement in the clinical signs or until there is evidence of hematopoietic disturbance, as indicated by a decline in the white blood cell count or in the platelet count. At that point, the dosage is reduced by 2 mg per day, and an attempt is made to taper the dosage of systemically administered corticosteroids that the patient may be taking. When this has been accomplished, the level of chlorambucil is then reduced gradually to a low maintenance level of 2 to 6 mg a day. This may need to be maintained for periods of 6 to 8 months. The number of side effects that can be antici-pated from chlorambucil therapy is relatively small, and in many ways it is the easiest of all of the immunosuppressive agents to administer on an outpatient basis. However, chlorambucil may occasionally cause serious and permanent bone marrow depression. It may also predispose to the development of leukemia, and it may cause sterility, particularly in males. When it is administered to young persons who may wish to pro-create at a later time, banking of sperm is advisable.

Other immunosuppressive regimens that might be considered include the combined use of cyclophosphamide and prednisone. Cyclophosphamide therapy may also be com-plicated by serious degrees of bone marrow depression and by other side effects includ-ing hemorrhagic cystitis and bladder carcinoma. In general, this agent is somewhat more difficult to administer on an outpatient basis.

The aim of all immunosuppressive therapy is to induce a permanent remission, if possible. This has been seen in a number of patients treated with chlorambucil and observed for periods of 8 to 10 years. Under these circumstances, it seems that the use of a potentially lethal agent was justified by the vision-saving results that it produced. Even when it is not possible to obtain a permanent remission, the use of an immuno-suppressive agent may make it possible to treat the patient with acceptable low doses of corticosteroids, retaining fairly good vision and freeing the patient from the annoyance of recurrent attacks. It is important to remember that if a decision is made to use im-munosuppressive agents, that decision must be made early enough to save vision. There is no point in treating a patient with potentially toxic agents if all of his retinal vascu-lature has already been obliterated by the ravages of the disease.

A number of other remedies have been suggested for the treatment of Behçet's disease. One of these, favored by Japanese ophthalmologists,[40] consists in the use of colchicine in doses of 1 to 2 mg a day. The rationale for this therapy is not exactly clear. The use of colchicine may paralyze the division of inflammatory cells in meta-phase, thereby reducing the number of cells that can respond to the chemotactic stimuli of Behçet's disease. This form of therapy would seem to have some merit during acute attacks of the disease, but maintenance therapy on colchicine could not be justified. Other authors[36] believe that Behçet's disease reflects excessive stimulation of the cholin-ergic portion of the autonomic nervous system. The use of atropine nitrate administered orally at dosages of 1 mg per day has been advocated. Still other authors[37] have related the progression of Behçet's disease to the availability of free oxygen radicals and have suggested vitamin E therapy as a remedy for this. It would seem that many of these latter forms of therapy are based on highly theoretical grounds, and such forms of therapy cannot be recommended until clinical trials prove their efficacy.

REFERENCES

1. Ahvonen, P., and Dickhoff, K.: Uveitis, episcleritis, and conjunctivitis associated with *Yersinia* infection, Acta Ophthalmol. **123**:209, 1974.
2. Ashton, N.: Vascular basement membranes in diabetes, Br. J. Ophthalmol. **58**:344, 1974.

3. Behçet's Disease Research Committee of Japan: Behçet's disease: guide to diagnosis of Behçet's disease, Jpn. J. Ophthalmol. **18:**291, 1974.

4. Bloch-Michel, E., Campinchi, R., Muller, J.Y., Binaghi, M., and Sales, J.: HLA antigens and uveitis, with special reference to Behçet's disease, chronic herpes simplex, toxoplasmosis, and recurrent acute anterior uveitis. In Silverstein, A.M., and O'Connor, G.R., editors: Immunology and immunopathology of the eye, New York, 1979, Masson & Co.

5. Bonamour, G., Grange, J.D., and Bonnet, M.: Retinal vein involvement in Behçet's disease. In Dilşen, N., Koniçe, M., and Övül, C., editors: Behçet's disease, Amsterdam, 1979, Excerpta Medica Foundation.

6. Burton-Kee, J.E., Mobray, J.F., and Lehner, T.: Different cross-reacting circulating immune complexes in Behçet's syndrome and recurrent oral ulcers, J. Lab. Clin. Med. **97:**559, 1981.

7. Curth-Ollendorff, H.: Recurrent genito-oral aphthosis and uveitis with hypopyon (Behçet's syndrome), Arch. Dermatol. **54:**179, 1946.

8. Denman, A.M., Fialkow, P.J., Pelton, B.K., Salo, A.C., and Appleford, D.J.: Attempts to establish a viral aetiology for Behçet's syndrome. In Lehner, T., and Barnes, C.G., editors: Behçet's syndrome, London, 1979, Academic Press, Inc.

9. Dilşen, N., Erbengi, T., Koniçe, M., Urgancioğlu, M., Gürsoy, E., Övül, C., and Ozdogan, E.: Type C virus-like particles in glomerular basement membrane in a case of Behçet's disease with amyloidosis. In Dilşen, N., Koniçe, M., and Övül, C., editors: Behçet's disease, Amsterdam, 1979, Excerpta Medica Foundation.

10. Evans, A.D., Pallis, C.A., and Spillane, J.D.: Involvement of the nervous system in Behçet's syndrome: report of three cases and isolation of virus, Lancet **2:**349, 1957.

11. Fink, M.E., and Finch, S.C.: Serum muramidase and granulocyte turnover, Proc. Soc. Exp. Biol. Med. **127:**365, 1968.

12. Fukuda, Y., Watanabe, I., Hayashi, H., and Kuwabara, N.: Pathological studies on Behçet's disease, The Ryumachi **20:**268, 1980.

13. Godfrey, W.F., Epstein, W., O'Connor, G.R., Kimura, S., Hogan, M., and Nozik, R.: The use of chlorambucil in intractable idiopathic uveitis, Am. J. Ophthalmol. **78:**415, 1974.

14. Hori, Y., Miyazawa, S., Miyata, M., Ishikawa, S., and Nishiyama, S.: Ultrastructural x-ray microanalysis of tissues in Behçet's disease. In Dilşen, N., Koniçe, M., and Övül, C., editors: Behçet's disease, Amsterdam, 1979, Excerpta Medica Foundation.

15. Hyman, N.M., and Sagar, H.J.: Behçet's syndrome: unusual multisystem involvement and immune complexes, Postgrad. Med. J. **56:**182, 1980.

16. Ikui, H., Tahara, Y., Nakamizo, K., Ueno, K., Iwaki, S., and Maeda, J.: Further studies on eyes with Behçet's syndrome, J. Clin. Ophthalmol. **14:**529, 1960.

17. Lehner, T., Almeida, J.D., and Levinsky, R.J.: Damaged membrane fragments and immune complexes in the blood of patients with Behçet's syndrome, Clin. Exp. Immunol. **34:**206, 1978.

18. Lehner, T., and Batchelor, J.R.: Classification and immunogenetic basis of Behçet's syndrome. In Lehner, T., and Barnes, C.G., editors: Behçet's syndrome, London, 1979, Academic Press, Inc.

19. Lehner, T., and Adinolfi, M.: Acute phase proteins, C9, factor B and lysozyme in recurrent oral ulceration and Behçet's syndrome, J. Clin. Pathol. **33:**269, 1980.

20. Levinsky, R.J., and Lehner, T.: Circulating, soluble immune complexes in recurrent oral ulceration and Behçet's syndrome, Clin. Exp. Immunol. **32:**193, 1978.

21. Mamo, J.G., and Azzam, S.A.: Treatment of Behçet's disease with chlorambucil, Arch. Ophthalmol. **84:**446, 1970.

22. Matsumoto, A., Hashimoto, T., and Shimizu, T.: Vascular permeability and lysosomal kinetics in Behçet's syndrome. In Dilşen, N., Koniçe, M., and Övül, C., editors: Behçet's disease, Amsterdam, 1979, Excerpta Medica Foundation.

23. Matsumura, N., Matsumura, Y., and Mizushima, Y.: Studies on cutaneous hyperreactivity and leukocyte chemotaxis in Behçet's disease. In Dilşen, N., Koniçe, M., and Övül, C., editors: Behçet's disease, Amsterdam, 1979, Excerpta Medica Foundation.

24. Merenlender, I.J., Schwartz, B., and Stafford, J.L.: Recurrent genital and oral ulceration with eosinophilia, Br. J. Dermatol. **73:**273, 1961.

25. Michelson, J.B., Michelson, P.E., and Chisari, F.V.: Subretinal neovascular membrane and disciform scar in Behçet's disease, Am. J. Ophthalmol. **90:**182, 1980.

26. Mortada, A., and Imam, Z.E.: Virus aetiology of Behçet's syndrome, Br. J. Ophthalmol. **48:**250, 1964.
27. Ohno, S., Sugiura, S., Aoki, K., and Ohguchi, M.: Studies on HLA antigens in Behçet's disease. In Dilşen, N., Koniçe, M., and Övül, C., editors; Behçet's disease, Amsterdam, 1979, Excerpta Medica Foundation.
28. Ostler, H.B., Schachter, J., and Dawson, C.R.: Ocular infection of rabbits with *Bedsonia* isolated from a patient with Reiter's syndrome, Invest. Ophthalmol. **9:**256, 1970.
29. Rosselet, E., Sandin, Y., and Jeanet, M.: Recherche des antigens HL-A dans la maladie de Behçet, Ophthalmologica **172:**116, 1976.
30. Sander, M.D.: Ophthalmic features of Behçet's disease. In Lehner, T., and Barnes, C.G., editors Behçet's syndrome, New York, 1979, Academic Press, Inc.
31. Schlaegel, T.F.: Current aspects of uveitis, Boston, 1977, Little, Brown & Co.
32. Sezer, N.: The isolation of a virus as the cause of Behçet's disease, Am. J. Ophthalmol. **36:**301, 1953.
33. Shimada, K., Kogura, M., Kawashima, T., and Nishioka, K.: Reduction of complement in Behçet's disease and drug allergy, Med. Biol. **52:**234, 1974.
34. Shimizu, T.: Clinicopathologic studies on Behçet's disease. In Dilşen, N., Koniçe, M., and Övül, C., editors: Behçet's disease, Amsterdam, 1979, Excerpta Medica Foundation.
35. Shimizu, K., Ishikawa, S., Miyata, M., Yoshida, H., and Kubo, H.: Relationship between the changes in serum copper levels and ocular attacks in Behçet's disease (an etiological consideration). In Dilşen, N., Koniçe, M., and Övül, C., editors: Behçet's disease, Amsterdam, 1979, Excerpta Medica Foundation.
36. Suyama, H., Fukuda, T., and Ishikawa, S.: The use of atropine methylnitrate in Behçet's disease, Proceedings of the Second International Conference on Behçet's Disease, Tokyo, 1982. (In press.)
37. Tanaka, K., Ohguchi, M., Ohno, S., Matsuda, H., and Sugiura, S.: Vitamin E treatment in Behçet's disease, Proceedings of the Second International Conference on Behçet's Disease, Tokyo, 1982. (In press.)
38. Tawara, J., Ichikawa, H., Akatsuka, K., Kumow, H., Jujio, K., and Shishido, A.: Nucleocapsid-like structures in the tissues of Behçet's disease patients, Jpn. J. Med. Sci. Biol. **29:**99, 1976.
39. Urgancioğlu, M., Saylan, T., Saracbaşi, Z., Atamer, T., and Tangun, Y.: Plasma fibrinolytic activity in Behçet's disease. In Dilşen, N., Koniçe, M., and Övül, C., editors: Behçet's disease, Amsterdam, 1979, Excerpta Medica Foundation.
40. Yamana, S., Yamamoto, M., Aoi, K., Miyake, S., and Ofuji, T.: Long term observation of patients with Behçet's disease treated with colchicine, Proceedings of the Second International Conference on Behçet's Disease, Tokyo, 1982. (In press.)

18

Ocular sarcoidosis

G. Richard O'Connor

Ocular sarcoidosis is a potentially serious disease of the eye that may ultimately produce highly destructive effects on all of the ocular tissues. Its incidence varies according to (1) geographic location, (2) the interests and referral pattern of the reporting ophthalmologist, and (3) the criteria selected for the diagnosis. Thus Schlaegel[17] reports that 2% of his large group of uveitis patients surveyed at the University of Indiana had ocular sarcoidosis, whereas a study of our series at the University of California in San Francisco showed that 78 out of 850 patients surveyed during the past 5 years (9.1%) had a presumptive or proved diagnosis of sarcoidosis. Still other reports, such as those of Simpson,[18] reflect special considerations in the diagnosis. Simpson reported on the case histories and laboratory findings of 39 well-defined cases of anterior granulomatous uveitis among a total of 334 uveitis charts that were reviewed. Thus he specifically rejected those patients whose primary manifestations may have been in the posterior segment of the eye. When comparing Simpson's cases with those seen during the past 5 years at the University of California, other important differences emerge. In Simpson's study, 100% of the patients were black; in our study, less than one third of the patients were black. In Simpson's study 31 of 39 (80%) of the patients had some abnormality shown in the chest x-ray film; in our series less than 10% had roentgenographic evidence of thoracic disease. Many of our patients, however, did have evidence of hilar or parenchymatous lung disease when tested by gallium scanning. Although there is general agreement that the best evidence of sarcoidosis is obtained from the examination of biopsy material, tissue specimens have not been obtained from the majority of cases reported in any series. Furthermore, there is nothing unique or absolutely characteristic in the histologic picture of sarcoidosis. The diagnosis is and probably shall remain a diagnosis by exclusion. Other granulomatous processes, such as bacterial or fungal infection or foreign body reactions, must be eliminated before a final diagnosis of sarcoidosis can be made. Simpson emphasized the importance of chest x-ray films, serum electrophoresis, and biopsies (including the Kveim test) in the diagnosis of sarcoidosis. These tests have not received equal emphasis in other studies reported by other authors.

Simpson reported that the eye can become involved at any time during the evolution of sarcoidosis, but in 80% of the patients in his series, the uveitis developed during a silent stage of sarcoidosis. I would agree with this finding. The majority of patients who

211

present with the signs of presumptive ocular sarcoidosis have no systemic complaints. We may do such patients a special service by alerting them to the existence of previously unsuspected pulmonary disease. If treatment can be administered before there is a serious restriction of vital capacity, many otherwise asymptomatic patients can be helped. On the other hand, a sizable number of patients with the established signs of systemic sarcoidosis (pulmonary, cutaneous, or osseous manifestations) will have mild signs of ocular inflammation without knowing about it. Thus 25% of a large group of patients with diagnosed pulmonary sarcoidosis seen by me at the National Institutes of Health in Bethesda, Maryland, were found to have mild signs of ocular inflammation, including small numbers of keratic precipitates, cells and flare in the anterior chamber, and even iris nodules. The majority of these patients had no specific complaints referable to their eyes but were examined in routine fashion so that occult eye disease could be detected.

CLINICAL MANIFESTATIONS OF OCULAR SARCOIDOSIS

Patients with presumptive ocular sarcoidosis most often present with the signs and symptoms of anterior uveitis. Occasionally this has an exposive onset, but much more often the disease is insidious in its onset. It may be accompanied by floating spots and by diminution of visual acuity, particularly if large numbers of dense keratic precipitates from in the visual axis.

Beginning with the external examination, patients with ocular sarcoidosis may show granulomatous lesions of the skin. These are often encountered on the lid margins or on the nose. They appear as papules of variable pigmentation, sometimes with crusting or scaling on their surfaces. They may incite a slight pigmentary reaction, or they may appear slightly lighter than the surrounding skin (Fig. 18-1). Examination of the conjunctiva may reveal the presence of opaque, gray-yellow slightly elevated lesions, particularly in the inferior nasal portion of the palpebral conjunctiva (Fig. 18-2). Such lesions often have the appearance of a confluence of three or four conjunctival follicles. However, sarcoid lesions are generally more opaque than follicles and lack the central superficial cap of fine vessels. The biopsy of suspicious conjunctival lesions has often been rewarding. A blind biopsy of the conjunctiva, however, is in our hands very unrewarding.

Examination of the cornea may show a number of revealing signs. Calcific band keratopathy may be seen with some regularity in juvenile forms of ocular sarcoidosis, and since sarcoidosis may also produce pauciarticular arthritis on occasion, juvenile sarcoidosis is sometimes mistaken for juvenile rheumatoid arthritis. In adults, calcific band keratopathy is usually not seen unless there is a concomitant hypercalcemia. In cases of active iridocyclitis the corneal endothelium may show large numbers of "mutton-fat" keratic precipitates. These are yellowish gray in color and often have a greasy appearance. This characteristic appearance comes from the agglutination of mononuclear cells, principally epithelioid cells, on the corneal endothelium. There is a characteristic tendency for large mutton-fat keratic precipitates to form on the periphery of the corneal endothelium. When these are viewed by gonioscopy, one can often seen fusion of these peripheral keratic precipitates with peripheral portions of the iris. It is likely that such formations give rise to the peripheral anterior synechiae so characteristic of ocular sarcoidosis. The heavy deposition of keratic precipitates on the inferior corneal epithelium

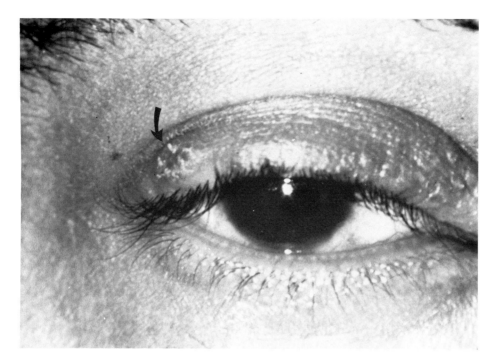

Fig. 18-1. Cutaneous lesions, *arrow,* on the eyelids of a patient suffering from sarcoidosis.

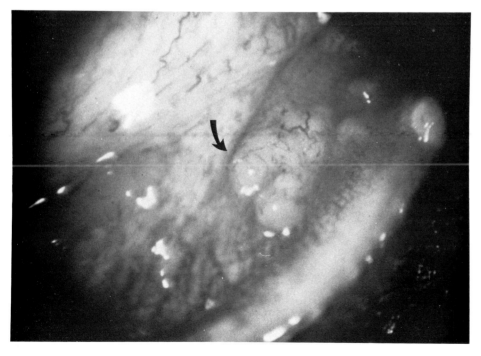

Fig. 18-2. Conjunctival nodules, *arrow,* on the inferior palpebral conjunctiva of a patient with biopsy-confirmed sarcoidosis.

may also give rise to a peculiar prismatic thickening of the inferior peripheral cornea. This may or may not be associated with the formation of an opaque membrane in this area. It should be emphasized that one does not always see mutton-fat keratic precipitates in presumptive ocular sarcoidosis. Depending on the stage of the disease in which the patient is first seen, the precipitates may be small and white and scattered diffusely over the corneal endothelium, or they may consist merely of individual cellular precipitates.

The iris may show nodules of various types. The most commonly seen nodules are so-called Koeppe's nodules on the pupillary margin. Although these were originally believed to be characteristic of granulomatous diseases, they have been seen in such conditions as Fuchs' heterochromic iridocyclitis, which is generally considered a nongranulomatous inflammation. Stromal nodules of the Busacca type are more characteristic of ocular sarcoidosis but are not frequently encountered. They represent granulomatous infiltrations in the iris stroma, sometimes superficial in their location and highly vascularized, and other times deep within the stroma where they are almost completely covered by the anterior mesodermal layers of the iris. Here again, there is nothing pathognomonic about Busacca nodules. They have been seen on numerous occasions as anterior complications of diseases such as toxoplasmic retinochoroiditis. Synechia formation is common in ocular sarcoidosis and may form particularly at the sites where Koeppe's nodules fuse with the anterior capsular surface of the lens. The lens itself may develop extensive opacity, either as a complication of the uveitic process or as a result of prolonged local and systemic corticosteroid therapy. Lens opacity seems to develop with greater frequency after synechia formation is established.

The vitreous body may be extensively infiltrated in cases of ocular sarcoidosis. The opacities vary in size from individual cells to large aggregates known as "snowballs." These snowballs appear similar to those seen in peripheral uveitis ("pars-planitis"), and it is a matter of record (19) that about 4% of patients initially diagnosed as "pars-planitis" eventually develop saroidosis. Histologic studies of these large snowball opacities have shown them to consist of floating granulomas with lymphocytes, epithelioid cells, and other mononuclear elements. When these large opacities settle on the inferior pars plana area, they may coalesce to form a "snowbank." This also has a striking resemblance to the snowbank formation seen in "pars-planitis."

The fundus may show a number of different signs, all of them potentially related to sarcoid. Vasculitis, principally periphlebitis (Fig. 18-3), is the most frequently encountered sign. This may produce thick aggregations of mononuclear cells around the exterior portions of retinal veins that have been fancifully described as "candle-wax drippings." Lesser degrees of periphlebitis are also encountered, however, and occasionally small retinal hemorrhages may be seen. These may be associated with actual invasion of the blood vessel wall by the granulomatous process. Focal retinochoroiditis, resembling that of toxoplasmosis in some respects, may be encountered in the fundus. Gass[10] has shown that these may consist of focal granulomatous processes that extend all the way through the retina into the underlying choroid.

Macular edema may be seen as a sequela of extensive inflammation of the retina and choroid. Under conditions of prolonged inflammation cystoid edema may form in the area of the foveola giving rise to a decrease in visual acuity or metamorphopsia. Such anatomic changes may occasionally result in a permanent loss of vision. The optic

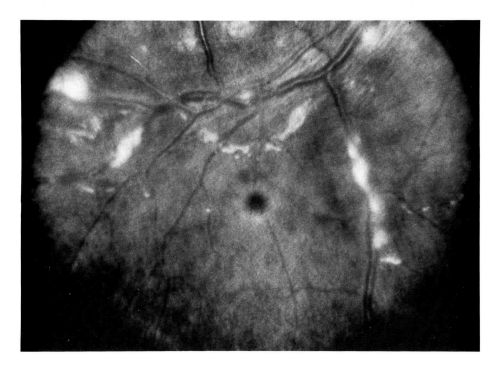

Fig. 18-3. Retinal vasculitis in a patient with ocular sarcoidosis.

nerve itself is relatively infrequently involved by sarcoidosis, and when it is involved, there is often evidence of simultaneous involvement of the brain. This has been nicely illustrated by Gould and Kaufman.[14]

PATHOGENESIS

The cause of sarcoidosis is essentially unknown. In many respects, the disease behaves like an infection. Several different infectious organisms, including *Mycoplasma*[16] and atypical mycobacteria from the soil,[4] have been indirectly implicated in the disease, but Koch's postulates have never been fulfilled for these organisms.

Histologically, the sarcoid lesion consists of a noncaseating granuloma of the tuberculoid type. Epithelioid cells are prominent in these lesions, and giant cells, which probably represent the fusion of epithelioid cells,[1] are also characteristically seen in the lesions. In addition, Tannenbaum et al.[20] have shown that lymphocytes of both T-cell and B-cell origin are present in the lesions. The persistence of epithelioid cells and giant cells in the lesions suggests a ''frustrated macrophage'' function in which macrophages are present in the lesion but are unable to complete their task of phagocytosis. Epithelioid cells clearly belong to a phagocyte line. A defect in collaboration beetween T lymphocytes and these specialized phagocytes may result in an incomplete removal of particulate or precipitated matter from the tissue.

There has been a great deal of speculation about the nature of possible antigenic substances in the lesion. One theory, reviewed by Cummings,[6] suggests that pine pollen may trigger the peculiar sequence of events seen in sarcoidosis. The prevalence of sarcoidosis in certain geographic areas has been correlated with the distribution of certain types of pine trees. The fact that sarcoidosis has a higher prevalence in certain southeastern states, where particular species of pine trees cast allergenic pollens into the air, may merely reflect relatively higher numbers of blacks in these areas or other factors causally related to the disease but as yet unidentified. Various types of immunologic abnormalities have been linked with sarcoidosis. These have been extensively reviewed and evaluated by Daniele et al.,[7] who found that specific T-cell defects could be correlated with the active stages of sarcoidosis. Specifically, there are decreased numbers of T lymphocytes in the circulating blood of sarcoid patients. The reason may be that T lymphocytes are specifically screened out of the circulation through the process of entrapment in enlarged lymph nodes, or the decrease may be associated with the specific activity of autoantibodies directed against T lymphocytes.[8] The T lymphocytes that remain in the circulation show increased numbers of "activated" T cells. This is indicated by an increased tendency to form rosettes with sheep red blood cells under certain conditions of temperature. Lymphocytes of sarcoid patients, when maintained in tissue cultures, show depressed proliferative responses to various common antigens and to nonspecific mitogens such as phytohemagglutinin. This may be reflected in the failure of sarcoid patients to manifest normal skin-test reactivity to such common antigens as those of *Candida, Trichophyton,* and mumps. On the other hand, the failure to manifest skin-test reactivity may reflect a decrease in the secretion of certain lymphokines by antigen-stimulated lymphocytes.

Within any population of T lymphocytes there are certain subpopulations that appear to be extremely important for immune regulation. Recently, these subsets of T lymphocytes have been shown to have different surface-membrane characteristics. The so-called suppressor T cells have receptors for the Fc segment of the IgG molecule, whereas the so-called helper T cells have receptors for IgM.[7] The ability to identify these receptors by monoclonal antibodies has allowed various investigators to determine that the numbers of helper T cells are decreased in sarcoidosis whereas the numbers of suppressor T cells are increased.

Soluble circulating factors in the serum of sarcoid patients also demonstrate significant deviations from the norm. Thus the serum of sarcoid patients, when incubated with lymphocytes of normal individuals, appears to suppress the proliferative responses of the normal lymphocytes to various common antigens and to nonspecific mitogens. Reference has already been made[8] to the existence of autoantibodies directed against T cells, and in this respect sarcoidosis bears a certain resemblance to systemic lupus erythematosus.

Other abnormalities in the serum of patients with sarcoidosis include the elevation of serum immunoglobulin levels. This applies particularly to the level IgG, as indicated in the early work of Simpson.[18] A failure in the regulatory mechanisms that ordinarily govern the production of immunoglobulins is reflected in polyclonal B-cell activation. This means that multiple clones of B lymphocytes may be stimulated into simultaneous production of immunoglobulins by a single environmental stimulus. Excess of immunoglobulin production in sarcoidosis is responsible for what used to be called an "inverted A/G ratio." That is to say, the normal ratio of albumin to globulins is reversed such that globulins are present in higher absolute amounts than albumin is. The variety of antibodies includes high titers of antibody to *Mycoplasma,* Epstein-Barr virus, rubella, parainfluenza, and herpes simplex.[3] In addition, sarcoid patients may show elevated levels of autoantibodies including rheumatoid factor and antinuclear antibody.[22] Yet, despite the high titers of antibodies to these agents, it is difficult to impugn any of them as the causative factor of sarcoidosis.

In addition to evidence for increased levels of immunoglobulins in the serum, there are high levels of circulating immune complexes of unknown origin in the serum of sarcoid patients. This was described by Hedfors and Norberg[15] in 1974 and has been substantiated by numerous other authors including Glikmann et al.[12] The nature of the antigen in these immune complexes has not been established, but the chromatographic work of Glikmann et al. indicates that it is a large molecular structure, most of which is eluted in the first elution peak from a Sephadex 200 column. By immunofluorescent techniques, deposits of immune complexes containing IgA, IgG, and IgM, as well as complement fragments, have been demonstrated in the granulomas of sarcoidosis.[11] It is possible that part of the "frustrated macrophage function" may be reflected in an inability to phagocytize these immune-complex deposits completely.

Prostaglandins may also play a role in the suppressor activity observed in sarcoidosis. It has been postulated that these prostaglandins are liberated from adherent monocytes. Removal of the adherent cell population from the peripheral blood mononuclear cells of patients with sarcoidosis results in a partial restoration of the responsiveness of these patient's lymphocytes to phytohemagglutinin.[13] Furthermore, the addition of indomethacin to mitogen-stimulated cultures increases the response of sarcoid lymphocytes, and this suggests that prostaglandins may be one of the soluble inhibitory factors involved in the impaired mitogenic responses of these patients.

DIAGNOSIS OF OCULAR SARCOIDOSIS

The diagnosis of ocular sarcoidosis is often presumptive at best. There is general agreement that the only firm diagnosis is a diagnosis established by biopsy. However, as noted earlier in this paper, the histologic picture of sarcoidosis is not absolutely characteristic or unique. Other granulomas of fungal, viral, or even foreign-body origin may mimic its appearance. The diagnosis therefore is mainly a diagnosis by exclusion.

Biopsy of certain tissues of the eye can be accomplished relatively easily. Biopsy of sarcoid lesions of the skin of the eyelids or of the conjunctiva may be performed relatively easily under local anesthesia, and on many occasions such biopsies have produced valuable information. Sarcoid granulomas of the conjunctiva appear most often on the palpebral conjunctiva, usually in the inferior fornix. Such lesions are generally irregular in shape, yellowish white in color, and covered by normal conjunctival epithelium. Sometimes there is evidence of vascular ingrowth into such nodules. They may be differentiated from follicles of the conjunctiva by the fact that they are more opaque in appearance and irregular in shape (Fig. 18-2). The histologic examination of such a nodule may reveal noncaseating granulomas of a morphologic pattern consistent with sarcoidosis.

Other tissues of the eye may lend themselves to biopsy examination, but there is usually little justification for intraocular biopsy unless surgery is required to relieve iris bombé or to remove a cataract. Under such circumstances, biopsy of the iris may reveal the typical noncaseating granulomas of sarcoidosis, particulary in areas that reveal nodules on gross examination. Recently Constable[5] has demonstrated the feasibility of chorioretinal biopsy for the purpose of making an accurate diagnosis. This, too, might be useful in making a diagnosis, but it hardly seems justified in view of the potential complications of the procedure.

In general, we are forced to rely upon indirect methods of diagnosis. In our clinic the diagnosis is generally based upon the presence of (1) two or more characteristic ocular signs, (2) characteristic hilar adenopathy or interstitial infiltration of the lungs on chest x-ray films, (3) abnormal biopsy findings from an extraocular site, (4) abnormal gallium scan results, and (5) serum abnormalities including elevated levels of angiotensin-converting enzyme, serum lysozyme, serum calcium, and serum IgG. The last finding is generally determined by immunoelectrophoresis.

The clinical characteristics of ocular sarcoidosis include (1) insidious onset, (2) the presence of mutton-fat keratic precipitates on the corneal endothelium, (3) iris nodules of either the Koeppe or Busacca type, (4) vitreous opacities, usually of the "snowball" type, (5) retinal vasculitis, usually a periphlebitis, (6) focal chorioretinal lesions of heterogeneous morphology, and (7) swelling or obvious infiltration of the optic nerve. The presence of ocular sarcoidosis is considered when two or more of these signs are present in any patient.

Relatively few of the patients seen in our clinic have had characteristic hilar adenopathy or other x-ray changes that would suggest pulmonary sarcoidosis. As mentioned earlier, this may be connected with the racial distribution of our patients or with other environmental factors that have not yet been identified. In this connection, it should also be noted that patients considered as serious candidates for sarcoidosis are generally tuberculin negative. This may have no special significance in view of the fact that most patients (in excess of 85%) show cutaneous anergy to a series of common microbial antigens.

The use of gallium 67 has permitted specialists in nuclear medicine to visualize infiltrates of a chronic inflammatory nature in various tissues of the body. This has been very useful in the detection of infiltrates commonly produced by sarcoidosis. It has also been useful in the detection of occult disease among patients who are otherwise asymptomatic. The so-called limited gallium scan performed in our clinic consists of an intravenous injection of gallium 67, followed in 2 days by monitoring of the patient's thorax and head with the scintillation camera. This allows the physician to visualize infiltrates in the lacrimal glands, the parotid glands, the axillary lymph nodes, and the hilar nodes. Pathologic changes in the hilar structures have thus become detectable long before x-ray films of the chest show evidence of infiltrative lesions. Infiltrations in the area of the lacrimal glands may indicate a potentially productive site for biopsy. Weinreb et al.[23] have recently demonstrated the value of limited gallium scanning, particularly in combination with tests for elevated levels of angiotensin-converting enzyme or serum lysozyme.

These latter two tests reflect excessive activity of macrophages and giant cells in parenchymal organs affected by granulomatous processes. They are not specific for sarcoidosis, and elevated serum levels of these products may be seen in such conditions as lepromatous leprosy or biliary cirrhosis. However, in combination with characteristic ocular signs, these tests may prove valuable as aids to the diagnosis.

In our experience abnormalities in the level of serum calcium are not frequently encountered among patients with sarcoidosis unless they have bony lesions attributable to this disease. Elevated levels of serum calcium may be encountered among adults who have calcific band keratopathy in association with chronic sarcoid uveitis.

As pointed out by Simpson,[18] the level of serum immunoglobulins, particularly IgG, may be elevated in patients with active inflammation attributable to sarcoidosis. This may be an indication of polyclonal B-lymphocyte stimulation. The test is variably positive among patients with confirmed sarcoidosis in our series.

Taken as a whole, the diagnosis of ocular sarcoidosis is mainly a clinical diagnosis. It may be supported by biopsy evidence or by laboratory studies that give indirect evidence of sarcoid involvement, but the clinical findings are the most important indicators of the disease. It is tempting to think that a genetic abnormality may predispose patients with sarcoidosis to some of the immunologic abnormalities described above. Although Brewerton et al.[2] found that among sarcoid patients the HLA-A1 antigen was increased among those with uveitis, there has been no general substatiation of this observation. On the other hand, patients with the HLA-B8 antigen are at a substantial risk for developing arthritis associated with sarcoidosis, especially if they also possess the DR3 antigen.[2] The meaning of these observations is still unclear. In the end it seems most likely that a combination of genetic and environmental factors will be found to be of ultimate importance in the etiology of sarcoidosis. Until such time as a definite immunogenetic marker for sarcoidosis can be established, the cost and inconvenience of HLA typing do not seem to be routinely justified.

TREATMENT

Once the diagnosis of sarcoidosis or presumptive sarcoidosis has been made, treatment should be administered according to the specific requirements of the patient. Patients who have evidence of pulmonary disease, as indicated by abnormal results in chest x-ray films or gallium scans, should be placed in the hands of an expert on pulmonary disease. Ventilatory function tests performed by such specialists often provide an important marker with regard to the progression of systemic disease. It is said that changes in the ventilatory capacity of a patient with pulmonary sarcoidosis are more accurate indices of the activity of the disease than chest x-ray films or other findings. In any case, the patient with a diagnosis or presumptive diagnosis of sarcoidosis is always at potential risk for the development of pulmonary signs. These generally require the use of systemic corticosteroids, which should be administered by an internist rather than by an ophthalmologist. With regard to the treatment of ocular sarcoidosis (in the absence of other serious signs of the disease) the treatment should be geared to the alleviation of specific ocular symptoms. In the case of ocular disease that manifests itself as an iridocyclitis alone, the treatment of choice is the local administration of corticosteroid drops. If the anterior chamber reaction is severe (4 + cells and flare), the hourly use of 1% prednisolone acetate drops may be indicated. This will generally have a profound effect on the cellular reaction in the anterior chamber and on the morphology of the keratic precipitates. Iris nodules may also "melt" under this therapy. Particular attention should be devoted to the prevention of synechia formation. During an attack of acute iridocyclitis long-acting cycloplegics such as atropine 1% should be applied two or three times a day as needed. If the iridocyclitis has reached a chronic stage, it is much more important to use short-acting dilators of the pupil, applied frequently during the course of the day. In patients with minimal activity, a single drop of a short-acting mydriatic (such as 1% tropicamide [Mydriacyl]) can be applied at bedtime. This will generally allow for the prevention of synechiae without causing the patient any serious disability.

Both the patient and the doctor must reconcile themselves to the fact that sarcoidosis of the anterior segment of the eye is a chronic disease. The anterior chamber rarely becomes absolutely free of cells and flare at any time. The potential for minor exacerbations of the disease is always there. Ophthalmologists are often disappointed that they cannot render their patients free of the signs of ocular inflammation, and patients often fail to understand that they cannot get over this disease in the same way that they can get over a pimple or a carbuncle. The aim of therapy is not to render the patient free of all signs of the disease; rather, the aim of therapy is to prevent vision-threatening complications. Synechia formation is one of these. The patient should be urged to inspect his pupil on a daily basis and to increase mydriatic therapy at the first sign of any pupillary irregularity. The patient should be urged to maintain his regular schedule of low-dose corticosteroid drop therapy even during times when he may not be having visual symptoms. Compliance with this mode of therapy is often hard to obtain, particularly among socioeconomic groups of lower status.

Secondary glaucoma is a very troublesome complication of sarcoidosis of the anterior segment. If the level of the intraocular pressure is 30 mm Hg or less, control of the pressure can often be achieved by the use of timolol maleate (Timoptic) combined with epinephrine or Propine (dipivalyl epinephrine) drops. Pilocarpine alone is not recommended for the control of glaucoma. Pilocarpine therapy often increases the irritation of the iris, and if pupillary constriction is obtained, synechia formation may result.

Many patients are obliged to take carbonic anhydrase inhibitors as well. Acetazolamide (Diamox) or methazolamide (Neptazane) are the most frequently used agents. Therapy with these drugs is fraught with multiple complications, including paresthesias, dizziness, and renal stone formation.

In many cases surgical treatment is required. The corneoiridic angle is usually open, but there may be extensive infiltration of the trabecular spaces with cells and debris. Peripheral anterior synechia formation is often encountered. Trabeculectomy is the operation of choice, but it often fails despite meticulous attention to surgical detail. Inflammatory deposits are often found in the newly made drainage channels, and scarring is the result. Peripheral iridoplasty has been performed on several cases in our institution, but the results have not been encouraging. The same is true of cryotherapy applied to the ciliary body. This generally produces too small an effect, or the eye is rendered hypotonous as a result of therapy that is too vigorous.

Sarcoid lesions of the posterior segment of the eye generally, though not always, accompany serious systemic lesions. For this reason, systemic therapy with corticosteroids is often required. Where this is not the case, lesions that are a threat to vision should be treated with injections of depo steroids. Cystoid macular edema, a common complication of the posterior lesions of sarcoidosis, can be greatly relieved by the use of posterior sub-Tenon's injections of Depo-Kenalog (triamcinolone acetonide). This form of therapy may also have a profound effect on the vitreous opacity. The retinal perivasculitis itself does not require therapy unless branch vein occlusion is threatened. Frequent inspection of the fundus must be made, for this complication often gives rise to hemorrhage in the vitreous.

Focal infiltrates of the retina and choroid may be treated by observation alone, particularly if they are small and peripheral. Those that threaten to impinge on the macula, the papillomacular bundle, or the optic nerve require treatment with large doses of systemic corticosteroids. For the average 70 kg patient, doses of 100 to 150 mg per day in divided doses are appropriate. After 1 week, the medication should be given on an alternate-day schedule, with twice the normal daily dose being given each morning at 8:00 A.M. Often it is necessary to administer small doses of corticosteroid on the alternate day, at least until one can be sure that a sustained anti-inflammatory effect is being maintained. The reason for this is clearly explained by Fauci,[9] who has analyzed both the successes and failures of the alternate-day steroid regimens. If an alternate-day regimen is to be used, it is important to administer prednisone or prednisolone rather than longer acting preparations such as dexamethasone. The principle benefit of alternate-day steroid medication is that the bloodstream is partially cleared of corticosteroid during certain periods. This gives the patient's adrenal glands a chance to function in their normal cyclic fashion.

Sarcoid infiltrations of the optic nerve are usually associated with similar infiltrations in the brain. These require the use of systemically administered corticosteroids in large doses.

Since sarcoidosis is a chronic disease that is characterized by exacerbations and remissions extending over many years' time, it is preferable to treat patients intermittently, rather than constantly, with corticosteroids. It is desirable to treat an exacerbation vigorously with relatively high dosage of corticosteroids for a few weeks and then to taper the medication to a null point or to a low maintenance dosage within 2 to 3 months. Even with intermittent systemic medication, the side effects may be very harmful. These include but are not limited to demineralization of bone, obesity, hirsutism, acne, gastric irritation, sleeplessness, and hypertension.

Because of the well-recognized acquired deficiency in cell-mediated immunity, attempts have been made to treat sarcoidosis with immunostimulating agents such as levamisole.[21] These have not met with success as far as the amelioration of the symptoms of sarcoidosis is concerned. It may well be that the depression of cell-mediated immunity is an epiphenomenon; that is, it is not directly connected with the pathogenesis of the lesions but is a secondary result of the disease. In this case, restoration of immune competence would not be expected to benefit the disease directly.

REFERENCES

1. Adams, D.O.: The structure of mononuclear phagocytes differentiating in vivo, Am. J. Pathol. **76:**17, 1974.
2. Brewerton, D.A., Cockburn, C., James, D.C.O., James, D.G., and Neville, E.: HLA antigens in sarcoidosis, Clin. Exp. Immunol. **27:**227, 1977.
3. Byrne, E.B., Evans, A.S., Fouts, D.W., and Israel, H.L.: Serological hyperreactivity to Epstein-Barr virus and other viral antigens in sarcoidosis. In Iwai, K., and Hosoda, Y., editors: Proceedings of the Fourth International Conference on Sarcoidosis, Baltimore, 1974, University Park Press.
4. Chapman, J.S.: Mycobacterial and mycotic antibodies in sera of patients with sarcoidosis: results of studies using agar double-diffusion technique, Ann. Intern. Med. **55:**918, 1961.
5. Constable, I.J., Chester, G.H., Horne, R., and Harriott, J.S.: Human chorioretinal biopsy under controlled systemic hypotensive anaesthesia, Br. J. Ophthalmol. **64:**559, 1980.
6. Cummings, M.M.: An evaluation of the possible relationship of pine pollen to sarcoidosis (a critical summary), Acta Med. Scand. **48**(suppl.):425, 1964.
7. Daniele, R.P., Dauber, J.H., and Rossman, M.D.: Immunologic abnormalities in sarcoidosis, Ann. Intern. Med. **92:**406, 1980.
8. Daniele, R.P., and Rowlands, D.T.: Antibodies to T-cells in sarcoidosis, Ann. N.Y. Acad. Sci. **278:**88, 1976.
9. Fauci, A.S.: Alternate-day corticosteroid therapy, Am. J. Med. **64:**729, 1978.

10. Gass, J.D.M., and Olson, C.L.: Sarcoidosis with optic nerve and retinal involvement: a clinicopathologic case report, Trans. Am. Acad. Ophthalmol. Otolaryngol. **73:**739, 1973.
11. Ghose, T., Landrigan, P., and Asif, A.: Localization of immunoglobulin and complement in pulmonary sarcoid granulomas, Chest **66:**264, 1974.
12. Glikmann, G., Nielsen, H., Pallisgaard, G., Cristensen, K.M., and Svehag, S.E.: Circulating immune complexes, free antigen, and α-1 antitrypsin levels in sarcoidosis patients, Scand. J. Respir. Dis. **60:**317, 1979.
13. Goodwin, J.S., DeHoratius, R., Israel, H., Peake, G.T., and Messner, R.P.: Suppressor cell function in sarcoidosis, Ann. Intern. Med. **90:**169, 1979.
14. Gould, H.L., and Kaufman, H.E.: Boeck's sarcoid of the ocular fundus, Am. J. Ophthalmol. **52:**633, 1961.
15. Hedfors, E., and Norberg, R.: Evidence for circulating immune complexes in sarcoidosis, Clin. Exp. Immunol. **16:**493, 1974.
16. Jansson, E.: Isolation of *Mycoplasma* from sarcoid tissue, J. Clin. Pathol. **25:**837, 1972.
17. Schlaegel, T.F.: Current aspects of uveitis, Boston, 1977, Little, Brown & Co.
18. Simpson, G.V.: Diagnosis and treatment of uveitis in association with sarcoidosis, Trans. Am. Ophthalmol. Soc. **66:**117, 1968.
19. Smith, R.E., Godrey, W.A., and Kimura, S.J.: Chronic cyclitis. I. Course and visual prognosis, Trans. Am. Acad. Ophthalmol. Otolaryngol. **77:**760, 1973.
20. Tannenbaum, H., Pinkus, G.S., and Schur, P.H.: Immunological characterization of subpopulations of mononuclear cells in tissue and peripheral blood from patients with sarcoidosis, Clin. Immunol. Immunopathol. **5:**133, 1976.
21. Veien, N.K.: Cutaneous sarcoidosis treated with levamisole, Dermatologica **154:**185, 1977.
22. Veien, N.K., Hardt, F., and Bendixen, G.: Humoral and cellular immunity in sarcoidosis, Acta Med. Scand. **203:**321, 1978.
23. Weinreb, R.N., Barth, R., and Kimura, S.J.: Limited gallium scans and angiotensin converting enzyme in granulomatous uveitis, Ophthalmology **87:**207, 1980.

19

Outer retinal ischemic infarction: a newly recognized complication of cataract extraction and closed vitrectomy

J. Donald M. Gass

Outer retinal ischemic infarction is a newly recognized complication of cataract extraction and closed vitrectomy.[2,3,7,8] The clinical features and animal model of this syndrome were presented at the 1981 American Academy of Ophthalmology.[3,7] The clinical features consist of the following: (1) acute loss of central, paracentral, and in some cases peripheral vision, discovered usually on the first postoperative day; (2) diffuse and patchy whitening of the outer retinal layers in the posterior fundus with sparing of the foveal area, which may simulate a central retinal artery occlusion (Fig. 19-1); (3) normal fluorescein angiographic retinal and choroidal appearance and circulation times; (4) a peculiar polygonal pattern of fluorescein staining of the pigment epithelium and outer retina in the area of retinal whitening (Fig. 19-2); (5) disappearance of the retinal whitening and the appearance in the same areas of mottling of the pigment epithelium (Fig. 19-3); (6) partial recovery of the visual field including the central field, but retention of permanent field loss corresponding to the zones of pigment epithelial derangement; and (7) preservation of a normal optic disc and normal retinal vessel caliber (Fig. 19-3).

How can we explain this remarkable ophthalmologic picture and sequence of events? It is postulated that during the use of intraocular volume-reducing devices before cataract surgery, during phakoemulsification, or during closed vitrectomy, that the intraocular pressure is elevated to a level sufficient to occlude the choroidal and retinal circulation for a time probably in excess of 30 minutes. The effects of oxygen deprivation on the retina is a product of the concentration of cells and their metabolic rate. On both counts the outer retina including the pigment epithelium is more susceptible to ischemic infarction than the inner. Because of the low concentration of cells, the foveal and peripheral retina are more resistant to ischemia than the pericentral and midportions of the retina. Temporary occlusion of both the choroidal and retinal circulation for a period of time, estimated to be 30 to 60 minutes, would be expected to cause relative ischemia of the entire retina, but it causes selective ischemic whitening and infarction of only the outer retina and pigment epithelium in the posterior fundus, with those tissues in the foveal area (cherry red spot) and the peripheral retina being spared. The peculiar mul-

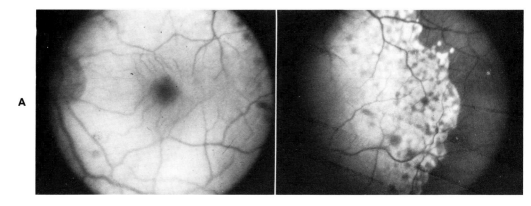

Fig. 19-1. One day after phakoemulsification, this 32-year-old man had bare light-perception vision. Note cherry red spot in **A** and peculiar pattern of outer retinal whitening in **B**.

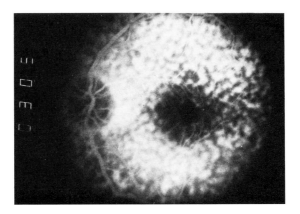

Fig. 19-2. Early angiogram (30 seconds) showing polygonal pattern of staining.

tifocal and multilobular pattern of whitening at the outer margins of the ischemic retina (Fig. 19-1) and the peculiar polygonal fluorescent staining pattern seen during the first 24 to 48 hours postoperatively (Fig. 19-2) are caused by variations in blood flow through the lily-pad angioarchitecture of the choriocapillaris. During the first few days postoperatively, the function of the ischemic but not infarcted retina in the fovea and peripheral retina begins to recover visual function. The patient may regain a small area of central visual field and good acuity in the midst of a dense broad area of a permanent ring scotoma. Within a matter of weeks, the necrotic outer retina disappears and a mottled pattern of remodeled pigment epithelium is left in the previous areas of infarction. The inner retina, because of its greater resistance to anoxia, is spared, and therefore the caliber of the retinal vessels and the appearance of the optic disc are unaffected.

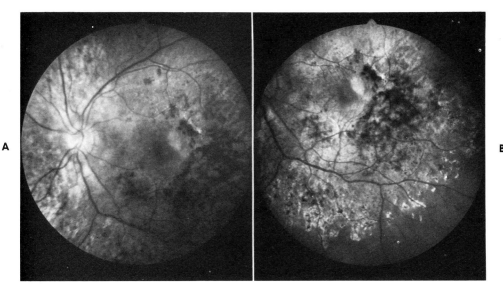

Fig. 19-3. Fourteen months after phakoemulsification. Visual acuity is 20/25. **A** and **B,** Compare Fig. 19-1.

The funduscopic picture just described is only one of a spectrum of ischemic pictures that may occur as the result of obstruction of intraocular blood flow caused by elevation of the intraocular pressure. At one end of the spectrum only a small zone of outer retinal whitening in the paracentral area may occur. At the other, a diffuse whitening of the entire inner and outer retinal layers may occur (combined choroidal and retinal artery occlusions) if the elevated pressure is maintained sufficiently long. The duration of occlusion required to produce these pictures in humans is not known and undoubtedly varies depending on the general physical status of the patient.

Parrish et al. produced an ordered range of ischemic pictures from one extreme to another, including that of outer retinal necrosis described above, experimentally in owl monkeys by perfusing the anterior chamber to artificially elevate and maintain the intraocular pressure just above the systolic ophthalmic artery pressure.[7] With perfusion between 60 and 90 minutes, the early and late ophthalmoscopic and angiographic changes of outer retinal ischemic necrosis in the human were reproduced in the monkey. Light and electron microscopy revealed necrosis of the outer retina and pigment epithelium in the areas of retinal whitening. Full-thickness retinal necrosis was produced by perfusion for 120 minutes.

In 1979, Diamond and Kaplan reported patchy pigment epithelial edema in the posterior pole postoperatively in 2 of 25 patients after combined lensectomy and closed pars plana vitrectomy for complications of vitrectomy.[2] Both patients had, in addition, scleral buckling procedures. The authors attributed these changes to choroidal ischemia caused by either a transient rise of intraocular pressure caused by the scleral buckling or decreased blood pressure of the patients. Elevation of intraocular pressure above systolic pressure with a scleral buckle would not be expected to last much more than 5 to 10 minutes and therefore would be unlikely to produce ischemic infarction. A more prolonged period of hypertension caused by excessive elevation of the infusion bottle would appear to be the greatest risk as a cause for retinal infarction during vitrectomy.

Recently Rosenblum et al. reported on three patients (including the case published by Gass et al.[3]), who noted loss of vision immediately after phakoemulsification.[8] All showed the typical findings of what we call "outer retinal ischemic infarction" and what these authors called "choroidal ischemia." They stated that the most likely cause was elevation of intraocular pressure during phakoemulsification. If the fundus changes are caused by sustained increase in intraocular pressure, the retinal changes are the result of both choroidal and retinal vascular insufficiency, since the level of intraocular pressure required to close arterial circulation in the choroid and retina is approximately the same.[1]

Other authors have reported visual loss caused by ocular compression, such as external eye pressure by a face rest during neurologic procedures,[5] and a combination of malpositioned anesthetic mask and surgical shock.[4,6] Most of these patients sustained severe permanent visual loss and a funduscopic picture of combined choroidal and central retinal artery obstruction (widespread pigment derangement, narrowing of the retinal blood vessels, and optic atrophy).

The fundus picture of acute outer retinal ischemic infarction may be misdiagnosed as a central retinal artery occlusion, particularly when it is observed immediately postoperatively in a patient who has had a retrobulbar injection of an anesthetic. Although profound visual loss, a cherry red spot, and retinal whitening are common to both, the sharp line of demarcation and irregular configurational borders of the areas of whitening, the round and polygonal islands of preserved retinal clarity within large zones of whitening, the neighboring isolated islands of retinal whitening, and preservation of a normal retinal circulation time angiographically are important clues that only the outer retina is infarcted. It is difficult in the early postoperative period to determine that the retinal whitening is largely confined to the outer retinal layers. The later findings, including pigment mottling, failure to develop optic atrophy and retinal vessel narrowing, and recovery of large areas of peripheral and often a central island of vision, are evidence that infarction was largely confined to the outer retina.

Although the precise cause of this peculiar fundus picture in patients after cataract extraction and vitrectomy is not established, the clinical and experimental data up to now suggest that it is caused by a sustained increase in intraocular pressure to levels above ophthalmic arterial pressure for periods of time, probably in excess of 30 minutes, either immediately before or during the course of surgery. Cautious use of techniques to lower intraocular volume preoperatively and careful monitoring of intraocular pressure during surgery should prevent his complication.

REFERENCES

1. Anderson, D.R., and David, E.B.: Sensitivities of ocular tissues to acute pressure-induced ischemia, Arch. Ophthalmol. **93:**267-274, 1975.
2. Diamond, J.G., and Kaplan, H.J.: Uveitis: effect of vitrectomy combined with lensectomy, Ophthalmology **86:**1320-1327, 1979.
3. Gass, J.D.M., and Parrish, R.: Outer retinal ischemic infarction: a newly recognized complication of cataract extraction and closed vitrectomy. I. A case report, Ophthalmology. (In press.)
4. Givner, I., and Jaffe, N.: Occlusion of the central retinal artery following anesthesia, Arch. Ophthalmol. **43:**197-201, 1950.

5. Hollenhorst, R.W., Svien, H.G., and Benoit, C.F.: Unilateral blindness occurring during anesthesia for neurosurgical operations, Arch. Ophthalmol. **52:**819-830, 1954.

6. Jampol, L.M., Goldbaum, M., Rosenberg, M., et al.: Ischemia of ciliary arterial circulation from ocular compression, Arch. Ophthalmol. **93:**1311-1317, 1975.

7. Parrish, R., Gass, J.D.M., and Anderson, D.R.: Outer retinal ischemic infarction: a newly recognized complication of cataract extraction and closed vitrectomy. II. An animal model, Ophthalmology. (In press.)

8. Rosenblum, P.K., Michels, R.G., Stark, W.J., and Taylor, H.R.: Choroidal ischemia after extracapsular cataract extraction by phacoemulsification, Ophthalmology **1:**263-270, 1982.

20

Pars plicata surgery in the child for pupillary membranes, persistent hyperplastic primary vitreous, and infantile cataract

Morton F. Goldberg
Gholam A. Peyman*

Surgery for the neonatal and infantile eye is considerably more complex than that in the adult. First of all, the small dimensions make atraumatic intraocular manipulations difficult, especially if there is any degree of microphthalmia. Second, the postoperative complications are often common but difficult to detect, and they frequently require multiple examinations or therapeutic maneuvers with the patient under general anesthesia.[3,15] Third, there is a compelling need to restore clarity of the media completely and as quickly as possible, followed by precise refraction and a patching regimen, in an attempt to prevent irreversible deprivation amblyopia. Repeated follow-up examinations are needed, both for evaluation of the anatomic status of the eye itself and for visual rehabilitation. Again, there is the necessity for frequent examinations under anesthesia, often for manipulations such as retinoscopy, keratometry, ultrasonography, intraocular pressure measurements, and multiple contact lens fittings.

The emotional and physical traumas to and social problems for the child and his entire family are considerable. Successful rehabilitation requires the following: (1) correct diagnosis, (2) an operable condition allowing creation of crystal-clear media and occurring in the presence of a normal macula and normal optic nerve, (3) modern, technically competent ocular surgery and general anesthesia, and (4) perhaps most importantly, a compulsively dedicated family and ophthalmic team for postoperative optical and amblyopia therapy.

GROWTH OF NEONATAL AND INFANTILE EYE

The major determinants of refractive error (axial length, corneal power, and lens power) change greatly, but in a compensatory fashion, under normal circumstances of postnatal growth. Interference with any of these major determining factors, as with

*M.D., Professor of Ophthalmology, Department of Ophthalmology, University of Illinois College of Medicine and University of Illinois Eye and Ear Infirmary, Chicago, Illinois.

surgical manipulations, may have profound but as yet largely unknown influences on the complex and active biologic processes known as compensatory emmetropization.[44] Clear retinal imagery appears to be important in the development of compensatory emmetropization,[22,63] and thus surgical intervention is often justified despite the unknowns involved.

Unlike that of the rest of the body, there is no pubertal spurt in the growth of the eyeball. There are, however, in the view of most investigators, two major growth phases, the infantile phase and the juvenile phase. The first and major growth phase occurs between birth and 3 years, and the second, slower and slighter period occurs between 3 and 14 years.[70]

Larsen[34] further divided the growth phases into an extremely rapid postnatal phase during the first half year, followed by a slower phase between 2 and 5 years, and finally an even slower phase until age 13 years, after which axial growth virtually ceases.

At birth, the average axial length of the normal globe is about 16 to 18 mm, enlarging to approximately 23 mm by 3 years of age.[10,70] Theoretically, this would account for about a 15-diopter shift[70] or greater,[74] if it were not for compensatory changes in the shape and size of the lens, cornea, and anterior chamber (compensatory emmetropization). Hirano et al. have shown ultrasonically that the overall axial length of the mature infant eye increases rapidly from birth until 4 to 5 months of age, slowing down therafter.[27] By way of contrast, the increase in axial length of the premature eye increases steadily until 12 months of age, after which growth is similar to that occurring in full-term babies. Between 3 and 14 years of age there is about a 0.1 mm increase in axial length per year, following which very little additional growth occurs.

Precise data on the dimensional changes occurring in the cornea, anterior chamber, and lens for the period between birth and 3 years are known to only a limited extent.[34] More such data are badly needed, both in the normal and abnormal eye, with and without surgery, especially when one considers that the critical or sensitive period for visual maturation occurs during this time and that intraocular surgical intervention for congenital or infantile eye diseases must have at least some (and probably a substantial) influence on maturation of the eyeball, emmetropization, and development of amblyopia. Most of the growth in corneal diameter, which averages about 10 mm in the newborn to about 11.8 mm in the adult,[11] has occurred by the end of the first year of life[70]; of this, the predominant expansion has been believed to occur in the second 6 months after birth.[11]

Of major concern has been the potential effect of removal of formed vitreous gel from the neonatal or infantile eye. The volume of the entire normal newborn globe is about 2.4 ml and that of the adult is about 6.9 ml, of which approximately 60% to 70% is vitreous. Most of the infantile growth spurt is attributable to enlargement of the vitreous.[34] It might be supposed, on theoretical grounds, that the semisolid infantile vitreous gel assists in the normal first and second phases of ocular growth. However, in a neonatal animal model, Zauberman and colleagues were unable to influence axial length or corneal diameter by performing total vitrectomy through a pars plana incision.[80] Furthermore, most immature human eyes subjected to vitrectomy surgery appear to enlarge relatively normally.

Unfortunately, however, a large number of reliable dimensional measurements of the various ocular components are not available after vitrectomy in children's eyes. The following case report indicates, nonetheless, that maturational enlargement can occur, despite extensive pars plicata lensectomy and vitrectomy, even in severe, congenital microphthalmia and even when complicated by the congenital rubella syndrome.

Case 1. A black male baby was born at 32 weeks' gestation with bilateral dense ("complete") cataracts as part of the rubella embryopathy syndrome. Corneal diameters were approximately 8 mm OU.

At 23 days of age his systemic condition permitted general anesthesia, and one of us (M.F.G.) performed pars plicata lensectomy and vitrectomy in the right eye with the Peyman Vitrophage. Vitreous was removed to the level of the retinal surface (Fig. 20-1). A week later, the same surgeon performed a limbal aspiration of the cataract in the left eye with the irrigating-aspirating handpiece of the Kelman Phacoemulsifier. The posterior lens capsule was left in situ. Soft contact lenses were fit 1 week postoperatively in both eyes, and multiple examinations with the patient under anesthesia with measurements of ocular dimensions and multiple refittings of contact lenses were carried out over the next 2½ years.

The initial postoperative course was unremarkable in both eyes, with development of crystal-clear media bilaterally. Within several months, however, the residual lens capsule in the left eye became translucent. The slight impairment in transparency of the ocular media was best appreciated during retinoscopy. This defect was not considered to be sufficiently dense to warrant another intraocular surgical procedure, but the patient developed a left esotropia of 24 to 30 prism diopters. The pupillary membrane allowed the fundus to be seen only in the immediate peripapillary region. Visual fixation was central but unsteady, bilaterally. Pendular nystagmus was constant though it improved whenever corrective lenses were in place.

The early postoperative refractive error was +39 D in the right eye and +40 D in the left. The baby's soft contact lenses were specially made (+45 D) to correct his refractive error for objects held within his own arms' length. A series of examinations with the patient under general anesthesia was carried out in order to verify the ocular dimensions and refractive errors, and adjustments of the lenses' power were repetitively made, eventually including correction for distance vision. After the loss of many contact lenses, the mother finally resorted to spectacles (with bifocals) for the child at age 2½ years.

Ocular dimensions remained remarkably symmetric; that is, despite the major differences in surgical technique, with vitreous removed from the right eye but not from the left, the corneal diameters, retinoscopic refractive errors, keratometric measurements, and ultrasonically determined axial lengths were virtually the same in the two microphthalmic eyes (Table 20-1).

The corneal diameters enlarged very little. Retinoscopy, however, showed progressive and symmetric diminution of hyperopic power, as would be expected if axial length were increasing during neonatal growth. The initial retinoscopic refractive errors of +39 D in the right eye and +40 D in the left decreased to +31 D in both eyes by 8 months of age, to +27 D in the right eye and +29 D in the left by 18 months of age, and to +19 D in the right and +18 D in the left eye by 24 months of age, after which the values remained about the same (Table 20-1). Concomitantly, the ultrasonically determined axial lengths enlarged symmetrically. Again, most of the growth occurred between birth and 8 months of age. Initial axial length measurements at 44 days of age were 11.5 mm in the right eye and 11.0 mm in the left. By 8 months of age, the axial lengths were 17.2 mm in the right eye and 17.4 mm in the left. At 24 months of age, the measurements were

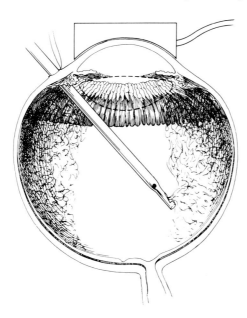

Fig. 20-1. Technique of pars plicata lensectomy and vitrectomy. A large central core of vitreous is removed routinely, along with the cataract.

18.4 mm in the right and 19.3 mm in the left eye, and at 30 months of age they were essentially unchanged at 19 mm in the right eye and 19.6 mm in the left (Table 20-1).

Fluorescein angioscopy was done with the patient under general anesthesia at age 18 months, and no cystoid macular edema was present in either eye.

At 30 months of age, the child could reach accurately for a 4 by 4 mm piece of paper at a distance of 1½ feet. His esotropia appeared alternating. At 33 months of age, the eyes appeared straight most of the time, with constant low-amplitude pendular nystagmus. The child's visual fixation was central and unsteady but equal with either eye.

Comment. The right eye had a pars plicata lensectomy and vitrectomy at 23 days of age, and the left eye had a translimbal extracapsular lens aspiration at 30 days of age by the same surgeon. Subsequent enlargement of the two eyes during the infantile phase of growth was symmetric despite removal of the vitreous gel from the right eye and despite initially severe bilateral microphthalmia and rubella infection. Enlargement of axial length in both eyes was substantial, from 11.0-11.5 mm at 44 days of age to 19.0-19.6 mm at 30 months of age. Prospective biometric data of this type have been previously reported only once.[14] There was a concomitant reduction of hyperopic power from +39-40 D at 44 days of age to +18.5-20 D at 30 months of age. Neonatal removal of the vitreous therefore did not substantially impede ocular growth. Interestingly, if one had relied solely on measurements of corneal diameter, one would have falsely concluded that substantial growth of the eyes had not occurred.

The eye subjected to the lensectomy and vitrectomy was clearly the preferred eye for most of the patient's life, ostensibly because of clearer media. The eye was also more easily and more accurately measured by retinoscopy, and its fundus was more easily and more completely examined by ophthalmoscopy because of the absence of a pupillary membrane.

Table 20-1. Case 1. Comparative effects of pars plicata lensectomy-vitrectomy (OD) and of extracapsular cataract aspiration (OS) on ocular biometry

Date	Age	Corneal diameter* (mm) OD H	OD V	OS H	OS V	Retinoscopy OD	Retinoscopy OS	Keratometry (D) OD	Keratometry (D) OS	Axial length (mm) OD	Axial length (mm) OS	Tonometry (mm Hg) OD	Tonometry (mm Hg) OS	Comments
1/21/79	Birth	≈8	≈8	≈8	≈8									
2/13/79	23 days	Surgery OD												
2/20/79	30 days	Surgery OS												
3/6/79	44 days													
5/16/79	4 months	9	8	9	8	+39 D	+40 D			11.5	11.0	5	5	Contact lens fitted for OD
9/79	8 months	9	8	9	8	+31 D	+31 D	44	44 × 42	17.2	17.4			Crystal clear media OU Soft contact lenses OU Poor fixation OU Pendular nystagmus
7/80	18 months					+27 D	+29 D					18	10	≈24 Δ left esotropia Slightly decreased red reflex OS (retinoscopy difficult) because of translucent lens capsule
1/81	24 months	9	9			+19 D	+18 D			18.4	19.3	7	18	
7/81	30 months	9	8.5			+20 D	+18.50 D	40 × 45.75	43.75 × 45	19.0	19.6	12	17	Fluorescein angioscopy shows no cystoid macular edema OU 30 Δ alternating esotropia Pendular nystagmus
10/81	33 months													Fixes centrally but unsteadily OU Multiple losses of contact lenses Spectacles being worn usually Eyes straight usually Pendular nystagmus OU

*H, Horizontal; V, vertical.

DEPRIVATION AMBLYOPIA

Of paramount concern to the ophthalmologist caring for an infant with cloudy ocular media is the possible development of irreversible deprivation amblyopia. Accordingly, clinical trends now suggest that intraocular surgery should be done as soon as possible; that such surgery should quickly, completely, and permanently restore transparency of the ocular media; and that intensively dedicated efforts at visual rehabilitation with contact lenses (or other devices) and with patching regimens must rank as high in order of priority as the surgery itself.[3,30]

Difficulties have arisen in the past with these rehabilitation programs because of difficulties in assessment of visual acuity in human infants. Any of three quantitative techniques (optokinetic nystagmus, preferential looking, and the visually evoked potential) can be utilized effectively by trained personnel in this endeavor,[8,30] along with the traditional clinical assessment of visual fixation and strabismus patterns.

Utilizing these techniques, one can demonstrate, even in unilaterally affected patients, that early surgery, followed by proper optical correction and frequent changes in the patching regimen, can result in symmetric vision.[3,13,30] The popular belief that congenital opacities in only one eye represent insoluble rehabilitative problems must be modified in view of these recent reports.

The precise timing of the critical or sensitive period for maturation of the visual pathways in the central nervous system is not known for the human.[3] Vaegan and Taylor[77] have suggested that restorative surgery and optical correction for such diseases as unilateral congenital cataract should be completed within the first 4 months of life. Results in humans reported by Jacobson et al.[30] are compatible with this idea. Beller et al.[3] have reviewed the older literature and have concluded that good visual results are rare in children 6 months or older. Accordingly, if the cataractous process is unilateral, they have restricted their operative attempts to infants 6 weeks of age or younger. Surgery will presumably do little good, however, if it leaves the ocular media less than completely transparent (such as opacification of the posterior lens capsule), or if the postoperative course is characterized by frequent complications and the necessity for additional operative procedures, or if optical rehabilitation cannot be effected immediately. The visual prognosis is also substantially worsened by the simultaneous presence of other congenital abnormalities in the same eye, as is often the case in persistent hyperplastic primary vitreous (PHPV).

TECHNIQUE OF SURGERY: TRANSCILIARY BODY ("POSTERIOR") APPROACH

With the foregoing considerations in mind, we generally use a transciliary body approach for congenital cataract, pupillary membrane, and carefully selected cases of PHPV. Although we occasionally utilize limbal incisions, with and without preservation of the posterior lens capsule, the so-called posterior approach to anterior segment lesions offers many advantages over the conventional anterior approach.

These advantages include the ability to perform the following maneuvers: (1) removal of opaque material in *all* axes through a single small sclerotomy, usually with a single intraocular instrument, even if some miosis occurs (Fig. 20-2); (2) the safe and complete removal of both the anterior and posterior lens capsules (This is desirable in neonates and infants in order to ensure quick, complete, and permanent restoration of crystal-clear media. If the posterior capsule is left in situ in a very young eye, it will almost

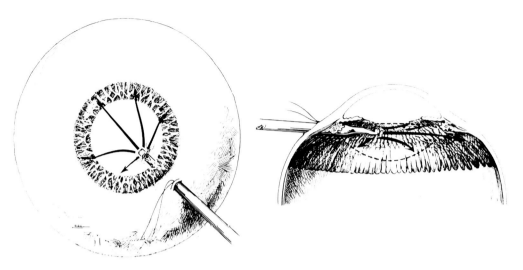

Fig. 20-2. Technique of pars plicata approach to neonatal cataract, pupillary membrane, or persistent hyperplastic primary vitreous. The posterior approach permits removal of opaque material in all axes through a single sclerotomy.

invariably become translucent or opacify,[26,32] thereby increasing the chance of deprivation amblyopia.); (3) the simultaneous repair, if necessary, of coexistent retinal lesions, such as retinal disinsertion, tear, or detachment associated with traumatic cataract or PHPV; (4) bimanual instrumentation, if needed, such as bipolar diathermy (as for operative hemorrhage) or a cutting-board (''chopping-block'') technique for cutting leathery or calcific tissue (Fig. 20-3); (5) atraumatic removal of the vitreous, especially when the cataract has been caused by perforating trauma involving penetration of the posterior lens capsule or when the cataract (or clear lens) is associated with ectopia lentis; and (6) use of an irrigating, surgical contact lens to bring the deep vitreous and fundus into focus with the operating microscope. Use of the contact lens and microscope permits removal of lenticular, membranous, or vitreous debris that falls into or is found within the deep vitreous or preretinal space (Fig. 20-4). The ability to operate safely in the deep vitreous and preretinal space is particularly helpful in PHPV (p. 238). The necessity to operate in the vitreous is illustrated by the following case report of cataract extraction in a child who proved, at the time of surgery, also to have severe vitreoretinal abnormality that was not detectable preoperatively.

> **Case 2.** A 13-year-old black girl was referred for treatment of uveitis and secondary mature cataract in the right eye (Fig. 20-5, *A*). This eye previously had normal vision and had been the better eye. She had had pain, redness, floaters, and greatly decreased vision in the right eye for the preceding 8 months. Her left eye had anisometropic amblyopia but was otherwise normal.
>
> Vision was perception and accurate projection of light in the right eye and 20/200 (6/60) in the left. Slitlamp examination of the right eye showed about two dozen small keratic precipitates, and 1 to 2+ band keratopathy. There were 2+ beam and 2+ cells in the anterior chamber. Extensive posterior synechiae to a mature, chalky white lens

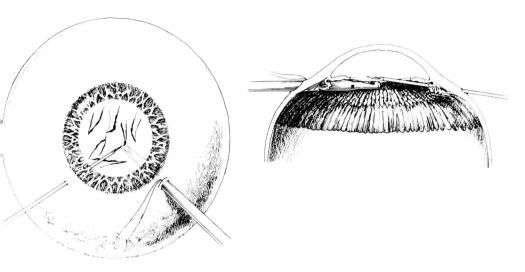

Fig. 20-3. Technique of pars plicata removal of leathery, taut, or calcific material using a ''chopping-block'' or ''cutting-board'' procedure. Ziegler knife (or needle) lacerates unwanted material into narrow triangular flaps and feeds it into mouth of vitrectomy instrument. If abnormal tissue resists cutting by the knife, it is minced between the tips of the two instruments. Both instruments are inserted through the pars plicata.

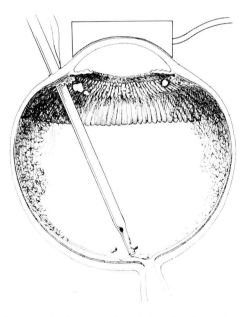

Fig. 20-4. Transciliary body approach allows use of surgical contact lens. Thus any debris falling into the deep vitreous or preretinal space can be visualized and then aspirated.

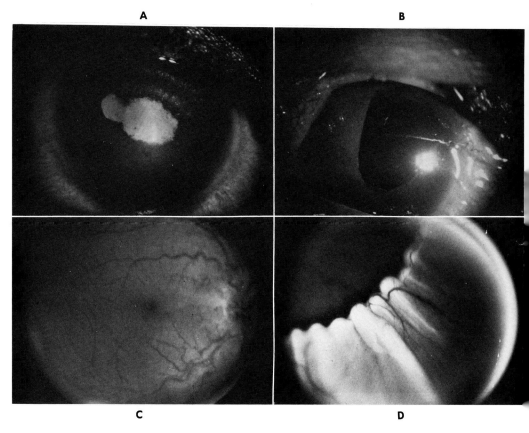

Fig. 20-5. Secondary cataract and posterior synechiae in 13-year-old girl. **A,** Preoperative appearance. **B,** Postoperative appearance. **C,** Postoperatively, the ocular media were clear, and the retina was attached. **D,** Postoperative appearance of many small meridional retinal folds on high, posterior scleral buckle. Retinal detachment procedure was performed at same time as lensectomy.

were present. B-scan ultrasonography showed no abnormalities in the posterior segment of the right eye.

The patient underwent a pars plana lensectomy and synechiectomy with the Vitrophage by one of us (M.F.G.). The posterior lens cortex was heavily vascularized. Once the lens was removed, the vitreous was found to be totally opaque with multiple membranes. These were also removed, and the macula and disc appeared relatively normal, except for some contracture of the internal limiting membrane over the macula. In the periphery, there was tractional elevation of the retina, which was pulled anteriorly into a vascularized cyclitic membrane. Because of this, a 360-degree buckling procedure was also performed at the same time.

The postoperative course was uneventful (Fig. 20-5, *B*). The media remained clear (Fig. 20-5, *C*), and the retina remained attached on a very high and posterior 360-degree buckle (Fig. 20-5, *D*). Two months postoperatively, her vision was 20/25 (6/7.5) with +9.00 sph +1.00 cyl × 135°.

Comment. Unexpectedly, opaque and vascularized vitreous membranes were encountered in a child's eye during pars plana lensectomy for a cataract secondary to severe uveitis. A peripheral tractional retinal detachment and vascularized cyclitic membrane were also seen after a vitrectomy was completed. They were treated with a simultaneous 360-degree scleral buckling procedure.

Simple lens extraction would clearly have failed to improve vision and would have had no favorable impact on the tractional retinal detachment. This patient's multiple problems were successfully treated at one operation utilizing a single pars plana sclerotomy.

Reduced complications

Complications of intracapsular and translimbal extracapsular cataract or membrane extractions that are eliminated or minimized by transciliary body surgery include the following[19]: unplanned rupture of the posterior lens capsule, scleral or corneal collapse, uncontrolled vitreous loss, intraoperative flattening of the anterior chamber, keratopathy from vitreous incarceration or adherence, pupillary block glaucoma, iris prolapse, detachment of Descemet's membrane, changing corneal astigmatism postoperatively, opacification of the posterior lens capsule, and so on.[19]

Pars plicata versus pars plana approach

To remain as far from the ora serrata as possible, we have been utilizing the pars plicata approach in young children for over 5 years.[59] This has proved to be free of complications specifically attributable to location of the sclerotomy incision. Bleeding from the ciliary processes, for example, has not occurred in over 32 eyes.[55]

We occasionally utilize transillumination for identification of the ciliary body but, in practice, make the sclerotomy incision 2 to 2.5 mm posterior to the corneoscleral limbus in almost all neonatal eyes, regardless of dimensions. If the microphthalmia is severe (corneal diameter of about 8 to 8.5 mm or less) and the palpebral aperture is also excessively small, despite lateral canthotomy, we have sometimes resorted to an anterior (limbal) approach. In almost all circumstances, however, the pars plicata approach has been highly satisfactory in young children's eyes, in that it offers all the advantages of the "posterior" approach while allowing one to avoid the anteriormost extension of the retina, even when the anteroposterior width of the pars plana is substantially narrower than normal.

Fears have been expressed[35,73] that severe PHPV or extensive cyclitic membranes may pull the retina so far anteriorly that an inadvertent and hidden retinal biopsy or tear might occur from a transciliary body approach. As yet, we have not experienced this complication with insertion of the vitrectomy instrument through the pars plicata. The chance of retinal trauma certainly seems greater with insertion through the pars plana rather than through the pars plicata, though we and others have not produced inadvertent retinal biopsy with incisions through the pars plana in older children and teen-agers.[42] On the other hand, the only cases of PHPV with inadvertent retinal biopsies that we have been able to identify occurred during translimbal operations. One of these operations utilized scissors and forceps through the limbus,[69] and the others employed a vitrectomy instrument and forceps through the limbus.[68] Another case of PHPV developed retinal detachment postoperatively despite translimbal use of a modern vitrectomy instrument.[42] Thus, although anterior displacement of the retina toward the ciliary processes can occur[38,39] in PHPV, the limbal approach has thus far not proved to be superior to that through the pars plicata. Because the advantages of the "posterior" approach outweigh those of the "anterior" approach (see previous discussion), we continue to operate through the pars plicata for most cases of PHPV and for infantile cataract and pupillary membranes.

CHOICE OF A VITRECTOMY INSTRUMENT FOR PUPILLARY MEMBRANES, PHPV, AND CATARACTS

Choice of a particular vitrectomy instrument depends largely on the surgeon's training and on the availability of specific hardware. We have found the wide-angle cutter of the Peyman Vitrophage[56] particularly suitable for cataracts, thick and leathery pupillary membranes, and the bulky tissue that often characterizes PHPV. The full-function capability of this instrument (infusion, suction, and cutting in a single instrument tip) has been convenient for anterior segment lesions in that only one sclerotomy has been necessary. This has been especially true in the small eyes of neonates, where space limitations sometimes make multiple sclerotomies cumbersome. The large cutting aperture of the wide-angle cutter (about 1×1.3 mm) usually permits rapid, safe, piecemeal removal of the unwanted tissues. The outer-tube diameter of about 1.8 mm is safe for almost all purposes.

For severely microphthalmic eyes, the conventional Vitrophage handpiece (outer-tube diameter about 1.8 mm; cutting aperture about 0.9×0.9 mm) or the Miniphage (outer-tube diameter about 1.07 mm; triangular cutting aperture about 0.7×0.7 mm) can be used with the Vitrophage console. An additional sclerotomy for a separate infusion port is usually necessary with the Miniphage. All these instrument handpieces are disposable, and one need not worry about blunting a blade edge against such tissues as calcific cataract or against another metal instrument if used in a cutting-board or chopping-block technique. Because Vitrophage cutting tips have not been previously used in other surgical procedures, the blades are always sharp and thus useful against such structures as leathery or elastic membranes.

In the presence of totally opaque material, such as moderately advanced PHPV, the blind insertion of a separate irrigating cannula through the ciliary body is potentially dangerous and represents a definite hazard for surgery with divided-function vitrectomy instruments. Nonetheless, a large variety of vitrectomy instruments (small and large; full function and divided function) have been successfully employed in surgery for infantile pupillary membrane, PHPV, and infantile cataract. Additional mechanical refinements will undoubtedly occur.

PUPILLARY MEMBRANES

The advent of extracapsular techniques of cataract surgery (including aspirations, phacoemulsification, phacofragmentation, and adult microsurgical extracapsular cataract expressions), with or without insertion of an intraocular lens, has substantially increased the incidence of reduced postoperative vision attributable to pupillary membranes. For example, as summarized a few years ago[54] Parks and Hiles[51] reported a 73% incidence of membrane formation (and a 6% incidence of vitreous loss) in 52 eyes that had undergone discission and aspiration. Ryan and von Noorden[65] reported a 23% incidence of secondary membranes (and 8% vitreous loss) in 75 cases having had discission and aspiration. Hiles and Waller[26] reported secondary or delayed capsulotomies in 66% of their aspiration group and 39% of their phacoemulsification group. The incidence of capsulotomy after phacoemulsification in children may eventually exceed 90%.[24]

When possible, a simple Ziegler type of discission should be utilized (translimbally) for opening a pupillary membrane.[33] Only when it appears too dense or the cataractous remnants are too extensive should one remove the debris through the pars plana or, in a young child's eye, through the pars plicata. The advantages of the "posterior" over the "anterior" approach, as discussed earlier in this chapter, are applicable. In the future, new sources of energy, such as Nd-YAG (neodymium in yttrium-aluminum-garnet) lasers, may allow creation of clear pupillary openings in such membranes, but for the present the automated vitrectomy instrument remains the surgical mainstay. In this regard, it has almost eliminated the use of translimbal punches (such as Holth punch) and scissors (such as Vannas scissors) though there may well be a role for automated microscissors (such as MPC scissors) inserted through a pars plicata or pars plana sclerotomy. Occasional translimbal insertions of scissors or of vitrectomy instruments may also be indicated, depending on the specific configuration of the abnormal tissue. The utility of the vitrectomy instrument in removing pupillary membranes is enhanced by its ability to handle coincident problems of vitreous removal in an atraumatic fashion, especially by the "posterior" approach. Removal of the vitreous eliminates a potential scaffold for regrowth of the membrane and minimizes current and future traction on the ciliary body and retina. Removal of the vitreous at the time of membranectomy (or of cataract extraction) also eliminates postoperative complications such as vitreocorneal adherence and pupillary block.

The success of this surgical procedure has been so great and the complication rate has been so low that dense pupillary membranes now constitute one of the chief indications for use of automated vitrectomy instruments.[52,53,60]

In our series of 400 consecutive cases of pars plana surgery, 27 cases were operated on for pupillary membranes and related diseases.[53] Vision improved or the ocular media cleared in 24 (89%). Failure to obtain improved vision occurred in one eye and was related more to preoperative underlying glaucoma and corneal edema than to complications of the surgery. The remaining two eyes were unchanged. The operation itself and the postoperative course were remarkably benign. We have thus expanded our experience with the pars plana and pars plicata approach. In 108 consecutive pupillary membranes treated in this fashion and followed for an average of 3.8 years (range: 1 to 7 years), there were no major operative complications.[31] Vision improved in 67.5% of eyes. In four cases (3.7%), postoperative visual acuity was worse because of glaucoma caused by previous blunt trauma. Similar beneficial results and comparable complication rates have also been reported by others.[76]

The technique of pars plana or pars plicata membranectomy is straightforward and permits surgical restoration of a clear pupil with relief of vitreous traction in most circumstances. In rare instances, an exceedingly dense cyclitic membrane, involving not only the ciliary body but also the pars plana, might transmit traction to the peripheral retina if approached through the pars plana or pars plicata.[76] An open-sky or other translimbal approach with scissors, a punch, or a vitrectomy instrument has thus been advocated by several surgeons. A translimbal approach with a vitrectomy instrument can be successful, but only when the pupillary membrane is relatively thin.[76] If the pupillary membrane is thick, intense and prolonged suction is necessary and may easily collapse the anterior chamber with rubbing of the corneal endothelium or iris on the vitrectomy instrument or with excessively rapid removal of material from the vitreous chamber.

Even for thin membranes, the transciliary body approach is more controlled than that through the limbus. Under most circumstances, the membranes can be rather easily and quickly removed with a full-function vitrectomy instrument by a single sclerotomy. Fiberoptic illumination is unnecessary in the anterior segment of the eye. If the membrane is too taut or too thick to be aspirated into the cutting aperture of the wide-angle Vitrophage, a second instrument, usually a Ziegler knife or a 20-gauge needle, is inserted 90 to 120 degrees away, and multiple slits are made in the membrane for creation of flaps of tissue that are narrow enough to be aspirated easily by the vitrectomy instrument. Whereas some surgeons recommend insertion of the second instrument through the limbus, we prefer a pars plana or pars plicata insertion with engagement and discission of the membrane from behind (Fig. 20-3). This location of the instrument allows maximum operative flexibility in the event that a deep vitrectomy, with use of a contact lens, is necessary for removal of debris or for preretinal manipulations. In addition, trauma to the cornea, iris, and pupil is avoided. Engaging the membrane from behind is a safe procedure that is visually controlled by the surgeon. In most circumstances the metal instrument can be seen through the translucent membrane. If the membrane is completely opaque, the Ziegler knife or similar other instrument is simply aimed from the sclerotomy toward the corneal apex until it perforates the pupillary membrane from behind. At that point, slow side-to-side or cruciate slashes create multiple openings in the membrane (Fig. 20-3). The vitrectomy instrument then aspirates the narrow flaps of tissue debris for piecemeal amputation and removal. The wide-angle cutter has been extremely useful in this situation, even for relatively taut and unyielding membranes. O'Malley[50] has described a rather complex multiple perforation or sieving technique for membranes too tough to be aspirated by the Ocutome. Multiple small holes are created, rendering the membrane flexible enough to be molded into the cutting aperture.

If the membrane is particularly dense, the two instruments can be used against each other for a chopping-block or cutting-board effect. In addition, the tip of the Ziegler knife or 20-gauge needle can be used to feed pieces of the membrane into the cutting aperture. This, of course, will blunt the knife edge of the vitrectomy instrument when the blade strikes the metal of the other instrument. Use of a disposable instrument, such as the wide-angler cutter of the Vitrophage, eliminates any such concern.

PERSISTENT HYPERPLASTIC PRIMARY VITREOUS (PHPV)
Varied clinical manifestations

The clinical manifestations of PHPV extend along a spectrum from minimal remnants of the fetal intraocular vascular system at one extreme, having no effect on vision, to abnormalities characterized by microphthalmia and in some cases absence of light perception at the other. At the severe end of the spectrum, there may also be absence of the pupillary light reflex and a nonrecordable electroretinogram. Associated malformations of the eye, such as retinal dysplasia, macular aplasia, and optic nerve hypoplasia or dysplasia, are distressingly common, even in eyes that appear almost normal in size and shape. These anomalies often nullify the visual results that are ordinarily expected of technically successful surgery.

The characteristic clinical appearance of a moderately affected eye with PHPV includes the following: the cornea is usually 1 to 1.5 mm smaller than normal. In addition, there may be prominent, radially oriented vessels in the iris that create tiny notches in

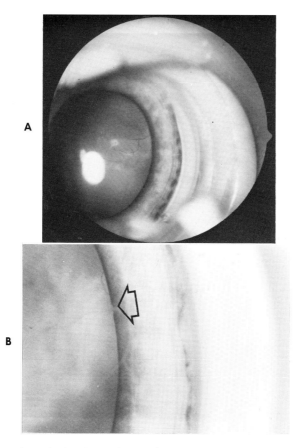

Fig. 20-6. Persistent hyperplastic primary vitreous. **A,** At low magnification, the pupillary notch from the iridohyaloid vessel is not seen. Retrolental fibrovascular tissue is visible through clear lens. **B,** At high magnification, tiny notch (atypical coloboma) can be seen, *arrow*, at location of iridohyaloid vessel.

the pupil (Fig. 20-6). These notches are best appreciated under the operating microscope.[41] The prominent vessels represent remnants of the fetal vascular system (the anterior portion of the tunica vasculosa lentis) and often pass posteriorly around the equator of the lens to anastomose with the retrolental fibrovascular tissue.[37,41] These radial iris (iridohyaloid or capsulopupillary) vessels should be sought in every case of congenital cataract or "pseudoglioma," and their detection should heighten the clinician's suspicion for the presence of PHPV (even if the retrolental fibrovascular tissue cannot be visualized behind an opaque lens). The orderly arrangement of these vessels should not be confused with rubeosis iridis, which can occur with PHPV, retrolental fibroplasia, or retinoblastoma.[45]

The configuration of the retrolental tissue, when visible, is often diagnostically helpful. The anterior end of the hyaloid artery in Cloquet's canal often can be seen as Mittendorf's dot, even when the entire retrolental space is occupied by abnormal white tissue. Mittendorf's dot appears just nasal to center as a denser white opacification (Fig.

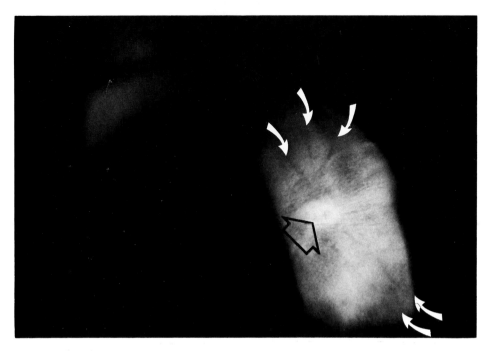

Fig. 20-7. Mittendorf's dot stands out as dense white oval, *open arrow,* in midst of retrolental white tissue in eye with persistent hyperplastic primary vitreous. Note dark radiating lines representing persistent embryonic blood vessels, *curved arrows.* Compare Fig. 20-8.

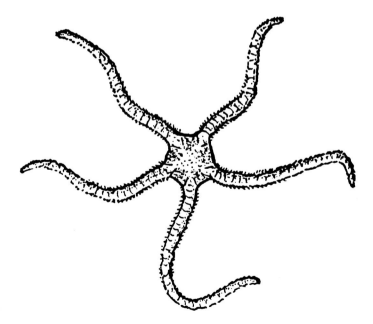

Fig. 20-8. Brittle star, a marine echinoderm, resembling Mittendorf's dot with radiating blood vessels in retrolental persistent hyperplastic primary vitreous. Compare Fig. 20-7.

20-7). It varies from 1 to about 3 mm in diameter and is largest when there is a great deal of abnormal tissue present. From this epicenter, a series of blood vessels often radiates to the periphery of the retrolental tissue, much like slightly curved spokes of a wheel. The overall appearance also resembles the so-called brittle star, a marine echinoderm with a central disc-shaped body and thin, wavy extremities (Fig. 20-8). The orderly arrangement of these blood vessels should be distinguished from the irregular nonradial vascularized retrolental mass sometimes observed in advanced retinoblastoma or retrolental fibroplasia.

If the media are not too opaque, indirect ophthalmoscopy will reveal the characteristic vascularized stalk extending to the disc or may show other posterior fundus problems, such as a falciform fold of the retina or, occasionally, fibrovascular tissue known as posterior hyperplastic primary vitreous.[62]

In the presence of opaque media, computed tomography has revealed the following set of characteristic findings[36]: (1) retrolental soft tissue can be demonstrated along Cloquet's canal; (2) the retrolental soft tissue becomes enhanced after administration of intravenous iodine contrast material; (3) there is increased density of the vitreous body; (4) in the retrohyaloid space there is layered, high-density fluid (blood), which shifts location in the decubitus position (this finding is apparently unique to PHPV and related diseases); (5) there is absence of ocular and orbital calcification; (6) microphthalmia can be demonstrated; and (7) the optic nerves, retrobulbar tissues, and other orbital structures appear normal.

Varied causes

PHPV represents an etiologically diverse group of diseases. There is a large idiopathic group of cases, which by themselves appear to represent different causations. Other causes include a primary autosomal recessive mutation, trisomy 13, and an X-linked recessive mutation known as Norrie's disease.[49] The single name of this heterogeneous group of disorders ("PHPV") thus represents a diagnostic oversimplification. Warburg has chosen to call these diseases congenital retinal nonattachment and falciform folds,[79] though this fails to recognize the commonly observed minimal expressions of persistence of the primary vitreous. Ohba has recently introduced the term "primary vitreoretinal dysplasia."[49] Because this name emphasizes the arrest in development of the retina and of the vitreous and because it can include both the milder and the severer forms of the disease, it is a useful designation. Furthermore, dysplastic rosettes frequently coexist with histologic remnants of the primary vitreous, not only in the PHPV syndrome, but also in the so-called retinal dysplasia syndrome, as observed in trisomy 13 and other diseases. Common usage, however, suggests that PHPV will remain the most frequently used clinical term, at least in North America.

The ophthalmologist must remember that the umbrella designation "PHPV" covers a broad array of clinical manifestations and diagnostic entities. It is not surprising that the natural course of this group of diseases is extremely varied. Therapeutic approaches should therefore be tailored to the individual case. It is widely assumed, however, that *all* eyes with PHPV have an inexorably downhill course, eventuating in blindness, phthisis, and enucleation. This supposition was originally advanced by Reese in his 1955 Jackson Memorial Lecture[64] after he realized that he had "not been able to discover a single recognizable case in an adult." Subsequently, a large number of eye surgeons have concluded erroneously that all cases of PHPV should have surgery as soon as the diagnosis is made in an effort to forestall repeated hemorrhaging or swelling of the lens, shallowing of the anterior chamber, and glaucoma. A slavish decision to operate in every case is unwise because, at the mild end of the disease spectrum, eyes will in fact survive without surgery to advanced childhood or adulthood with vision as good as, if not better than, those subjected to intraocular surgery. At the opposite end of the spectrum, severe PHPV can be associated with enough retinal dysplasia that an absence of light perception is present from birth onward. Such eyes generally are severely microphthalmic, and surgery, with its local and systemic risks, is generally contraindicated. Cosmetic improvement can be achieved with a shell prosthesis. The following case reports illustrate the benign and the severe clinical courses.

Case 3. A 23-month-old white female was referred for evaluation of a white "dot" in the right pupil and turning in of this eye since 2 weeks of age. Ocular fixation was central and steady bilaterally. There were about 32 prism diopters of right esotropia.

With the patient under general anesthesia, the following findings were noted: the right cornea measured 11.5 mm horizontally and 10.5 mm vertically. The left cornea measured 11 mm horizontally and 11.5 mm vertically. Cycloplegic retinoscopy showed -14.00 sph $+1.50$ cyl $\times 60°$ in the right eye and $+0.75$ sph in the left. The right fundus was albinotic, the optic disc was tilted, and no well-defined macula or foveal pit could be seen (Fig. 20-9). From the disc, a vascularized stalk extended through the vitreous and inserted into a retrolental fibrovascular membrane. The left fundus and anterior segment were entirely normal. Ocular pressures were also normal.

Immediately behind the nasal aspect of the clear right lens, the white vascularized membrane extended from about 1:30 to 3:30 o'clock. The membrane, which touched the posterior lens capsule, just barely encroached on the visual axis (Fig. 20-10). A densely white, circular opacity, representing Mittendorf's dot, was seen in the central part of the membrane (Fig. 20-10). An iridohyaloid vascular anastomosis[41] was present in the 2 to 3 o'clock axis (Fig. 20-6, *B*). The anterior chamber was normally deep, and there was no centripetal dragging of the ciliary processes.

Over the course of the next 10 years, one of us (M.F.G.) has treated the right eye with a contact lens and constant pupillary dilatation with 10% phenylephrine hydrochloride (Neo-Synephrine). Intermittent patching of the left eye (for prolonged periods of time during the first few years of life) was also carried out. There has always been a clear ophthalmoscopic view of the right macular region through the dilated pupil (Fig. 20-9). At 10 years of age, vision was 12/400 (4.2/120) in the right eye and 20/25 (6/7.5) in the left. There was no change in the physical status of either eye.

Comment. Mild PHPV was present in one eye. Therapy included pupillary dilatation, contact lens fitting, and intermittent occlusion of the other eye. The visual axis was unobstructed with the pupil dilated. The child was followed prospectively for 10 years and developed vision in the eye with PHPV that was as good as, if not better than, most eyes having undergone surgery. Despite minimal microcornea and minimal PHPV, the involved eye had such severe congenital abnormalities of the optic disc and macula that they appeared incompatible with better vision.

Case 4. A 5-month-old Palestinian Arab boy was referred for evaluation of poor vision and bilateral leukokoria. Several maternal male relatives were also congenitally blind (Fig. 20-11), but there was no family history of mental retardation, psychosis, or deafness.

Physical abnormalities were confined to the eyes. There was no visual fixation bilat-

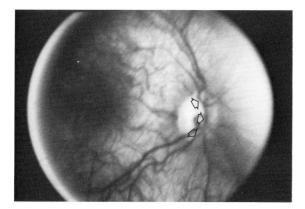

Fig. 20-9. Persistent hyperplastic primary vitreous with visual axis clear enough to take fundus photograph. Note tilted disc, *arrows,* albinotic fundus, and absence of well-defined macula or foveal pit.

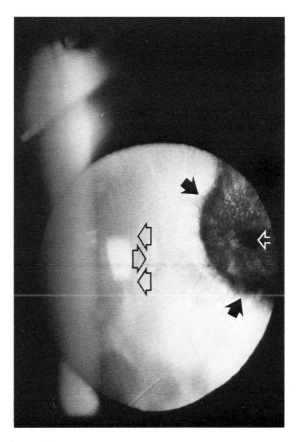

Fig. 20-10. Persistent hyperplastic primary vitreous with clear visual axis, *open black arrows.* The retrolental membrane is seen through pupil as a dark disc, *solid arrows,* because of retroillumination. Within the retrolental membrane is a more opaque, smaller ovoid structure, Mittendorf's dot, *open white arrow.*

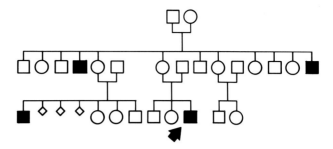

Fig. 20-11. Pedigree of family with Norrie's disease. Note X-linked inheritance. *Arrow,* Proband (case 4).

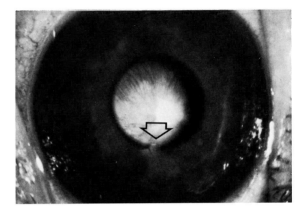

Fig. 20-12. Appearance of eye of case 4. Note retrolental white fibrovascular tissue as well as missing portion of pupillary sphincter, *arrow,* through which an iridohyaloid vessel passed.

erally, but the pupils were slightly reactive to light. Pendular nystagmus was present.

With the patient under general anesthesia, the corneal diameters were found to be 9 mm horizontally and 9.5 mm vertically in the right eye and 10 mm horizontally and 10 mm vertically in the left. Applanation pressures were 6 mm Hg in the right eye and 16 mm Hg in the left. The right anterior chamber was shallow, and the left was flat. There was a missing portion of the pupillary sphincter in the left eye, through which a prominent, radial iridohyaloid vessel extended (Fig. 20-12). The lenses were clear in both eyes. Both retrolental spaces had opaque, vascularized grayish white and yellow masses of tissue. No fundus reflex was present in either eye. Blood was intermixed with the mass in the right eye.

In the left eye, a translimbal lensectomy, vitrectomy, and partial excision of the retrolental mass were performed in the hopes of improving vision and deepening the anterior chamber. The abnormal mass of tissue seemed to fill the vitreous cavity, extending posteriorly to the optic nerve and fundus. Only about one fourth to one third of the tissue could be excised through the tranlimbal incision. Histologic examination of the surgical specimen showed a small piece of retinal tissue.

Postoperatively, both eyes have remained free of pain and inflammation. Neither has apparent light perception. The right anterior chamber is flat, and the left is deep. The corneal diameters and pressures are approximately unchanged.

Comment. A blind male baby with Norrie's disease underwent translimbal lensectomy, vitrectomy, and partial excision of abnormal retrolental and intravitreal tissue. The surgical approach did not allow removal of all the abnormal intravitreal tissue, which appeared to fill the vitreous cavity. Despite the translimbal approach, a biopsy of the retrolental mass contained retinal tissue.

It would appear that the intravitreal and retrolental anomalous tissue was so extensive that no form of surgery could provide clear ocular media or useful vision. One year later, both the operated and the unoperated eyes were blind, but otherwise they were free of symptoms.

SURVIVAL OF EYES WITH PHPV TO ADULTHOOD

Contrary to widespread opinion, several eyes have survived to adult life without surgery. Even Reese, in his Jackson Lecture, cites the details of five such cases culled from the older literature.[64] The ages of these patients ranged from 12 to 31 years. Subsequent to Reese's landmark publication, similar instances have appeared in the ophthalmic press. A few of these unoperated eyes have had some vision and no glaucoma, others have been blind but pain free, and others have eventually developed painful glaucoma requiring enucleation during adulthood. We, for example, reported the clinical and angiographic features of one such case, a patient 18 years of age, in 1978.[18] Spontaneous resorption of most of the lens had occurred. Spaulding and Naumann reported a woman whose eye survived until 22 years of age, when enucleation for painful glaucoma was finally required.[72] Histopathologic examination revealed macular degeneration, a partial macular hole, and preretinal gliosis. Mason and Huamonte,[40] in our institution, removed the opaque material from a similar 29-year-old man. He had no change in visual function postoperatively, despite technically excellent surgery, which resulted in clear ocular media. A hypoplastic optic nerve and an ectopic macula were detected once the opacities of the media had been removed. Gitter[20] described a 45-year-old patient with an asymptomatic eye showing spontaneous lens resorption. Spaulding also reported a man who lived without symptoms to 71 years of age before glaucoma required enucleation.[71] The common denominator of many eyes that survive beyond 10 years of age without surgery is partial or complete spontaneous resorption of the lens, allowing the anterior chamber angle to remain open despite some anterior shifting of the iris because of contracture or swelling of the retrolental fibrovascular tissue. Such eyes have survived without surgery even with pronounced centripetal dragging of the ciliary processes.[18]

In view of the fact that data from only a few more than 100 cases of PHPV have appeared in the literature, these 10 eyes may represent a rather substantial percentage that survived for considerable periods of time without surgery. It is also possible that additional asymptomatic cases are not reported, because they either are misdiagnosed or have not been followed up because of the affected patients or their physicians having concluded that their congenital anomaly or poor vision is beyond help and therefore not worthy of close attention.

It could be argued that early operative intervention might not only preserve the eye but also provide good vision. This point of view seems unduly optimistic, except for unusual instances. Eyes with PHPV, particularly those that appear severe enough to warrant surgery, often have coincident blinding anomalies of the optic nerve or macula that are untreatable. In addition, problems associated with deprivation amblyopia are extremely difficult to overcome. Sadly, this is true of children even when the only abnormality is congenital unilateral cataract. The problem of visual rehabilitation is compounded to an extreme degree when microphthalmia and congenital anomalies of the macula and optic nerve are superimposed.

If one reviews the published reports of the postoperative visual status in eyes with PHPV, one must conclude that substantial visual improvement is extremely rare.[21,40,61,69] Smith and Maumenee, for example, reported six cases of their own and collected 32 cases from the literature.[69] In their personal series only one eye had 20/200 (6/60) vision postoperatively, whereas four eyes could see hand motion or had poor fixation or both, and one had questionable light perception. It is important to note that surgery was not successful in one of six eyes, even though the surgical goal was limited to salvaging the globe. In the 32 cases culled from the literature, one eye obtained acuity of 15/20 (4.5/6) and one eye obtained 20/200 (6/60) vision. The remainder saw only hand motions or less. Complications such as severe hemorrhage, glaucoma, synechiae, iris bombé, vitreous loss, and retinal detachment occurred in a small number of cases.

Because the technical ease of operating on PHPV with vitrectomy instruments far surpasses that attending conventional instrumentation (scissors, punches, and so on), one might have supposed that the percentage of eyes with good vision postoperatively would have increased with the advent of this methodology. This has proved to be so in only exceptional cases, despite technically excellent surgery.[40,47,48,58,61] For example, Eifrig et al. reported that one of five cases with PHPV obtained visual acuity of 20/100 (6/30).[12] Pollard, in the largest personal series available, reported 20 cases with excellent anatomic but ''quite poor'' visual results. Only four cases ''have a chance at useful vision.'' The remainder have only hand-motions to light-perception vision, and one has a phthisic eye after surgery. Pollard emphasized the common occurrence of a falciform retinal fold or abnormal pigmentation affecting the macula. Similar macular defects have been noted by Fung,[16] Gass,[17] Mason and Huamonte,[40] Nankin and Scott,[47] and ourselves.[18,41] Nankin and Scott reported seven patients, four of whom had extraction of their abnormal tissue with a vitrectomy instrument. Only one eye obtained useful vision (20/60: 6/18). A translimbal cataract aspiration, followed by a discission of the residual membrane over a year later, was done in this case. The remainder of the eyes had uncentral, unsteady, or unmaintained fixation. Operative results in most other reported cases have also failed to demonstrate substantial visual improvement.[1,17,40,42,68]

SURGICAL INDICATIONS

In view of the fact that some eyes do survive to adulthood without surgery and there are generally poor visual results in eyes having modern, uncomplicated microsurgery, including that with vitrectomy instrumentation, what can one conclude about the proper surgical indications for PHPV?

If retinoblastoma cannot be excluded from the differential diagnosis of a patient with opaque white retrolental tissue, enucleation, rather than intraocular surgery, is indicated. Fortunately, with the advent of computed tomography and enhanced diagnostic awareness, this type of diagnostic problem has largely ceased to exist.[36]

If the particular instance of PHPV is at either end of the spectrum of clinical severity, intraocular surgery is generally contraindicated (Fig. 20-13). For example, if the visual

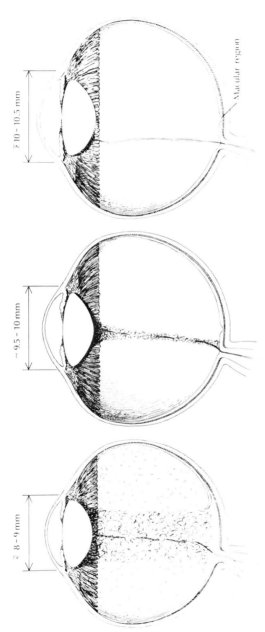

Fig. 20-13. Spectrum of eyes with persistent hyperplastic primary vitreous (severe at left; mild at right). Eyes at either end of clinical spectrum generally do not warrant surgery. Surgical decision-making is complex for eyes located in middle of spectrum.

axis is unobstructed or, at the opposite end of the spectrum, there is no perception of light, surgery generally has no merit. For the cases located somewhere in the middle of this spectrum, however, surgical decision-making can be complex. Operation on all such cases is overly aggressive, and withholding of surgery from all such cases is overly conservative. In the past, an aggressive approach to early surgery in such cases has been recommended because the unoperated prognosis appeared so bad. The goal was preservation of the eye, even if useful vision was considered unobtainable. The specific indications for surgery under these circumstances have included a shallow anterior chamber, a swollen cataractous lens, progressive traction on the ciliary processes, and ensuing complications, such as hemorrhage and glaucoma.[69] We believe it is appropriate, however, to question the applicability of this philosophy to all cases. Are the risks of general anesthesia and of sympathetic ophthalmia offset by the minimal utility of preserving a microphthalmic eye, which will neither see well nor look normal? In many cases, the answer is no.

An assessment of visual function and potential must be made through use of the electroretinogram, visual evoked response, pupillary reflexes, and, where feasible, ophthalmoscopy. Intraocular pressure should be measured with the patient under general anesthesia, and gonioscopy should be performed. Computed tomography and ultrasonography are helpful. If there is no chance of useful vision (such as, the vitreous chamber being filled with abnormal embryonic tissue), withholding intraocular surgery, even if the anterior chamber angle is compromised and the pressure is elevated, is a reasonable alternative. Rather than risk sympathetic ophthalmia in the only useful (contralateral) eye, palliation for the glaucoma or enucleation for the eye with painful PHPV would appear acceptable under these circumstances. If the condition is bilateral (which fortunately occurs in only a minority of cases), intraocular surgery in at least one eye does seem justified, even if the chance of useful vision appears remote. In this situation simple lensectomy should salvage the eye, even if the intravitreal tissue is left alone,[61] and a translimbal approach would have the advantage of avoiding any anteriorly displaced retinal tissue completely. Any type of lens-aspiration procedure should suffice. If necessary, later removal of the retrolental tissue can be considered.

If the microphthalmia is minimal, if there is preoperative evidence of visual function, if the ocular condition is *demonstrably* progressing (shallowing of anterior chamber, closing of the anterior chamber angle, active hemorrhaging, and so on), if the ophthalmologist anticipates that surgery is technically feasible and offers a reasonable chance of obtaining some useful vision (hand motions or better), and if the parents understand the limited goals involved in this type of surgery, a recommendation to operate is justified. Depending on circumstances, lensectomy alone or lensectomy with removal of intravitreal tissue will be indicated. If there is no demonstrable progression and the anterior chamber angle and intraocular pressure are normal, however, watchful waiting with scheduled, frequent follow-up visits is more desirable, in our view. Pupillary dilatation or optical iridectomy may also be indicated, as in case 3 (p. 244). Surgery is clearly not justified, however, when the visual axis is reasonably clear and the anterior chamber angle is not compromised (Figs. 20-9 and 20-10).

If the patient demonstrates spontaneous resorption of a lens late in childhood or as an adult,[18,40] operative removal of the remaining abnormal tissue is unlikely to improve vision because of preexisting deprivation amblyopia. Since the anterior chamber angle is usually in no danger of closure in such cases, surgery is also usually contraindicated because one cannot justify intervention on grounds of salvaging a globe threatened with secondary angle-closure glaucoma.

SURGICAL TECHNIQUE

If a decision to remove only the lens or perform only a sector iridectomy has been made, we prefer the conventional translimbal approach. If a decision to remove both the lens and the retrolental tissue has been made, we generally utilize the pars plicata approach with the wide-angle cutter of the Vitrophage. Bipolar or unipolar diathermy should be available in the event substantial bleeding occurs.[1] The surgeon should be aware that the abnormal tissue may extend all the way from the retrolental space to the disc. Preoperative ultrasonic and computed tomographic studies help in establishing the extent of this tissue. The surgery, itself, has been largely free of complications,[40,58] but occasionally the tissue may bleed extensively[1] or may be very difficult to cut.[42,78]

Advocates of the anterior (translimbal) approach argue that anteriorly displaced retina[64] may be injured with a pars plana insertion of a vitrectomy instrument.[43,47,61,73] Of course, this may occur. In actuality, however, the only cases with inadvertent retinal biopsy we have been able to identify in the literature were operated translimbally (see also case 4, p. 244).[68,69] Other translimbal procedures have been complicated by postoperative retinal detachment.[42] In our own experience[42,58] through the pars plicata, and in most others' through the pars plana,[12,76] the retina has not been displaced far enough anteriorly by contracted retrolental fibroglial tissue to cause a problem in the surgical field. Such displacement, however, certainly occurs sometimes to the pars plicata[38,39] and must be considered whenever the posterior lens capsule is removed, regardless of other aspects of the surgical approach. Thus the fundus should be carefully inspected at the end of the operation for detection and cryotherapy of any peripheral retinal breaks. Other proponents of the translimbal approach[47] argue that the commonly associated microphthalmia makes the posterior approach technically more difficult than the anterior one. Any limbal incision, however, no matter how extensive, provides poor operative exposure for removal of retrolental tissue, particularly when the tissue extends all the way to the disc and when the deep vitreous chamber often contains old and fresh hemorrhagic debris.[64] Using an operating microscope, it is generally impossible to obtain a clear view of the fundus under these conditions. A pars plicata incision, on the other hand, allows use of an irrigated, surgical contact lens, thereby providing the opportunity to bring the fundus into focus, unlike the situation that prevails in the translimbal operation. Furthermore, if massive bleeding from a transected hyaloid artery occurs, the posterior approach will permit visualization of the bleeder and underwater diathermy, whereas the limbal approach may prohibit successful management and lead to loss of the eye. The other arguments advanced earlier in the chapter for the posterior approach through the pars plicata also apply to surgery for PHPV.

If the eye is very malformed and the retina is dragged onto the pars plana or all the way to the pars plicata,[64] a transciliary body approach to the retrolental tissue certainly could be dangerous. It is also unlikely that a limbal approach with a small incision and a vitrectomy instrument will be more helpful (see case 4). Under these extreme circumstances, an open-sky microsurgical dissection conceivably might help,[67] but avoiding surgery altogether (or confining it to less aspiration) may well be wiser and kinder for the patient and the patient's family. Unfortunately, the exterior configuration of the globe and the size of the cornea are not always accurate indications of the extent of intraocular abnormalities.

INFANTILE CATARACT
Indications for surgery on infantile/neonatal cataracts

Although this is an exceedingly controversial area, decision-making can be simplified if one categorizes infantile and neonatal cataracts within one of the following groups[23]: bilateral and complete, bilateral and incomplete, unilateral and complete, unilateral and incomplete, and those associated with other ocular or systemic anomalies. Cataracts that are acquired well after the neonatal and infantile periods generally have a better prognosis for vision, especially if they are induced by trauma,[25] and will not be considered here in detail, except for noting that the improved visual outlook justifiably enhances the surgeon's confidence and broadens the indications for surgery.

Neonatal and infantile cataracts are considered complete when no fundus details are ophthalmoscopically visible, even with full dilatation of the pupil.[23] Effective retinal stimulation is thus impossible. Incomplete cataracts are those in which some visual stimulation of the developing retina is assumed to be possible because some of the lens is free of cataractous changes. In other words, the cataract affects only part of the lens, such as only the nucleus, only the periphery, or only the central portion of the anterior capsule.

For bilateral and complete cataracts, early bilateral lens extraction appears to offer the best chance for subsequent equal retinal and central nervous system maturation. Surgery on the first eye can be accomplished as soon as general anesthesia is considered safe, perhaps at about 1 week of age or even earlier, to be followed by surgery on the second eye about 1 week thereafter. The chance of obtaining improved symmetric vision still exists, however, if surgery is delayed by 3 to 4 months.[30] Further delays appear inadvisable on the basis of experience to date. As soon as possible postoperatively, contact lens fittings are instituted, and frequent evaluations of refractive status, fixation patterns, strabismus, and visual acuity[3,30] are then pursued assiduously. Spectacle correction is provided so that the infant can have focused images at times when the contact lenses are lost or cannot be worn.

For bilateral and incomplete cataracts, the decision for or against surgery becomes more difficult. In general, the two eyes should be treated similarly so that image-size disparities do not occur. Avoiding aniseikonia and deprivation amblyopia must remain major goals. If one cataract, however, is almost complete and the other is only minimally developed, one might argue that the patient should be treated as in the unilateral, complete cataractous situation described below. If the cataracts are symmetric but minimal, the ophthalmologist may best be advised to follow the patient's visual behavior, fixation patterns, ocular alignment, and clarity of the fundus reflex before making a decision to operate. If possible, the visual acuity should be measured quantitatively. Accommodation should be preserved if possible. Therefore, if pupillary dilatation is necessary, a trial with sympathomimetics alone is worth undertaking if one bears in mind the possibilities of systemic toxicity. If this trial is unsuccessful, a cycloplegic agent such as atropine can be utilized, with appropriate correction for near vision. If neither course appears successful, optical iridectomy can be considered. It should be emphasized, however, that these approaches rarely result in normal vision. Crawford has found that the median visual acuity of patients with central lens opacity was 20/60 (6/18) after optical iridectomy but 20/30 (6/9) after surgical aspiration.[7] He thus recommends optical iridectomy only for patients with mental retardation who might have difficulty postoperatively with aphakic spectacles or contact lenses.

Bilateral and incomplete cataracts may be progressive, and careful monitoring of physical findings is necessary. Combined deprivation and strabismic amblyopia is common. An initially conservative approach should be converted to a surgical one when the cataracts become sufficiently dense. In this regard, it is worth emphasizing that visual acuity in children with bilateral and incomplete cataracts depends more on the *density* of the center of the cataract than on the size (linear dimensions) of the lens opacity.[7]

Unilateral, complete cataracts represent a distressing condition because of the difficulties in successful rehabilitation caused by deprivation and strabismic amblyopia. Many of these eyes have associated anatomic abnormalities of the retina and optic nerve or varied degrees of microphthalmia. Many may represent subclinical or minimal expressions of persistence of the embryonic vascular system.

The results of surgery of such eyes have been so poor in the past that many authorities have recomended that surgery not be done at all.[23] Recently, however, Beller, Hoyt, and their colleagues have reported extremely favorably results in a small group of patients having surgery within 6 weeks of birth (5 to 41 days).[3] Postoperatively, binocular total occlusion was maintained until a contact lens was successfully fitted, generally within 4 days of surgery. Retinoscopy was repeated monthly. Because of repeated contact lens loss as well as change of refractive power, the average number of contact lenses required by each infant in the first year of surgery was nine. Patching and strabismus surgery were then performed as necessary. Visual acuities ranged from 20/20 (6/6) to 20/80 (6/24) in eight eyes, despite microphthalmia in four. None of the patients had any binocular interaction. Somewhat similar findings have been reported by Jacobson et al.[30] and by Enoch et al.[14] in a few patients who had undergone intensive postoperative rehabilitation programs. These results are extraordinarily good and demonstrate that a dedicated team of visual rehabilitation specialists can salvage such eyes if they and the patient's family are devoted to the task of a very large number of examinations and therapeutic sessions, often requiring general anesthesia, during the infant's first few weeks and months of life.

For incomplete, unilateral cataracts, surgical indications are somewhat similar to those for incomplete, bilateral cataracts. If strabismus develops and does not respond to nonsurgical therapy, surgical intervention can be carried out, to be followed by contact lens and occlusive therapy and so on. If the methodologies are available, actual visual acuity should be measured quantitatively and utilized in the decision-making process.

The role of intraocular lenses in childhood aphakia management remains highly experimental and controversial.[29] Major problems exist because such eyes are often small, because they have major growth phases still to occur, and because the long-term effect of any intraocular lens on such eyes is simply not known, regardless of location in front of, at, or behind the pupil.

Hiles has explored this problem in some depth[25] and has reserved use of an intraocular lens (IOL) for the following: (1) traumatic cataracts associated with corneal scars preventing use of a contact lens, (2) a previously unsuccessful trial of contact-lens fitting after otherwise successful cataract surgery (that is, secondary lens implantation), and (3) unilateral cataracts operated on between 1 and 9 years of age. In addition to the totally unknown biologic consequences of chronic implantation of an intraocular lens (such as corneal endothelial decompensation), there is the obvious dilemma of choosing a suitable optical power for an implant in an eye that will continually change its total refractive power during the critical, sensitive period of visual maturation and thereafter. The problem is compounded when microphthalmia is present. Hoffer has outlined three possible alternatives[28]: (1) the IOL power should produce emmetropia at the time of implantation, (2) the IOL should be replaced in adulthood with one of lesser power, or (3) the initial IOL power should be suitable for adult life. There are obvious disadvantages to all three, especially the second one, because it requires a dangerous additional operation. Although Hiles[25] advocates the third choice, with additional spectacle correction or contact lens correction utilized during childhood, it would seem that such a lens combination will not provide the optimal optical image for the eye during its critical period of visual maturation. Thus, if any IOL surgery is to be done, the first choice might be best. For the time being, however, the results of Beller et al.[3] Enoch et al.,[14] and Jacobson et al.[30] suggest that IOLs are not usually necessary, even in demanding rehabilitative circumstances (unilateral, complete cataract) and their use in children should be considered experimental and thus held in abeyance by all except qualified investigators.

In an effort to avoid the problems of IOL implantation in infancy, Morgan et al. have suggested the use of epikeratophakia grafts for unilateral aphakia.[46] This procedure also has its limitations and must also be considered experimental at the present time.

Surgical history

The history of surgery for infantile and juvenile cataracts is replete with one new technique after another. Simple discissions gave way to linear extractions and then to a variety of aspirating techniques through small incisions, once the soft consistency of these cataracts became widely known.[33] The rather high incidence of operative and postoperative complications in the chronologically earlier techniques has been the driving force behind technical innovation in this surgical area.[15]

A major advance in the early 1960s was the one-needle "push-pull" aspiration of the cataract through a single, small limbal incision, as advocated then by Maumenee.[33] This one-stage procedure, utilizing a blunt, bent, thin-walled 19-gauge needle and a 2-ml syringe for manual aspiration and irrigation, eliminated many of the problems associated with linear extractions and with two-stage discissions and aspirations, such as wound dehiscences, incomplete removal of cortex, prolonged inflammation, and phthisis.[66] This technique was enhanced through use of an operating microscope, which provided improved vision of the anterior and posterior capsules and cortical remnants. The unfortunate occurrence of a major rubella epidemic in the mid-1960s provided an opportunity for this technique to be widely used. Despite its obvious advantages, many operations failed because of postoperative complications such as pupillary block, opacified pupillary membranes, anterior and posterior synechiae, secluded and occluded pupils, and inadvertent laceration of the posterior lens capsule with incarceration of vitreous in the limbal wound. The magnitude of some of these complications is quantitated elsewhere in this chapter in the section devoted to pupillary membranes.

With the development of phacoemulsification and phacofragmentation in the mid- to late 1960s and thereafter, the ease and finesse of aspiration and irrigation increased substantially. Kelman has noted that "whereas phacoemulsification in senile cataracts is more difficult than the conventional technique, phacoemulsification and aspiration of the congenital cataract is easier to perform than current methods of irrigation-aspiration."[32] There have been additional microsurgical refinements, such as more convenient irrigating and aspirating devices, more complete removal of equatorial lens cortex, polishing of the posterior lens capsule, and purposeful posterior capsulotomy at the time of lens aspiration.[4,6,19] Nonetheless, complications related to the pupil, synechiae, glaucoma, and vitreous prolapse into the anterior segment have continued to occur.

Vitrectomy instrumentation

Accordingly, the advent of vitrectomy instruments, which could not only irrigate and aspirate, but also cut lens capsule, iris, and vitreous, presaged a major technical advance. It became apparent that if moderately hard lenses could be cut and aspirated during a vitrectomy procedure in adults, softer infantile and juvenile cataracts would be eminently amenable to similar techniques.

The translimbal approach has appealed to many surgeons, even when using vitrectomy instrumentation, for traditional reasons and because of a desire to avoid operating through the ciliary body or in the vitreous. This technique, however, has been associated with vitreous being incarcerated in the wound in about 23% of cases[75] and may possibly be responsible for cystoid macular edema. Concerns for the posterior approach have largely proved to be unfounded, and the general advantages of the posterior approach through the pars plicata, as outlined earlier in this chapter, are quite applicable to surgery for infantile and juvenile cataracts. In addition, there are several specific advantages to the posterior approach for neonatal and infantile cataracts.

For example, these cataracts tend to be extremely soft and, in some cases such as rubella infection, completely liquefied. A controlled anterior capsulectomy is therefore often impossible translimbally because the first tear in the anterior capsule may liberate opaque milky fluid into the anterior chamber, not only obscuring the view, but also causing the posterior capsule to move forward rapidly. Repeated attempts at engaging the anterior capsule can often result in inadvertent lacerations of the anteriorly displaced posterior capsule and intermixing of vitreous with cataractous remnants. Furthermore, the small size of the infantile cornea and anterior chamber and their ready collapsibility also contribute to technical difficulties with aspirating instruments inserted translimbally. Instrumentation allowing infusion and aspiration through one or more small and relatively watertight incisions has made translimbal cataract aspiration somewhat safer. However, O'Malley has noted that "the texture of the cornea and the relatively small volume of the anterior chamber do not permit a desirable *range* of suction and manipulation with the 20-gauge instruments via the limbus without causing intermittent hypotony or anterior chamber collapse."[50] He has recently recommended a one-handed technique through the pars plicata[50] with a separate infusion terminal. We have employed a single full-function instrument, the Vitrophage, through a single pars plicata incision, and follow-up study now exceeds 5 years in several children.[55] There has been an extremely low rate of complications, with a lack of pupillary block, secondary membranes, vitreocorneal adhesions, and retinal detachments. Together with the extremely clear media, this lack of important surgical complications suggests strongly that the advantages of the posterior approach through the pars plicata, in which the cornea, posterior lens capsule, and vitreous can all be managed atraumatically, outweigh those of the anterior approach through the limbus. As yet, sufficient postoperative visual acuity and angiographic data are unavailable, and a conclusion about the relative merits of the pars plicata lensectomy vitrectomy procedure must be held in abeyance.

Pars plicata approach

The pars plicata procedure is simplified if one utilizes a full-function vitrectomy instrument that requires only a single scleral incision. Fiberoptic illumination and a separate infusion terminal are not necessary. As pointed out by Aaberg and Machemer,[35] Douvas,[9] Girard,[19] Calhoun and Harley,[5] and others, some anterior vitrectomy is unavoidable with the posterior approach and, in our view, would actually appear to be desirable in terms of preventing future pupillary block (with secondary glaucoma) and vitreocorneal adherence (with corneal decompensation). We have thus purposefully extended the vitrectomy component of the operation so that a large core of vitreous is removed from the level of the lens to the fundus, extending to the equatorial region for 360 degrees (Fig. 20-1). The peripheral vitreous "skirt" and vitreous base are left intact. This procedure appears to minimize tangential vitreous contraction and also the chance of late migration of collapsed vitreous gel into the pupil or against the cornea. The chances of postoperative pupillary block glaucoma and of corneal decompensation thereby appear to be reduced. Whether or not inclusion of this moderately extensive deep vitrectomy in the cataract-extraction technique proves to be useful remains to be seen. Thus far, it has been free of complications, and even neonatal microphthalmi have enlarged well during their subsequent infantile growth phase (see case 1, p. 230).

The detailed technique of lens cutting and aspiration is reasonably straightforward.[54,55] A 3.5 to 4 mm scleral incision is made with a Beaver 64 blade to the external surface of the pars plicata region of the ciliary body (2 to 2.5 mm peripheral to the limbus). A 5-0 polyglactin 910 (Vicryl) or 4-0 polyfilament (Supramid) mattress suture is placed across the incision after light cauterization or diathermy of the exposed ciliary body. Care should be exerted so that heat-induced shrinkage of the scleral lips does not occur. A Beaver 52-s blade is then inserted through the sclerotomy into the lens, and a slow sweeping cut is made through the nucleus. If the knife blade easily penetrates the center of the lens (the usual circumstance in children's eyes), the lens substance is soft enough to be aspirated and cut with the wide-angle cutter of the Vitrophage without any further maneuvers. If moderate resistance is encountered (rare in children's eyes), the lens fragmentor[57] (a pneumatic minijackhammer) is inserted, and the lens nucleus is pulverized. The wide-angle cutter is then inserted for aspiration, cutting, and removal of the lens debris. If the knife blade cannot penetrate the nucleus at all (extremely rare in children's eyes), the lens can be removed through the limbus by cryoextraction, and its remnants are then removed through the sclerotomy with the wide-angle cutter. Alternatively, a second instrument, such as a 20-gauge needle can be inserted 120 to 170 degrees away, and a "lollypop"[35] or "cutting-board" technique can be utilized to crush and fragment the lens between the two instruments.

Another technique for hard nuclei involves use of the Shock phacofragmentor or other such devices.[35] Removal of the cataract itself begins in its center. An attempt is made to maintain the integrity of the anterior and posterior capsules until the nucleus and most of the cortex are removed. Integrity of the anterior capsule will prevent collapse of the anterior chamber if strong suction is required on the nucleus. An intact posterior capsule will prevent premature or excessively strong suction on vitreous strands and will also prevent migration of lens debris into the deep vitreous. Eventually the capsules are removed. This is easily and rapidly achieved with the wide-angle cutter. With the Ocutome, the capsules, particularly the anterior one, may be difficult to aspirate, and O'Malley has suggested a multiple-sieving technique for this problem.[50]

To remove residual cortex in the equatorial capsular "bag," it is usually necessary to indent the sclera overlying the equator of the lens. First, the eye is softened by increasing the suction or by lowering the infusion bottle. Indentation of the globe overlying the lens equator can then be carried out with a cotton-tipped applicator, and if necessary, the globe is simultaneously rotated toward the direction of the material to be aspirated (Fig. 20-14). The material is engaged by suction, and the tip of the instrument is withdrawn 1 to 2 mm away from the ciliary processes before activation of the cutting mechanism. The cortical remnants near the sclerotomy are removed last of all as the instrument is withdrawn. Care is taken to stop the suctioning, cutting, and infusion before the ciliary processes are encountered by the tip of the vitrectomy instrument as it leaves the eye.

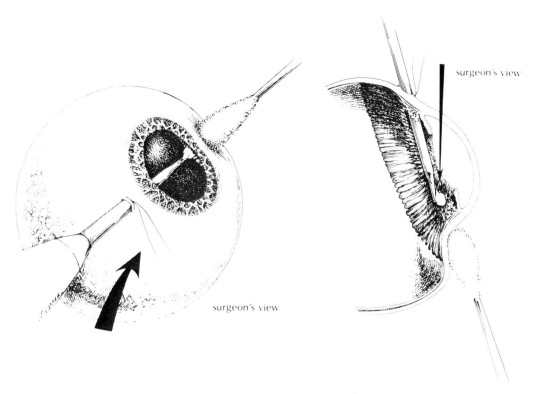

Fig. 20-14. For removal of equatorial portions of cataract, globe is indented over pars plicata and rotated toward the direction of the material to be aspirated.

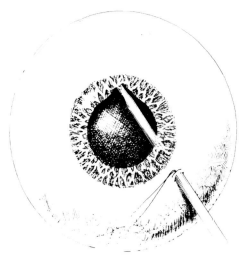
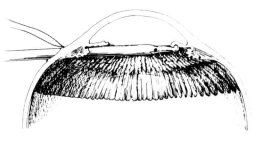

Fig. 20-15. Pars plicata sector iridectomy in case of small pupil.

After removal of the lens and anterior vitreous, the irrigated fundus contact lens is utilized for visualization of the deep vitreous, as described above. Any lens debris (Fig. 20-4) on the surface of the retina or in the deep vitreous is aspirated, cut, and removed.

Iridectomies to prevent pupillary block are usually not necessary and are not performed at the time of lens aspiration, unless the pupil fails to dilate (as in some cases of Marfan's syndrome, posterior synechiae, and so on) or becomes small or refractory to mydriatics. If an iridectomy is required, it can be performed, as suggested by O'Malley,[50] with the vitrectomy instrument passing anteriorly from the posterior scleral incision through the pupil to excise iris from its anterior surface. We have found it more convenient and less traumatic to the iris to perform either peripheral or, more usually, sector iridectomies by approaching the iris from its posterior surface (Fig. 20-15).

At the end of the operation, the fundus and sclerotomy are inspected with the indirect ophthalmoscope, and retinal breaks, if any, are frozen. Up to now, we have experienced none at the time of surgery for neonatal and infantile cataracts. The sclerotomy can also be treated with cryotherapy before the procedure is terminated.

Results

The foregoing technique reliably and reproducibly creates clear media immediately or, if any corneal edema or iris bleeding had occurred, within several days.[55] We have performed over 32 such procedures for infantile and juvenile cataracts, and follow-up study has ranged from 6 to 74 months. Early complications have been limited to three cases of transient corneal edema, one case of mild iris bleeding associated with sector iridectomy, one eye with a 5-day period of hazy vitreous caused by the presence of blood, and two eyes with transient elevation of intraocular pressure. No permanent sequelae resulted. There were no detectable differences between those eyes with and without rubella infection. There was no severe or persistent intraocular inflammation, entry-site dialysis, early or late retinal detachment or pupillary block, and no instance of hazy media requiring secondary surgery of any sort. The only late complication known thus far was bilateral cystoid macular edema in one patient with Down's syndrome.

With passage of time, it is inevitable that long-term complications such as retinal detachment will occur in some of these patients.

Because of the necessity of treating deprivation amblyopia as soon as possible, the foregoing technique appears particularly desirable. A one-stage procedure is used to create clear media that subsequently do not become translucent or opaque during the critical period of visual maturation. The complication rate is minimal, and secondary operations have thus far not been necessary. Difficult postoperative decision-making about the clarity (or lack thereof) of the media is eliminated, and retinoscopies, which are often inaccurate in the presence of small pupils or cloudy media and require frequent examinations under general anesthesia, are enhanced substantially.

Visual rehabilitation

There remains the need for rapid contact-lens fitting and a treatment regimen for amblyopia. Refer to the exemplary program promulgated by Beller et al.[3] and to those of Jacobson[30] and Enoch et al.[13,14] The avoidance of limbal surgery and the absence of an opacifying lens capsule makes these complex and difficult ministrations easier than they might otherwise be. Even when retinoscopy is limited by a small pupil, one can apply the ultrasonic refractive technique of Belkin and Levinson[2] in which the refractive error is calculated by subtraction of the corneal dioptric power (determined by keratometry or by trial fitting with contact lenses) from the total dioptric power of the eye. The total dioptric power of the aphakic eye *(F)* is calculated as follows:

$$F = n/f \times 1000$$

where n is the eye's refractive index (1.33) and f is the total axial length in millimeters.

ACKNOWLEDGMENTS

Art work was provided by Linda Warren, and photographic assistance was provided by Norbert Jednock. Editorial services were provided by Maxine Gere.

REFERENCES

1. Barber, J.C.: Management of anterior intraocular opacities with the roto-extractor, South. Med. J. **70:**286, 1977.
2. Belkin, M., and Levinson, A.: Ultrasonographic refraction of aphakic infants and children, Doc. Ophthalmol. **43:**147, 1977.
3. Beller, R., Hoyt, C.S., Marg, E., and Odom, J.V.: Good visual function after neonatal surgery for congenital monocular cataracts, Am. J. Ophthalmol. **91:**559, 1981.
4. Benson, W.E., Blankenship, G.W., and Machemer, R.: Pars plana lens removal with vitrectomy, Am. J. Ophthalmol. **84:**150, 1977.
5. Calhoun, J.H., and Harley, R.D.: The roto-extractor in pediatric ophthalmology, Trans. Am. Ophthalmol. Soc. **73:**292, 1975.
6. Coleman, D.J.: Phakoemulsification with vitrectomy through the pars plana, Ophthalmic Surg. **6:**95, 1975.
7. Crawford, J.S.: Conservative management of cataracts, Int. Ophthalmol. Clin. **17**(4):31, 1977.
8. Dobson, V., and Teller, D.Y.: Visual acuity in human infants: a review and comparison of behavioral and electrophysiological studies, Vision Res. **18:**1469, 1978.
9. Douvas, N.G.: Microsurgical pars plana lensectomy, Trans. Am. Acad. Ophthalmol. Otolaryngol. **81:**371, 1976.
10. Duke-Elder, S., and Cook, C.: Embryology: normal and abnormal development: system of ophthalmology, St. Louis, 1963, The C.V. Mosby Co., vol. 3.

11. Duke-Elder, S., and Wybar, K.C.: The anatomy of the visual system. In System of ophthalmology, St. Louis, 1961, The C.V. Mosby Co., vol. 2, p. 94.
12. Eifrig, D.E., Lockhart, D.L., Berglund, R.D., and Knobloch, W.H.: Pars plana vitrectomy, Ophthalmic Surg. **9:**76, 1978.
13. Enoch, J.M., and Rabinowicz, I.M.: Early surgery and visual correction of an infant born with unilateral lens opacity, Doc. Ophthalmol. **41:**371, 1976.
14. Enoch, J.M., Rabinowicz, I.M., and Campos, E.C.: Postsurgical contact lens correction of infants with sensory deprivation amblyopia associated with unilateral congenital cataract, J. Jpn. Contact Lens Soc. **21:**95, 1979.
15. François, J.: Congenital cataracts, Springfield, Ill., 1963, Charles C Thomas, Publisher.
16. Fung, W.E.: Vitrectomy in the management of persistent hyperplastic primary vitreous. In McPherson, A., editor: New and controversial aspects of vitreoretinal surgery, St. Louis, 1977, The C.V. Mosby Co.
17. Gass, J.D.M.: Surgical excision of persistent hyperplastic primary vitreous, Arch. Ophthalmol. **83:**163, 1970.
18. Gieser, D.K., Goldberg, M.F., Apple, D.J., Hamming, N.A., and Kottow, M.H.: Persistent hyperplastic primary vitreous in an adult: case report with fluorescein angiographic findings, J. Pediatr. Ophthalmol. Strabismus **15:**213, 1978.
19. Girard, L.J.: Pars plana lensectomy by ultrasonic fragmentation: results of a retrospective study, Trans. Am. Acad. Ophthalmol. Otolaryngol. **88:**434, 1981.
20. Gitter, K.A., editor: Current concepts of the vitreous including vitrectomy, St. Louis, 1976, The C.V. Mosby Co.
21. Gloor, B.P.: Persistierender hyperplastischer primärer Glaskörper: Differentialdiagnose und Probleme der chirurgischen Therapie, Klin. Monatsbl. Augenheilkd. **166:**293, 1975.
22. Gollender, M., Thorn, F., and Erickson, P.: Development of axial ocular dimensions following eyelid suture in the cat, Vision Res. **19:**221, 1979.
23. Hiles, D.A., and Biglan, A.W.: Indications for infantile cataract surgery, Int. Ophthalmol. Clin. **17**(4):39, 1977.
24. Hiles, D.A.: Phacoemulsification of infantile cataracts, Int. Ophthalmol. Clin. **17**(4):83, 1977.
25. Hiles, D.A.: Indications, techniques, and complications associated with intraocular lens implantation in children. In Hiles, D.A., editor: Intraocular lens implants in children, New York, 1979, Grune & Stratton, Inc.
26. Hiles, D.A., and Waller, P.H.: Phacoemulsification versus aspiration in infantile cataract surgery, Ophthalmic Surg. **5:**13, 1974.
27. Hirano, S., Yamamoto, Y., Takayama, H., Sugata, Y., and Matsuo, K.: Ultrasonic observation of eyes in premature babies. VI. Growth curves of ocular axial length and its components, Acta Soc. Ophthalmol. Jpn. **83:**227, 1979.
28. Hoffer, K.J.: Selection of lens power for implantation in infants and children, J. Am. Intraocular Implant Soc. **1**(2):49, 1975.
29. Jaffe, N.: Foreword. In Hiles, D.A., editor: Intraocular lens implants in children, New York, 1979, Grune & Stratton, Inc.
30. Jacobson, S.G., Mohindra, I., and Held, R.: Development of visual acuity in infants with congenital cataracts, Br. J. Ophthalmol. **65:**727, 1981.
31. Juarez, C.P., Peyman, G.A., Raichand, M., and Goldberg, M.F.: Secondary pupillary membranes treated by the pars plana–pars plicata approach: results of 108 cases, Br. J. Ophthalmol. **65:**762, 1982.
32. Kelman, C.D.: Congenital cataract: phacoemulsification. In Kwitko, M.L., editor: Surgery of the infantile eye, New York, 1979, Appleton-Century-Crofts.
33. King, J.H., Jr., and Wadsworth, J.A.C., editors: An atlas of ophthalmic surgery, Philadelphia, 1981, J.B. Lippincott Co.
34. Larsen, J.S.: The sagittal growth of the eye. IV. Ultrasonic measurement of the axial length of the eye from birth to puberty, Acta Ophthalmol. **49:**873, 1971.
35. Machemer, R., and Aaberg, T.A.: Vitrectomy, ed. 2, New York, 1979, Grune & Stratton, Inc.
36. Mafee, M.F., Goldberg, M.F., Salzano, T., Valvassori, G.E., Nabawi, P., and Capek, V.: Computed tomography in the evaluation of patients with persistent hyperplastic primary vitreous (PHPV), Radiology. (Submitted for publication.)
37. Mann, I.: Persistence of capsulopupillary vessels as a factor in the production of abnormalities of the iris and lens, Arch. Ophthalmol. **11:**174, 1934.

38. Mann, I.: Congenital retinal fold, Br. J. Ophthalmol. **19:**641, 1935.
39. Manschot, W.A.: Persistent hyperplastic primary vitreous, Arch. Ophthalmol. **59:**188, 1958.
40. Mason, G.I., and Huamonte, F.U.: PHPV in an adult managed by vitrectomy, Arch. Ophthalmol. **10:**93, 1979.
41. Meisels, H., and Goldberg, M.F.: Vascular anastomosis between the iris and persistent hyperplastic primary vitreous, Am. J. Ophthalmol. **88:**179, 1979.
42. Michels, R.G.: Vitreous surgery, St. Louis, 1981, The C.V. Mosby Co.
43. Michels, R.G., Machemer, R., and Mueller-Jensen, K.: Vitreous surgery: history and current concepts, Ophthalmic Surg. **5:**13, 1974.
44. Mittelman, D.: Geometric optics and clinical refraction. In Peyman, G.A., Sanders, D.R., and Goldberg, M.F., editors: Principles and practice of ophthalmology, Philadelphia, 1980, W.B. Saunders Co.
45. Moazed, K., Albert, D., and Smith, T.R.: Rubeosis iridis in "pseudogliomas," Surv. Ophthalmol. **25:**85, 1980.
46. Morgan, K.S., Werblin, T.P., Asbell, P.A., Loupe, D.N., Friedlander, M.H., and Kaufman, H.E.: The use of epikeratophakia grafts in pediatric monocular aphakia, J. Pediatr. Ophthalmol. Strabismus **18**(6):23, 1981.
47. Nankin, S.J., and Scott, W.E.: Persistent hyperplastic primary vitreous, Arch. Ophthalmol. **95:**240, 1977.
48. Offret, H., Saraux, H., Limon, S., and Lefrançois, A.: Vitréophagie par la pars-plana de deux cas de persistance de vitré primitif, Arch. Ophtalmol. **37:**473, 1977.
49. Ohba, N., Watanabe, S., and Fujita, S.: Primary vitreoretinal dysplasia transmitted as an autosomal recessive disorder, Br. J. Ophthalmol. **65:**631, 1981.
50. O'Malley, C., and Boyd, B.F.: Closed-eye endomicrosurgery (ab-interno microsurgery). In Boyd, B.F., editor: Highlights of ophthalmology, New York, 1981, Arcata Book Group, vol. 1.
51. Parks, M.M., and Hiles, D.A.: Management of infantile cataracts, Am. J. Ophthalmol. **63:**10, 1967.
52. Peyman, G.A., and Diamond, J.: The Vitrophage in ocular reconstruction following trauma, Can. J. Ophthalmol. **10:**419, 1975.
53. Peyman, G.A., Huamonte, F.U., Goldberg, M.F., Sanders, D.R., Nagpal, K.C., and Raichand, M.: Four hundred consecutive pars plana vitrectomies with the Vitrophage, Arch. Ophthalmol. **96:**45, 1978.
54. Peyman, G.A., Raichand, M., and Goldberg, M.F.: Surgery of congenital and juvenile cataracts: a pars plicata approach with the Vitrophage, Br. J. Ophthalmol. **62:**780, 1978.
55. Peyman, G.A., Raichand, M., Oesterle, C., and Goldberg, M.F.: Pars plicata lensectomy and vitrectomy in the management of congenital cataracts, Ophthalmology **88:**437, 1981.
56. Peyman, G.A.: Wide-angle cutter Vitrophage, Ophthalmic Surg. **7**(3):96, 1976.
57. Peyman, G.A., and Sanders, D.R.: Vitreous and vitreous surgery. In Peyman, G.A., Sanders, D.R., and Goldberg, M.F., editors: Principles and practice of ophthalmology, Philadelphia, 1980, W.B. Saunders Co.
58. Peyman, G.A., Sanders, D.R., and Nagpal, K.C.: Management of persistent hyperplastic primary vitreous by pars plana vitrectomy, Br. J. Ophthalmol. **60:**756, 1976.
59. Peyman, G.A., Sanders, D.R., Rose, M., and Korey, M.: Vitrophage in management of congenital cataracts, Albrecht von Graefes Arch. Klin. Exp. Ophthalmol. **202:**305, 1977.
60. Peyman, G.A., and Swartz, M.: Management of dense secondary membranes with the Vitrophage, Albrecht von Graefes Arch. Klin. Exp. Ophthalmol. **195:**155, 1975.
61. Pollard, Z.F.: Diagnosis and treatment of persistent hyperplastic primary vitreous, Perspect. Ophthalmol. **5:**27, 1981.
62. Pruett, R.C., and Schepens, C.L.: Posterior hyperplastic primary vitreous, Am. J. Ophthalmol. **69:**535, 1970.
63. Rabin, J., van Sluyters, R.C., and Malach, R.: Emmetropization: a vision-dependent phenomenon, Invest. Ophthalmol. **20:**561, 1981.
64. Reese, A.B.: Persistent hyperplastic primary vitreous: the Jackson memorial lecture, Am. J. Ophthalmol. **40:**317, 1955.
65. Ryan, S.J., and von Noorden, G.K.: Further observations on the aspiration technique in cataract surgery, Am. J. Ophthalmol. **71:**626, 1971.
66. Scheie, H.G.: Aspiration of congenital or soft cataracts: further experience, Am. J. Ophthalmol. **63:**3, 1967.

67. Schepens, C.L.: Clinical and research aspects of subtotal open-sky vitrectomy: Jackson memorial lecture, Am. J. Ophthalmol. **91:**143, 1981.
68. Scuderi, G., Balestrazzi, E., and Ranieri, G.: Destructive and conservative treatment of persistent hyperplastic primary vitreous and retinal dysplasia, Ophthalmologica **172:**346, 1976.
69. Smith, R.E., and Maumenee, A.E.: Persistent hyperplastic primary vitreous: results of surgery, Trans. Am. Acad. Ophthalmol. Otolaryngol. **78:**911, 1974.
70. Sorsby, A.: Biology of the eye as an optical system. In Duane, T.D., editor: Clinical ophthalmology, Philadelphia, 1981, Harper & Row, Publishers.
71. Spaulding, A.G.: Persistent hyperplastic primary vitreous humor: a finding in a 71-year-old man, Surv. Ophthalmol. **12:**448, 1967.
72. Spaulding, A.G., and Naumann, G.: Persistent hyperplastic primary vitreous in an adult, Arch. Ophthalmol. **77:**666, 1967.
73. Stark, W.J., Taylor, H.R., Michels, R.G., and Maumenee, A.E.: Management of congenital cataracts, Ophthalmology **86**(suppl.):1571, 1979.
74. Tait, E.C.: Refraction and heterophoria. In Harley, R.D., editor: Pediatric ophthalmology, Philadelphia, 1975, W.B. Saunders Co.
75. Taylor, D.: Choice of surgical technique in the management of congenital cataract, Trans. Ophthalmol. Soc. U.K. **101:**114, 1981.
76. Treister, G., and Machemer, R.: Pars plana approach for pupillary membranes, Arch. Ophthalmol. **96:**1014, 1978.
77. Vaegan, and Taylor, D.: Critical period for deprivation amblyopia in children, Trans. Ophthalmol. Soc. U.K. **99:**432, 1979.
78. van Selm, J.: Surgery for retinal dysplasia and hyperplasia of the persistent primary vitreous, Trans. Ophthalmol. Soc. U.K. **89:**545, 1969.
79. Warburg, M.: Aetiological heterogeneity and morphological similarity in congenital retinal non-attachment and falciform folds, Trans. Ophthalmol. Soc. U.K. **99:**272, 1979.
80. Zauberman, H., Warshavsky, R., and Burde, R.: Experimental control of eye growth, Metab. Ophthalmol. **2:**403, 1978.

21

Ocular *Toxocara canis* infection: clinical and experimental features

Robert C. Watzke

*T*oxocara canis is so commonly present in puppies and cats that one may assume almost a 100% prevalence.[8] The primary source of infection in humans is soil contaminated with embryonated eggs. The source of these eggs is the intestinal tract of infected puppies and lactating bitches. Adult dogs are not infective because *T. canis* larvae do not produce eggs in adult dogs. Only in pregnant bitches do the larvae achieve maturity, cross the placental tissue, infect fetal pups and begin producing embryonated eggs. Eggs are excreted by bitches and puppies, often in enormous numbers.

The eggs are not immediately infective but must develop for about 3 weeks. These eggs can withstand drying, freezing, and prolonged exposure, and since they are widely distributed in the soil, human infection is probably widespread.[8]

One enigmatic feature of *T. canis* infection in the human is the difference in clinical features of early childhood infection and ocular infection. Typically a childhood infection gives the signs of visceral larva migrans with fever, eosinophilia, pneumonitis, spleno-megaly, hepatomegaly, malaise, and weight loss. Ocular infection occurs in older children and young adults without any signs of systemic toxocariasis. There is uaually a history of pica in young children with visceral larva migrans, but very seldom such a history in young adults.

A possible explanation of this finding is that one contracts the condition in early childhood and the ocular infection later because of subsequent migration of a larva into the eye. We know that larvae can live in subhuman primates for years and our recent studies indicate that this is probably true in humans.[1]

Larvae migrate through vessels but can also migrate at will through any tissue. Larvae could enter the eye along the optic nerve or through or along posterior ciliary arteries or the central retinal artery. They are able to migrate within the eye at will and produce a variety of pathologic responses.

CLINICAL FORMS OF *TOXOCARA CANIS* OCULAR INFECTION
Ednophthalmitis

A typical form of ocular toxocariasis is an indolent endophthalmitis. Typically a child is noticed to have decreased vision in one eye with leukokoria. The vitreous is

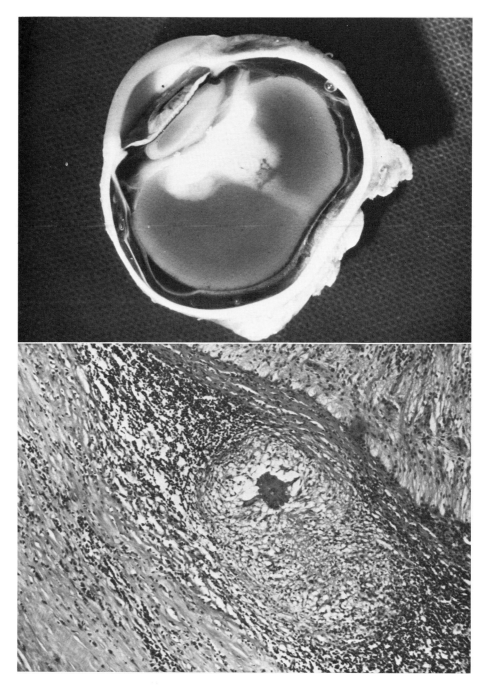

Fig. 21-1. A, Cross section of enucleated eye of 6-year-old child with leukokoria. **B,** The retrolental mass contains a *Toxocara canis* larva surrounded by chronic inflammatory cells. Serum ELISA (enzyme-linked immunosorbent assay) titer was negative.

opaque and there are signs of a chronic uveitis. The eye is often suspected of containing retinoblastoma and is enucleated. In such an eye, there is behind the lens an inflammatory mass consisting of detached retina and organized granuloma surrounding a fragmented larva (Fig. 21-1).

Peripheral granuloma

In the peripheral granuloma form of ocular toxocariasis there is cellular inflammation of the vitreous and the patient complains of decreased central vision and floaters. Onset is very insidious, and the condition may mimic that of peripheral uveitis or "pars-planitis." There is an organized, white mass in one quadrant at the vitreous base covering the pars plana and peripheral retina. There are signs of preretinal traction in this area, and there may be a slight dragging of the fovea, preretinal membrane formation in the posterior pole, and cystoid macular edema. The peripheral mass is more circumscribed and does not cover the entire lower pars plana as it does in the typical cases of peripheral uveitis.[10]

Diffuse unilateral subacute neuroretinitis (unilateral "wipe-out" syndrome)

The clinical features and cause of diffuse unilateral subacute neuroretinitis have been described by Gass et al.[5] Since it is the subject of Chapter 8, I do not describe it here.

Optic neuritis

In 1970 Bird described a unilateral severe papillitis and uveitis caused by *Toxocara* larva invasion of the nerve head.[4] I have reproduced this condition by intravitreal inoculation of *Toxocara* larvae in the primate.

THE ELISA TEST

Previous serologic tests for *Toxocara canis* have been inaccurate because of cross-reactions with other roundworms, particularly *Ascaris*. The enzyme-linked immunosorbent assay (ELISA) test provides a much more specific test for the presence of antibodies to *Toxocara,* particularly when *Ascaris* antibodies are previously absorbed.

This test is quite specific for previous exposure to *Toxocara canis*. However, titers are low in ocular toxocariasis, and a significant number of clinically uninfected patients will have positive titers. The Communicable Disease Center in Atlanta, Georgia has approached this problem by chooing a titer that is specific enough to diagnosis 95% of ocular *Toxocara* infections and sensitive enough to select 75% of patients with the disease. This titer is 1:32.[7]

Unfortunately, patients with ocular toxocariasis frequently have a lower titer. Indeed, it appears that a patient with pathologically proved ocular toxocariasis may have a "negative" titer.[9] For example, the patient who had *Toxocara* endophthalmitis and whose eye is depicted in Fig. 21-1 had a "negative" titer.

I believe that any titer is significant, and when sending serum for ELISA testing, I ask that all titers be reported. Given the frequency of low titers in the general population, because of the frequency of exposure to this parsite and lack of "high" titers in patients with the ocular form of the disease, we must still depend on our clinical judgment in making the diagnosis of ocular toxocariasis.

There is clinical evidence that titers from the vitreous or subretinal fluid in patients with ocular *Toxocara* infections will be higher than that of the serum.[3] The cause for this is not known, but it may represent local antibody production. In certain cases, vitreous aspiration may be necessary to substantiate the diagnosis. Certainly, if vitrectomy is performed on these eyes, ELISA testing should be performed on the vitreous or subretinal fluid.[6]

EXPERIMENTAL STUDIES OF OCULAR *TOXOCARA* INFECTION IN PRIMATES

Because of the puzzling inconsistencies seen in the clinical evaluation of patients with ocular *Toxocara* infection, we have studied the various features of this disease in a primate model. This research, done with Dr. John Oaks, Associate Professor of Anatomy at The University of Iowa College of Medicine, has been underway for the past 4 years. Specific details of the method and results are being reported in separate publications and are summarized here.

Materials and method

Briefly, the methods consisted in the collection of embryonated *Toxocara canis* eggs from puppies and the hatching of these eggs in vivo. These larvae were then injected by various routes in rabbits in preliminary experiments and then in a total of 32 young cynomolgus monkeys. The pathologic state of the ocular infections and its time relationship, the mobility of the larvae over a long period of time, the route of exit from the eye, the ELISA titers produced by systemic and ocular injection of small amounts of larvae, and the influence of previous sensitization to *Toxocara* larvae upon the ocular inflammatory response were studied. The results are briefly summarized.

Mobility and pathologic effects of *Toxocara* larvae

The best route for production of ocular toxocariasis was intravitreal injection of adult *Toxocara* larvae in the amount of 50 to 100 larvae. Retrobulbar injection did not produce any sign of intraocular inflammation though larvae were subsequently found in the brain. Intracarotid injection of larvae was similarly negative. Larvae were so motile that they did not appear to remain in the retinal or choroidal vasculature and produce an ocular infection.

Clinical features of experimental toxocariasis

Intravitreal injection of 50 to 100 larvae produced a variable uveitis during the first week. Larvae then showed a remarkable ability to either incite typical signs of ocular infection or to move throughout ocular tissue without any inflammation whatsoever.

Lesions produced by intravitreal injection consisted of perivasculitis, retinal hemorrhages, white-centered retinal hemorrhages, and white retinal inflammatory nodules (Fig. 21-2 and 21-3).

This type of response reached its peak within the first 2 weeks. After that, the uveitis gradually cleared, the retinal hemorrhages and perivasculitis resolved and only a few chronic granulomas remained. Many eyes became clinically normal; others continued to have a few retinal granulomas with mild cellular vitreal reaction. Occasionally granulomas appeared after a latent period during which the retina and vitreous were clinically normal. No eyes were lost from overwhelming uveitis or inflammation.

No larvae were seen in the fundus or vitreous on gross or slitlamp examination of

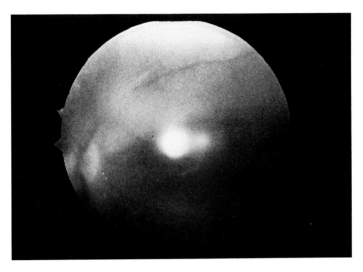

Fig. 21-2. Fundus of monkey 11 weeks after intravitreal injection of *T. canis* larvae. Vitreous is cellular. Two contiguous retinal granulomas are present in center.

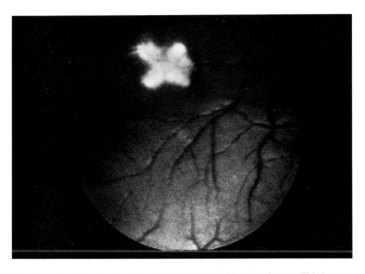

Fig. 21-3. Fundus of monkey 1 week after intravitreal injection of *T. canis* larvae. This is a segmental intense perivasculitis.

primate eyes. Immediately after intravitreal injection, a few larvae could be seen in the anterior vitreous with a contact lens of 40 magnification. The adult larvae were just barely visible even under these circumstances.

Pathologic features of experimental ocular toxocariasis

At 3 days larvae could be seen in the vitreous surrounded by eosinophils and lymphocytes. Perivasculitis consisted of a lymphocytic inflammation of the coats of retinal

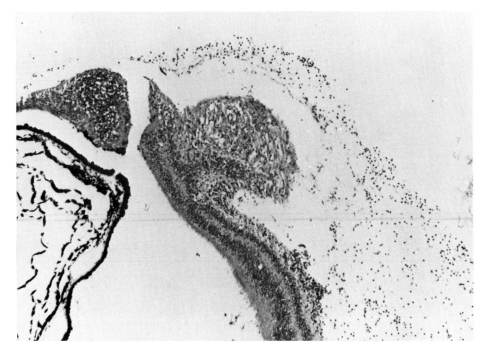

Fig. 21-4. Peripheral retina 30 days after intravitreal injection of *T. canis* larvae. There is a superficial retinal mass composed of chronic inflammatory cells with cells in the adjacent vitreous. (Hematoxylin and eosin, 100×.)

vessels. Retinal hemorrhages consisted of extravascular hemorrhage in the retina at all layers surrounding nests of chronic inflammatory cells without larvae being visible on serial sectioning. Granulomas at 1 month consisted of lymphocytes and eosinophils arranged around a larva. However, some granulomas did not contain larvae (Fig. 21-4). It was impossible to tell if larvae were dead or living by histologic appearance. After 30 days, the cellular reaction often consisted of giant cells and lymphocytes.

Most surprising was the finding of larvae within retinal tissue and the optic nerve without any inflammatory reaction around these larvae. These larvae appeared to have all anatomic characteristics of living larvae. The larvae were found both within and outside of vessels, and they were found at every level of the retina and choriocapillaris and in the optic nerve. For example, one larva was found deep in the substance of the optic nerve at 30 days (Fig. 21-5). In another eye, 10 months after intravitreal injection, a normal-appearing larva was found in the retina without any inflammatory response. Yet, other portions of the retina were found to have granulomas.

Another eye at 1 year showed a larva within a fibrous capsule within the retina with minimal inflammatory response.

Influence of previous sensitization

The type of ocular reaction was the same whether a monkey had been previously sensitized by intraperitoneal injection of live larvae or was unsensitized.

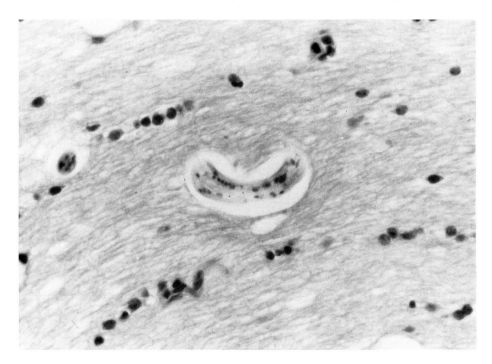

Fig. 21-5. Optic nerve 30 days after intravitreal *T. canis* larvae injection. A larva is present without cellular reaction or signs of necrosis. (Hematoxylin and eosin, 100 × .)

ELISA titers

Intraperitoneal injection of live larvae in primates produced the expected eosinophilia and a positive ELISA titer. Serum ELISA titers produced by intravitreal injection of live larvae were invariably low.

Causes of ocular inflammatory response

In our first series of six monkeys our controls were intravitreal injection of culture medium in the fellow eye of each monkey. This invariably caused no visible or pathologic response except for an occasional vitreous cell during the first week.

In a later series we injected a culture medium that had supported larvae and from which larvae were then removed. These eyes developed perivasculitis and uveitis, but no retinal hemorrhages or granulomas.

In a third series of experiments we injected larvae that were killed by boiling and from which all culture medium had been washed. These eyes developed only a mild uveitis.

Finally, six eyes were injected with 50 to 100 intravitreal larvae and then examined after killing the monkeys at periods up to 1 year. The eyes were opened and the granulomas located under the dissecting microscope. The retina containing the granulomas was excised and examined by transillumination. Larvae could be seen in these granulomas. These larvae were definitely motile and alive.

DISCUSSION

What does this research tell us about ocular toxocariasis?

Toxocara larvae can move into and out of the eye along tissue planes at will without inciting any inflammatory response. Even larvae within granulomas are motile up to 1 year and probably longer. Granulomas are not necessarily evidence of death of the larvae.

Some antigenic fraction of the larvae produce uveitis and vasculitis. Retinal hemorrhages probably are attributable to the transient activity and are not an immune response to the larvae.

The long latent period between the signs of ocular toxocariasis and visceral larva migrans is caused by the permanent infestation and occasional ocular migration of *Toxocara* larvae that have infected the patient in childhood. Ocular infection is probably a chance occurrence. Larvae are freely motile for several years and, in fact, may be permanent inhabitants of humans.

The ELISA test, though it is quite specific, cannot be depended on being diagnostic of ocular infection. If a patient has ingested *T. canis* larvae in childhood, his titer may decline to a very low level after several years. Yet, the larvae are still motile and if at any time during is adult life, one enters the eye and produces an ocular inflammation, one would not expect the titer to become appreciably elevated.

An exception to this might be intravitreal levels of ELISA-titer levels that seem to be increased after ocular infection. We are currently examining this.

Pathologic proof of ocular toxocariasis is difficult. It takes meticulous search of many serial sections to find a fragment of one larva. If the larva has not been "trapped" by the inflammation, the cause of the uveitis or chorioretinitis in an enucleated eye may never be found. Certainly the usual studies of a pathology laboratory would be inadequate.

The words of Beaver on the parasite-host relationship in 1969 are still pertinent. "When a larva that has caused extensive inflammation is seen lying immobile in an encapsulating granuloma, there is a tendency to conclude that it has been trapped and immobilized by the host defenses which eventually will destroy it. In certain instances, however, in view of the long persistence of the larva before and after encapsulation, and the eventual lack of inflammation around the encapsulating tissue, it is not illogical to interpret the reaction as being under the control of the parasite, induced by it to provide for its comfort and needs in long survival."[2]

When we consider the numbers of dogs and cats throughout the world, their proximity to humans, the exposure that all of us have to embryonated eggs, the ability of larvae to live for years in humans, their mobility, and finally the difficulty of demonstrating the presence of larvae by pathologic examination, does it not seem possible that many types of ocular and systemic inflammatory disease could be caused by this parasite?

REFERENCES

1. Aljeboori, T.I., Stout, C., and Ivey, M.H.: *Toxocara canis* infections in baboons. II. Distribution of larvae and histopathologic responses, Am. J. Trop. Med. Hyg. **19:**815-820, 1970.
2. Beaver, P.C.: The nature of visceral larva migrans, J. Parasitol. **55:**3, 1969.
3. Biglan, A.W., Glickman, L.T., and Lobes, L.A.: Serum and vitreous *Toxocara* antibody in nematode endophthalmitis, Am. J. Ophthalmol. **88**(5):898-901, 1979.
4. Bird, A.C., Smith, J., and Curtin, V.C.: Nematode optic neuritis, Am. J. Ophthalmol. **69:**72, 1970.
5. Gass, J.D.M., Gilbert, W.R., Guerry, R.K., and Scelfo, R.: Diffuse unilateral subacute neuroretinitis, Trans. Am. Acad. Ophthalmol. **85:**521-545, 1978.

6. Hagler, W.S., Pollard, Z.F., Jarrett, W.H., and Donnelly, E.H.: Results of surgery for ocular *Toxocara canis,* Ophthalmology **88:**1081-1086, 1981.
7. Pollard, Z.F., Jarrett, W.H., Hagler, W.S., Allain, D.S., and Schantz, P.M.: ELISA for diagnosis of ocular toxocariasis, Trans. Am. Acad. Ophthalmol. **86:**743-749, 1978.
8. Schantz, P.M., and Glickman, L.T.: Medical intelligence, current concepts in parasitology, N. Engl. J. Med. **298:**436-439, 1978.
9. Searl, S.S., Moazed, K., Albert, D.M., and Marcus, L.C.: Ocular toxocariasis presenting as leukocoria in a patient with low ELISA titer to *Toxocara canis,* Ophthalmology **88:**1302, 1981.
10. Wilkinson, C.P., and Welch, R.B.: Intraocular *Toxocara,* Am. J. Ophthalmol. **71:**921, 1971.

22

Pattern recognition of ocular tumors

D. Jackson Coleman
Mary E. Smith*

Ultrasound has achieved widespread recognition for its value in the evaluation of ocular tumors. In the 20 years since its inception, ophthalmic ultrasound has become a widely applicable technique similar in importance to the slitlamp in routine patient management. In conjunction with photographic and angiographic studies, ultrasonography is the primary tool for the diagnosis and evaluation of ocular tumors.

In view of the changing approach to the management of ocular tumors, particularly malignant melanomas, many patients are observed for extended periods of time to ascertain growth or stability patterns. Ultrasonography thus serves the dual role of initial diagnostic aid and subsequent documentation technique as a patient is followed either before or after treatment.

Our laboratory has long advocated a combined B- and A-scan system[2,3] that emphasizes overall pattern recognition rather than isolated features derived from either of these two display techniques. This pattern-recognition scheme encompasses not only the basic topography obtained from B-scan[1,5] or A-scan amplitude as relied upon by standardized echography,[4] but also includes variations in tumor shape and contour and associated ocular changes viewed as a whole with A-scan texture, pattern, and amplitude.

In addition, the kinetic nature on both B and A scans is viewed as an integral part of the examination rather than a singularly definitive feature. Thus the term "pattern recognition" implies a system of varied components in a scheme using constantly shifting emphasis, where one factor may be of emphasized assistance in arriving at a particular diagnosis but certainty of diagnosis is augmented when one takes all features into consideration.

Conventional pattern-recognition techniques are summarized in the following list of specific features associated with both B and A scans. In addition, the amplitude character of the A scan can be appreciated on B scan when gray scale, color encoding, or isometric viewing are used.

*Senior Research Associate in Ophthalmology, Department of Ophthalmology, Cornell University Medical College, New York, New York.

Conventional ultrasound techniques
B scan for pattern recognition
   Location
   Shape, size
   Related pathologic states
A scan for characterization
   Amplitude
   Pattern
   Textural relationships

OCULAR TUMOR PATTERNS

The differential diagnosis of ocular tumors comprises four main categories: malignant melanoma, metastatic carcinoma, choroidal hemangioma, and subretinal hemorrhage. The varying modes of treatment for these tumors are so disparate that a certainty of identification is required before one initiates treatment or continues observation. We have attempted to classify these four major groups of ocular tumors according to the outline in Table 22-1, describing areas of similarity that indicate further analysis and those features we believe are characteristic of each group.

The acoustic features used in identifying malignant melanoma of the choroid are summarized as follows:

Malignant melanoma
Pattern
   Convex
   Collar button
   Tissue replacement
   Absorption and shadowing
Character
   Pronounced amplitude attenuation
   Spontaneous vascular movement
   Frequency variation

A typical malignant melanoma at the posterior pole, with a convex configuration, is shown in Fig. 22-1. The relation of the mass to other intraocular structures (lens, optic nerve) is well shown, as is the relative size of the mass in relation to the globe. The accompanying A-scan pattern is that characteristically seen in malignant melanoma, with a rapidly diminishing slope identified between the two reference points of the leading edge of the tumor and the posterior sclera. This rapidly decaying slope is produced by the absorption and attenuation of sound as it traverses this relatively homogeneous tumor tissue. With linear amplifiers, the decay slope shows an exponential decline, whereas logarithmic amplifiers produce a relatively straight decline. Vessels and septa may produce some irregularity or "texture" in the A scan. Vessel-wall movement may produce variable amplitude echoes seen in real time on the A scan as "spontaneous" movements. These are commonly seen in melanomas but rarely in other vascular tumors.

To analyse optimally the intraocular tumor patterns, one must position the sound beam so that it simultaneously maximizes the leading edge of the tumor and the underlying scleral echo. This technique of aligning the sound beam normal (or perpendicular) to the tissue examined is important in all aspects of ultrasonography, but particularly essential

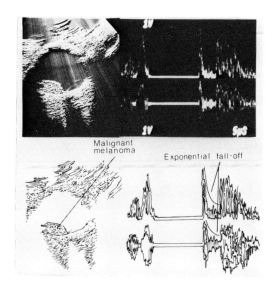

Fig. 22-1. Malignant melanoma shown on B scan, *left,* and A scan, *right*. The diagrams illustrate the B-scan solid convex appearance and the characteristic exponential falloff on the A scan.

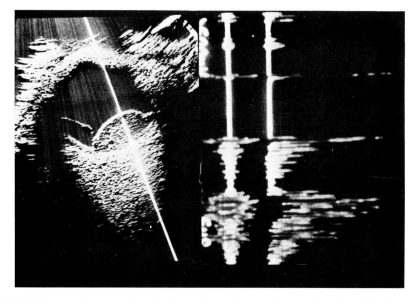

Fig. 22-2. Malignant melanoma and associated retinal detachment on B scan with an intensified line or vector enhanced to show the position of the simultaneous A scan.

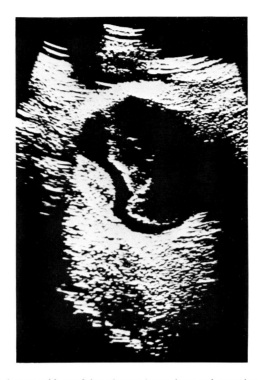

Fig. 22-3. Malignant melanoma with overlying vitreous hemorrhage and retraction of the posterior vitreous into a vitreous veil formation.

in A-scan tumor analysis (Fig. 22-2). Information obtained from an obliquely aligned section greatly reduces the value of A-scan pattern analysis.

Secondary ocular changes, such as vitreous hemorrhage or retinal detachment affecting both examination and ultimate identification are usually well demonstrated, as shown in Fig. 22-3. The homogeneous nature of malignant melanoma can be appreciated on B scan, and when the homogeneous nature of the tumor is pronounced, additional acoustic features, such as an acoustic quiet zone can be seen (Fig. 22-4). When the quiet zone replaces a high amplitude area such as choroid, a tissue-replacement phenomenon called "choroidal excavation" (Fig. 22-5) can be seen. This irregular dip in the normal choroidal curvature, indicative of a tumor that is replacing the normal choroid, is characteristically only seen in malignant melanoma. Amplifier design can reduce the value of the choroidal-excavation sign, since a low-amplitude tumor section must be able to replace a high-amplitude choroid in order to be appreciated. Logarithmic amplifiers (which compress dynamic range) will often elevate lower-amplitude patterns of tumors so that the acoustic tissue-replacement feature is no longer visually apparent on B scan. When large malignant melanomas are examined, two acoustic features may be seen (Fig. 22-6). The first is a vacant area in the posterior portion of the tumor, the "acoustic quiet zone" previously described produced by both lack of discrete interfaces (homogeneity) and attenuation of the sound by more anterior portions of this highly absorbent tumor. The second is a

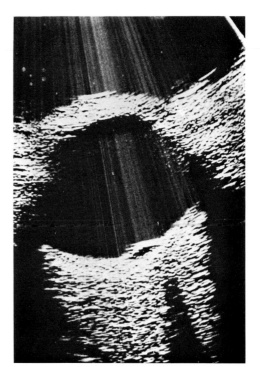

Fig. 22-4. Malignant melanoma with hollow appearance or acoustic quiet zone caused by low-amplitude echoes. (See also Fig. 22-7.)

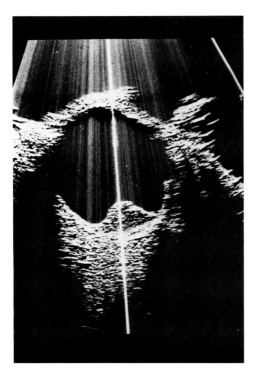

Fig. 22-5. Scan of malignant melanoma with choroidal excavation produced by replacement of the choroid of solid tumor, resulting in a ''dip'' in the normally smooth curve of the posterior pole.

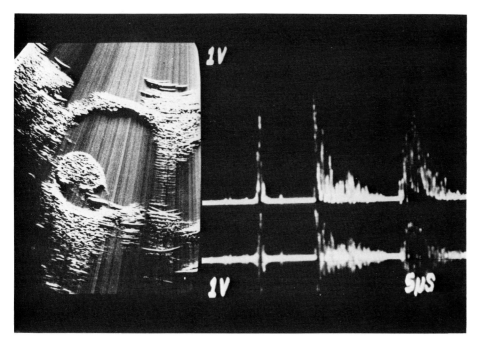

Fig. 22-6. Scans of malignant melanoma demonstrating a collar-button anterior lobe and a clear posterior "acoustic quiet zone" produced by homogeneous tissue. The orbital area posterior to the mass shows the shadowing effect of absorption of sound by the tumor.

defect in the retrobulbar fat behind the tumor, and "shadowing" is also caused by the solid nature of the tumor.

As discussed in B-scan patterns, the degree of internal tissue homogeneity will also influence the acoustic pattern on A scan. Melanomas with a high degree of homogeneity will demonstrate a more precipitous drop to base line with accompanying low-level internal echoes (Fig. 22-7). The internal A-scan pattern should be viewed as a whole, since isolated high-amplitude peaks within the tumor may represent small vascular channels throughout the mass, appearing in some sections and not others, and should not detract from the recognition of the overall tissue signature.

Many malignant melanomas also assume somewhat predictable and recognizable topographic patterns that are shown well on both B and A scans. Notably, a break in Bruch's membrane or a collar-button configuration will present as a mushroom-shaped, narrow-necked tumor mass on B scan (Fig. 22-8). The A scan through this tumor will present a variation from the characteristic rapidly diminishing slope and will, in many instances, show a well-circumscribed mass of high-amplitude echoes anterior to a lower-level region representing the posterior part of the tumor. This pattern correlates with the histologic pattern seen in these tumors upon enucleation where the anterior portion of the tumor is more highly vascularized whereas the posterior portion is of a more homogeneous cellular composition.

Tumors that are situated at the equator or more anteriorly can be difficult to evaluate

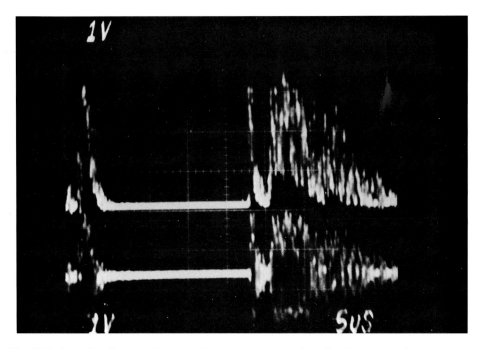

Fig. 22-7. Scan of malignant melanoma with precipitous drop to base line in an extremely homogeneous tumor. (See also Fig. 22-4.)

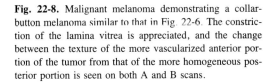

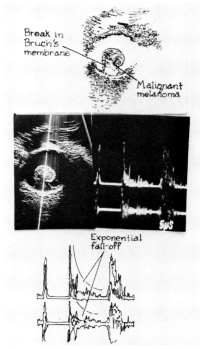

Fig. 22-8. Malignant melanoma demonstrating a collar-button melanoma similar to that in Fig. 22-6. The constriction of the lamina vitrea is appreciated, and the change between the texture of the more vascularized anterior portion of the tumor from that of the more homogeneous posterior portion is seen on both A and B scans.

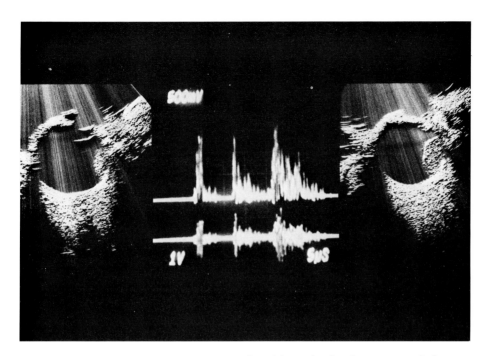

Fig. 22-9. Malignant melanoma at the equator requires globe rotation for adequate portrayal of tumor.

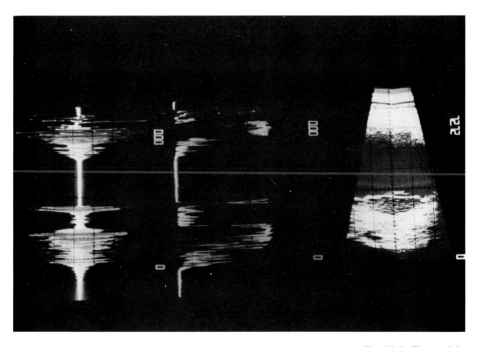

Fig. 22-10. Contact B and A scans of the same malignant melanoma as shown in Fig. 22-9. The handpiece containing the transducer may be more sharply angulated to obtain perpendicular alignment to the tumor. Note that the A-scan pattern is similar in both techniques.

with the immersion technique as the orientation of the transducer becomes more awkward (Fig. 22-9). A contact method can provide a greater degree of maneuverability when one is depicting these tumors (Fig. 22-10). Although contact scanners have inherently less resolution and sensitivity than immersion systems because of transducer-design constraints and loss of sound in the enclosed water-bath membrane, the overall patterns are generally identical.

GROWTH AND REGRESSION OF MALIGNANT MELANOMAS

Ultrasonography is essential in following patients to document growth before definitive treatment and in comparison with subsequent ultrasonic examinations. All efforts should be made to duplicate the original scan plane, and great care taken to achieve a maximum anterior-to-posterior diameter to document growth, both on initial and subsequent examination. Dramatic changes in tumor size and shape can be well shown on the B scan (Fig. 22-11). For documentation of more subtle progression of tumor growth, reliance should be placed on an electronic measuring technique. We have used a system that automatically converts time into distance by using a presumed velocity of sound in tumor tissue, and although small variations in tumor-height measurement can be produced

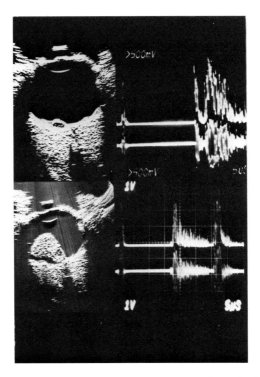

Fig. 22-11. B- and A-scan ultrasonogram of the same patient on initial examination, *top,* and 16 months later, *bottom.* Growth is well documented with ultrasound and is regarded as reliable when 0.5 mm of change is noted. In this case, the anterior to posterior height of the tumor was measured at 4.04 and 14.21 mm, respectively.

by variation in scan plane or involuntary movement, a documented change of 0.5 mm or more is considered significant with this technique.

In subsequent surgical management, this technique has proved extremely useful in the calculation of radiation dose in the cobalt-plaque application. Subsequent to cobalt-plaque treatment, the tumor can then be monitored at selected intervals for documentation of the efficacy of treatment as portrayed by reduction in the anterior-to-posterior height of the tumor (Fig. 22-12).

METASTATIC CARCINOMA

Similar to malignant melanoma, metastatic carcinoma can present as an isolated convex mass emanating from the choroid and appearing on both B and A scans as a solid tumor. The characteristics of metastatic carcinoma are listed as follows:

> *Metastatic carcinoma*
> Pattern
>   Convex
>   Placoid
>   Associated serous retinal detachment
> Character
>   Sustained moderate amplitude
>   Difficulty in maximizing leading edge

The A-scan pattern in metastatic carcinoma, however, differs drastically from that seen in malignant melanoma and characteristically presents a series of sustained moderate-

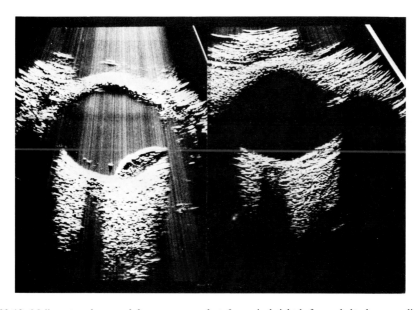

Fig. 22-12. Malignant melanoma, *left,* was measured at 6 mm in height before cobalt plaque application. Eight months after treatment, a reduction in size to 2.85 mm was documented, *right.*

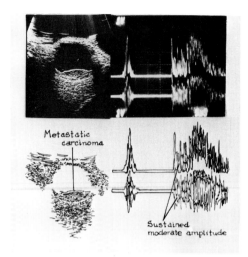

Fig. 22-13. Metastatic carcinoma with solid B-scan appearance, *left.* The A scan, *right,* shows a sustained amplitude of approximately 50% of scleral echo height. The characteristic heterogeneous cell and septal pattern produces the sustained echoes.

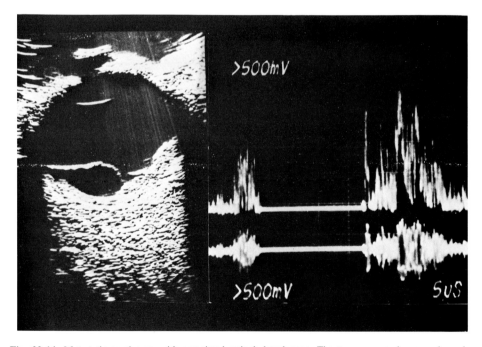

Fig. 22-14. Metastatic carcinoma with associated retinal detachment. The tumor mass shows an irregular anterior surface noted at times in these tumors.

amplitude internal echoes on A-scan analysis (Fig. 22-13). Variations in the B-scan pattern of metastatic carcinoma have also been observed, however, and at times these tumors will present as a placoid elevation very similar in structure and texture to normal choroid. A well-defined leading edge of these tumors is not easily identified, and there may be difficulties in maximizing the leading edge of tumor for optical A-scan analysis. These low-lying posteriorly located choroidal tumors are also often seen in association with serous retinal detachment (Fig. 22-14). Depending on the elevation of the overlying detachment, again difficulty can be encountered in identification of the leading edge of the tumor. Similar to the documentation technique used in following malignant melanomas after local irradiation, metastatic carcinoma of the choroid can be followed after external-beam radiation for evaluation of the efficacy of treatment.

HEMANGIOMA

B- and A-scan characteristics of choroidal hemangioma are summarized as follows:

Choroidal hemangioma

Pattern
    Convex
    Placoid
Character
    Sustained, high amplitude
    Coarse texture

Choroidal hemangiomas present a similar B-scan appearance; that is, a solid elevated lesion appears at the posterior pole. However, in many instances these tumors will assume a plateau-shaped configuration that may be helpful in their differentiation. In addition, secondary retinal detachment is seen quite frequently in these patients. The A-scan pattern produced by choroidal hemangiomas is that of a discrete well-defined leading edge of tumor with sustained, higher-amplitude internal echoes, at times approximately 85% to 95% of scleral echo height (Fig. 22-15). Additionally, depending on or in relation to the orientation of intratumor vascular formation, the internal A-scan pattern may

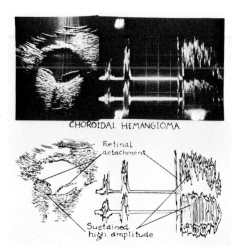

Fig. 22-15. Choroidal hemangioma of the choroid, with a shallow overlying retinal detachment, shows sustained high-amplitude echoes on the A scan, nearly 90% of scleral echo height.

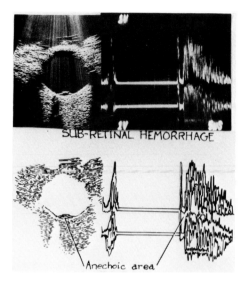

Fig. 22-16. Subretinal hemorrhage produces a B-scan pattern resembling the small malignant melanoma seen in Fig. 22-4. The A scan shows the same sharp drop to base line as seen in Fig. 22-7, but the base line is flat as compared to the low but solid echoes seen in the case of homogeneous malignant melanoma.

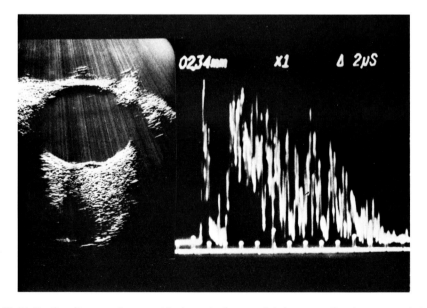

Fig. 22-17. Small malignant melanoma with electronically expanded A scan to allow better appreciation of the internal echo pattern and more accurate identification of the echoes and measurement.

present a more coarse texture produced as the sound beam transverses large vascular channels within the tumor. Texture is better appreciated on the radio frequency (RF) trace than on the video display.

SUBRETINAL HEMORRHAGE

The following is an outline of subretinal hemorrhage:

> **Subretinal hemorrhage**
> Pattern
> > Discrete, disciform elevation
> Character
> > Low-to-absent internal pattern

This type of hemorrhage will characteristically produce a well-circumscribed local elevation of the retina with an anechoic area internally, appreciated on B-scan. The corresponding A-scan pattern will produce an isolated, high-amplitude peak originating from the retina with extremely low level to no echo response from the internal section of this lesion (Fig. 22-16). This pattern can be most difficult to differentiate acoustically from that produced by extremely homogeneous small malignant melanomas (Figs. 22-4 and 22-7), and for adequate evaluation of the internal A-scan pattern, electronic magnification of the section of the A scan representing the tumor is recommended (Fig. 22-17).

CILIARY BODY TUMORS

Anteriorly located tumors can be identified with ultrasonic techniques (see the following outline), and their location, in relation to other anterior ocular structures such as the iris ciliary body and lens, can be well documented.

> **Ciliary body tumors**
> Pattern
> > Relation to iris, lens, and ciliary body
> > Posterior extent
> Character
> > Leading edge masked
> > Solid versus cystic

The posterior extent of these tumors is well shown with ultrasonography and can be of great clinical assistance, since the posterior edge of such a tumor may be poorly visualized on ophthalmoscopic examination. Differentiation between solid or cystic tumors of the iris and ciliary body is a diagnosis easily made on both B and A scans (Fig. 22-18). In the instance of a solid ciliary body tumor, however, A-scan tissue analysis can be more difficult than that with some posterior tumors because the aforementioned principles of A-scan analysis are no longer applicable. First, in most instances, the eye must be rotated and the transducer beam carefully aligned so that the maximum anterior-to-posterior diameter of the tumor can be shown (Fig. 22-19, *A* and *B*). When this orientation is achieved, the tissue-analysis technique or the maximization technique (mentioned on the bottom of p. 273) is reversed in that the scleral echo is now more anteriorly located, and the sound beam traverses sclera before passing through tumor tissue itself, with the posterior border of the tumor being the point of comparison. Since

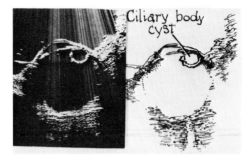

Fig. 22-18. Ciliary body cyst shows characteristic hollow internal appearance.

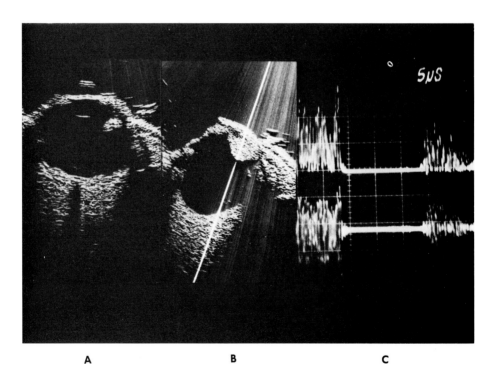

A   B   C

Fig. 22-19. Solid tumor of the ciliary body (malignant melanoma). The globe has been rotated to bring the tumor into perpendicular alignment with the transducer, and the accompanying A scan shows the higher amplitude internal echoes produced by traversal of the sclera anteriorly.

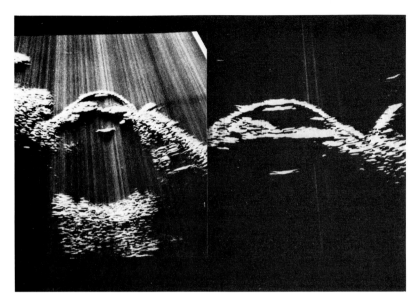

Fig. 22-20. Iris tumor shows as solid mass in the anterior chamber. Electronic expansion of the display and adjustment of the focal zone allows better definition of the mass.

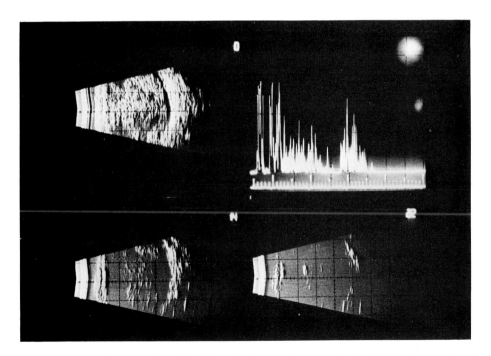

Fig. 22-21. Attenuation study of a child with retinoblastoma, demonstrating the highly reflective internal echoes from calcium deposits. Echoes from the tumor are still evident at lowered sensitivity and persist even after the scleral echoes have disappeared.

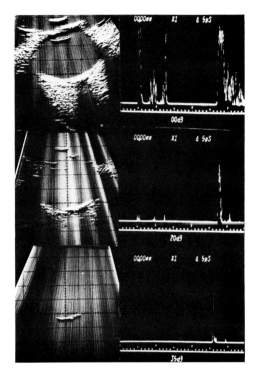

Fig. 22-22. Choroidal osteoma with high reflective portion of the posterior pole still evident with 35 dB of attenuation.

the sclera is an exceptionally high reflector acoustically, trailing echoes produced by this high-amplitude complex may mask the initial pattern of the tumor (Fig. 22-19, *C*). Small lesions of the iris can be demonstrated acoustically. However, because of the minimal size of these lesions, exact acoustic differentiation can rarely be obtained (Fig. 22-20).

Tumors, in other than the four major types mentioned in the classification above, may also be well demonstrated with ultrasound, and variations in ultrasonic techniques may aid in their recognition and diagnosis. Most notably, the calcium particles contained in retinoblastoma can be studied with ultrasonic techniques by reduction of the sensitivity of the instrument to the point that these are the sole reflectors within the tumor mass (Fig. 22-21). In a similar manner, the density of choroidal osteoma can be well appreciated by reduction of the attenuation (Fig. 22-22).

COMPUTERIZED ACOUSTIC TUMOR ANALYSIS

Visual recognition of acoustic patterns can be greatly augmented by the use of sophisticated mathematical evaluation of the power spectrum of ocular tumors. The main strength of this analytic method lies in the use of computerized evaluation of range-gated "sections" of tissue that can be analyzed independently to create such reproducible tissue features as thickness, spectral slope (Fig. 22-23), and attenuation (Figs. 22-24 and 22-25) constants.

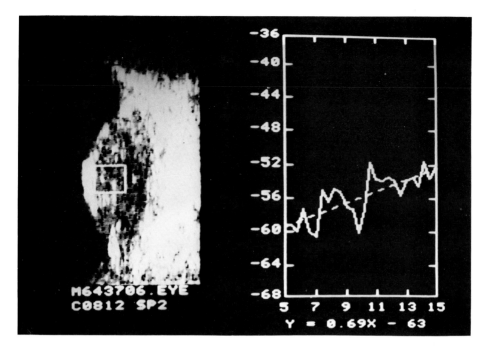

Fig. 22-23. Computerized analysis technique for intraocular tumors. The display on left is a 7.5 mm section including the posterior pole and a malignant melanoma. Boxes 2 mm in width may be placed in any section of the tumor to produce the power spectrum shown on the right. The amplitude levels are depicted on the ordinate in decibels and frequency range on the abscissa over a range of 5 to 15 MHz. The equation shown at the bottom of the screen is the straight-line slope and amplitude intercept at 0.00 MHz scale base.

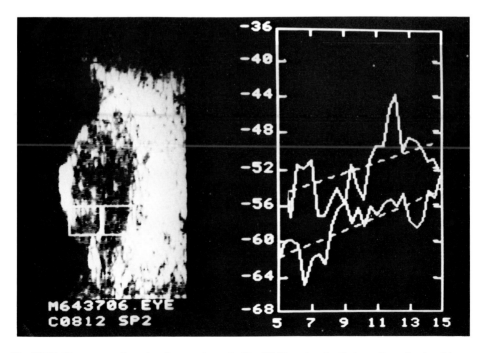

Fig. 22-24. The same malignant melanoma shown in Fig. 22-23 analyzed with two adjacently placed boxes. The difference in the resulting spectra on the right is caused by the attenuation of sound by the tumor tissue.

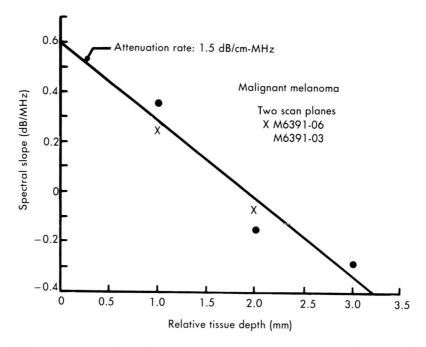

Fig. 22-25. Attenuation curve derived from different planes of a malignant melanoma. This attenuation coefficient is a reliable and reproducible range of values that helps to distinguish between different types and subtypes of tumor tissue.

Our program, along with Dr. Frederic Lizzi and the Riverside Research Institute, has analyzed well over 200 tumors with this technique. We are compiling, through an iterative program, statistics on reliability and weighting of functions that can lead to an even more defined tissue diagnosis with ultrasound.

REFERENCES

1. Bronson, N.R., II, Fisher, Y.L., Pickering, N.C., and Trayner, E.M.: Ophthalmic contact B-scan ultrasonography for the clinician, Westport, Conn., 1976, Intercontinental Publications, Inc.
2. Coleman, D.J., Konig, W.F., and Katz, L.: A hand-operated ultrasound scan system for ophthalmic evaluation, Am. J. Ophthalmol. **68**(2):256-263, 1969.
3. Coleman, D.J., Lizzi, F.L., and Jack, R.L.: Ultrasonography of the eye and orbit, Philadelphia, 1977, Lea & Febiger.
4. Ossoinig, K.C.: Standardized echography: basic principles, clinical applications and results. In Dallow, R.L., editor: Ophthalmic ultrasonography: comparative techniques, Int. Ophthalmol. Clin. **19**(4):127-210, Winter 1979.
5. Purnell, E.W.: Intensity modulated (B-scan) ultrasonography. In Goldberg, R.E., and Sarin, L.K., editors: Ultrasonics in ophthalmology: diagnostic and therapeutic applications, Philadelphia, 1967, W.B. Saunders Co.

23

Subretinal neovascularization in senile macular degeneration

J. Wallace McMeel
Marcos P. Avila*
Alexandre E. Jalkh‡

Among the types of deterioration associated with senile macular degeneration, the occurrence of subretinal neovascularization produces the most profound loss of vision. However, it is the one aspect of senile macular degeneration that lends itself most readily to a specific therapy, laser photocoagulation. Except for treatment of subretinal neovascular lesions away from the fovea, there has been an inordinate hesitation in treating this disease entity. This has been related to a combination of factors, which include a photocoagulation system that in most instances has been less than optimal, an underutilization of available diagnostic techniques, and unduly high expectations with regard to the objectives of the photocoagulation treatment.

A recognition of these factors and a synthesis of a new mode of treatment has been the prime contribution of Dr. Clement Trempe.[14] For several years he has used central visual fields to detect the nonseeing areas. By evaluating the scotoma size before and after treatment, he was able to detect further enlargement or shrinkage of the scotoma and to correlate it thereafter with the best visual acuity.

In 1940, the association of drusen and disciform macular detachment was recognized.[5] Recent studies demonstrate the histopathologic changes at levels of Bruch's membrane, retinal pigment epithelium, and drusen.[3,5,8,12,13] High-risk factors regarding the development of senile disciform macular degeneration are well known. These factors include greater numbers of drusen, their rapidly increasing number, extensive retinal pigment epithelium changes, and senile disciform macular degeneration in one eye.[2,4] The incidence of development of second-eye involvement in patients with senile disciform macular degeneration in one eye was found to be 12% to 15% per year[6] or 35% in 3½ years.[4]

Since the first fluorescein description by Gass[3] the features of this disease entity have been well recognized. Other degenerative changes that may ultimately be associated with subretinal neovascularization are central serous retinopathy, retinal pigment epithelial

*M.D., Vitreo-Retina Fellow, Retina Associates and Retina Foundation, Boston, Massachusetts.
‡M.D., Assistant Clinical Scientist, Eye Research Institute of Retina Foundation, Harvard Medical School, Boston, Massachusetts.

decompensation, and retinal pigment epithelial detachment. Among these the differential diagnosis may be difficult because in some instances fine networks of new vessels may actually be present at these sites of fluorescence.[13]

NATURAL COURSE OF SENILE MACULAR DEGENERATION

It is frequently stated that the natural course of senile macular degeneration may give patients an aggravating loss of central vision but they should not worry about

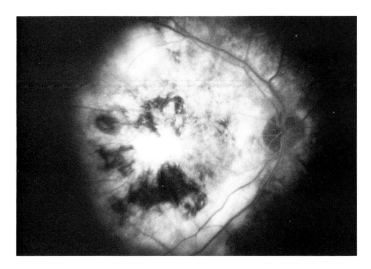

Fig. 23-1. From 77-year-old woman monochromatic photograph of right eye with green light showing senile disciform macular scar with hemorrhage, exudate, and elevation of retinal pigment epithelium and retina.

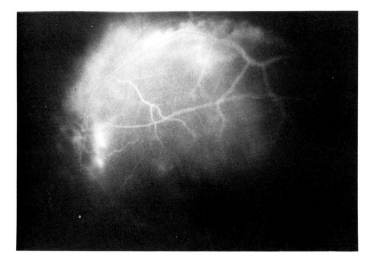

Fig. 23-2. Fluorescein angiogram of left eye showing serous detachment of sensory retina secondary to large area of new vessels involving the posterior pole.

profound loss of vision. Our experience indicates that the visual prognosis may be more ominous than this statement would imply. Although infrequent, the consequences can be disastrous, including massive vitreous hemorrhage after choroidal hemorrhage (Figs. 23-1 and 23-3). We reviewed cases of submacular neovascularization treated with photocoagulation that already has submacular neovascularization and its sequelae in the other eye. A high percentage of the untreated eyes had a profound degree of visual loss. Not only was the visual acuity at a count-fingers or hand-motions level in many of them, but also the central scotoma was 20 degrees or greater. In most of these instances, in addition to the subretinal fibrovascular scar, there was an extensive collection of subretinal fluid, producing a large detachment of the neurosensory retina.

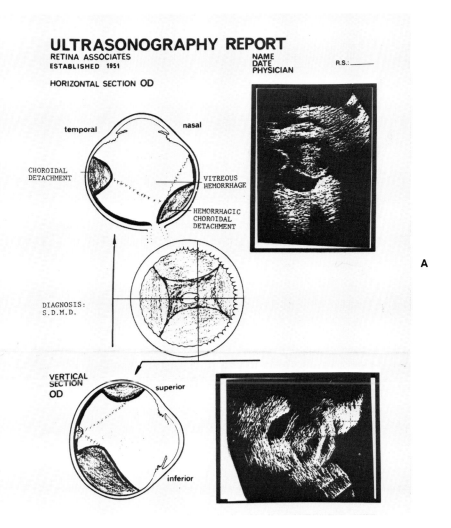

Fig. 23-3. Ultrasonography of each eye of this patient 15 months after the fluorescein in Fig. 23-1. **A,** Right eye demonstrates massive vitreous hemorrhage and hemorrhagic choroidal detachment secondary to the senile disciform macular degeneration. *Continued.*

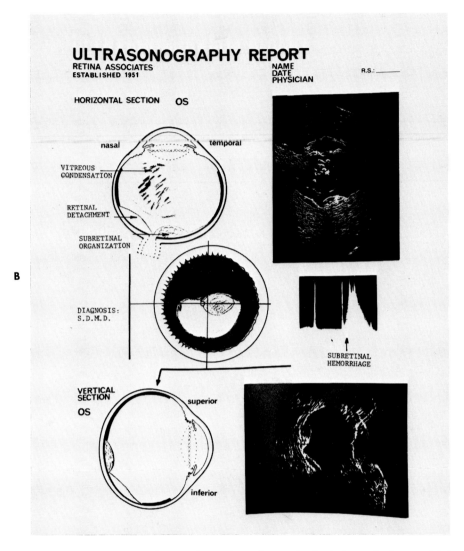

Fig. 23-3, cont'd. B, Left eye shows a vitreous hemorrhage and subretinal organization associated with detachment of sensory retina. Ultimately both eyes became phthisic and had no light perception.

PHOTOCOAGULATION TREATMENT

The earlier results of photocoagulation attribute a failure rate of 25% to 50% to the therapy.[1,4,9] Better results were achieved by Hirose and McMeel in 1976.[7] Recent reports give a rate of 93% of subretinal neovascularization closure by use of argon green (514.5 nm) and krypton yellow lasers.[14]

The purpose of the photocoagulation treatment is to destroy the subretinal neovascularization that has entered the inner sanctum of the eye by growing through breaks in Bruch's membrane. Once these vessels are destroyed, serous and hemorrhagic outflow from these vessels should cease, and the potential impetus for further fibrotic tissue development is also minimized. Also it is possible that the scar produced by the photocoagulation may plug up the defect in Bruch's membrane and cauterize the small vessels of the choriocapillaris. This may further deter repeat ingrowth.

BASICS OF MACULAR PHOTOCOAGULATION

Knowledge of the biophysical characterists of the various wavelengths and the relationship to the role of absorbing pigments is important in understanding the interaction of these two major factors in laser-burn production. Five wavelengths are available in the two types of lasers now in clinical usage by ophthalmologists. The argon laser has 70% of its energy in the band at the 488 nm wavelength. This is blue light and, as such, is particularly absorbed by the xanthophyll (yellow) pigments in the lens and macula. The green wavelength of the argon laser is 514.5 nm. This wavelength is absorbed only about 20% as much by the xanthophyll pigments as the blue wavelength of argon is. Good absorption by both hemoglobin and oxyhemoglobin occurs at this wavelength. The krypton green (530 nm) has a maximum of absorption by hemoglobin, as the yellow wavelength does at 568.1 nm. Green and yellow wavelengths each contain only about 10% of the total energy output of the krypton. Therefore, a laser of over 10 watts is necessary to obtain sufficient power to create retinal burns when each wavelength is used alone. The red wavelength of the krypton laser (647 nm) accounts for 70% of the energy production. The minimal degree of scattering because of its longer wavelength permits it to reach the absorbing pigment, melanin, with a minimum of prior scattering or absorption by xanthophyll or hemoglobin pigments. The red light of the krypton can penetrate through flat hemorrhage on the surface of the retina without secondarily burning the neurofiber layer. The only pigment within the eye to absorb red to any significant degree is melanin, which lies at the level of the retinal pigment epithelium and the choroid. This permits an optimal relative absorption of energy at this level.

The other facets of creating optimal laser burns is an understanding of the location of the intraocular pigments that absorb the particular laser. Macular xanthophyll, with its predilection for absorption of blue light, lies mainly in the superficial layers of the retina in the fovea.[10,11,14] Therefore this is the portion of foveal retina tissue that first becomes edematous and then opaque when treated with blue-containing laser light. Once it does this, it significantly decreases the energy to pass on to the pigment epithelium, where the melanin of the retina pigment epithelium and hemoglobin of the subretinal new vessels lie. Not only does this superficial opacification over the fovea prevent subsequent energy delivery to the structures needing it the most, but persistence of this opacification for 2 to 3 weeks after photocoagulation with the blue light prevents visualization of the neovascular network by fluorescein angiography.

Hemoglobin is not a significant factor as regards absorption of green or yellow laser energy until the laser light penetrates to the level of the new vessels in the subretinal neovascular membrane. An important consideration is the direct absorption of heat in the vessels themselves. The green wavelength of argon and krypton and the yellow wavelength of krypton are both highly absorbed by hemoglobin in these vessels.

Melanin is the only one of the three pigments that absorb red light. Thus photocoagulation with the krypton red creates a burn well localized to the pigment epithelium and choroidal melanosomes. The heat absorbed by melanin secondarily affects the adjacent subretinal neovascularization. An unevenness of melanin pigmentation can be seen in several situations. Patients with a generally light complexion may be more likely to have a mottling of melanin, particularly those in the older age groups, than those with a dark complexion. It is precisely these age groups that one deals with, however, in treating senile macular degeneration with subretinal neovascularization. This creates an uneven pattern of energy absorption, increasing the risk of hemorrhage. Highly myopic patients also are more likely to have relative depigmentation, in which instance there is a dearth of energy absorption at the desired level. These considerations put red light in a middle position between the undesirable blue wavelength and the highly desirable green and yellow wavelengths.

INDICATIONS FOR PHOTOCOAGULATION

The purpose of photocoagulation of subretinal new vessels at the macula is to destroy the network of subretinal new vessels with a minimum involvement of overlying neurosensory retina and an optimal capability for early follow-up examination. The indications for photocoagulation include a history of demonstrable visual loss, a demonstrable network of subretinal new vessels on fluorescein angiography, and visible borders to this network, particularly in the region of the fovea itself. If an undue portion is obscured by subretinal hemorrhage, photocoagulation may have to be postponed until it clears. These characteristics of the lesion should indicate a relatively recent onset rather than one of long standing. Characteristics that suggest a relatively recent onset are edema and recent hemorrhage and exudates along the junction of slightly elevated or edematous retina and the adjacent normal retina. Highly elevated thinned neurosensory retina with subretinal fibrovascular scars represent long-standing lesions that are poor candidates for treatment. There should also be an absence of hazy media, from either lens opacities or vitreous hemorrhage, an anticoagulated state, or a nonacceptance of either the proposed risks or limited visual prognosis.

PREOPERATIVE WORK-UP

The work-up includes a pertinent family history with regard to progenitors that may have had loss of central vision and query into a history of visual loss in the other eye. In addition to optimal visual acuities, a central visual field is obtained on each eye. An autoplot is used, with 1:1000 and 6:1000 white isopters being measured. Fundus photographs and fluorescein angiograms are obtained. A composite is then made with a posterior pole drawing that is composed of the information in the color photograph, the fluorescein angiogram, and the scotoma revealed by the central visual field.

Before photocoagulation, certain checks, safeguards, and referral to documentation should be reviewed. A vision taken the day of treatment should be recorded. A central field and fluorescein angiograms recently obtained should supply the information for the composite referral diagram. The composite is adjacent to the ophthalmologist as he treats for immediate reference. A treatment plan should be made before the photocoagulation is begun. A good, sharp fluorescein angiogram in the arterial venous stage with clear filling of the abnormal vessels may serve as a reference device in lieu of the composite drawing. This angiogram can be projected onto a screen behind the patient or be in a viewer handy to the photocoagulator. Checking the fundus with indirect ophthalmoscopy just before the treatment reassures the ophthalmologist in regard to the clarity of the media and the capability of delivering his laser treatment.

INSTRUMENT PREPARATION

A check of the instrumentation may save subsequent embarrassment. The focus of the oculars should be checked when a sharp image of the reticle is obtained. Younger ophthalmologists will need to use the fogging technique. The pedal mechanism should be tested and the image of the laser beam on the wall should be inspected. An eccentric crescentic beam might not deliver sufficient or predictable enough energy levels to safely treat in the macula. If a laser using multicolors is used, this check also determines the wavelength of laser light being used.

TECHNIQUE OF PHOTOCOAGULATION

The patient is prepared by dilatation of the pupil with a standard short-acting mydriatic solution. This is usually given in two or three doses approximately 1 hour before treatment. Topical anesthesia, Proparacaine, is instilled into the eye just before insertion of the contact lens. Retrobulbar anesthesia has been used only twice in our personal experience of over 5000 treatments. A Goldmann three-mirror contact lens is then placed on the eye. Its bulk and slight pressure exerted by the ophthalmologist as he holds the lens tends to splint any ocular movement. A test spot may be made outside the macular area. If a 50 μm spot is to be used, a power setting of 50 milliwatts (mW) is used. For spot sizes of 100 to 250 μm an initial power setting of 100 mW is used. If there is no reaction to this amount, the burns are made in increments of 30 to 50 mW, depending on the degree of haziness of the media. Once one produces a grayish burn that develops almost immediately, that is the power setting desired.

The physical parameters of the photocoagulation may vary because of the size, placement, or characteristics of the neovascularization lesion or of the degree of haziness of the ocular media. The spot size required varies from 50 to 250 μm. When larger vessels are noted in the network, larger spot sizes are used. The power settings have varied from 50 to 300 mW. Higher power settings are needed if there is haziness of the ocular media or if there is slight elevation of the retina overlying the lesion. The duration of the burn is usually between 0.2 and 0.5 second to avoid hemorrhage, and the longer burns are placed if the patient's eye stays immobile. Burns are placed in a contiguous manner. In some instances, each area is covered three or four times. The routine on termination is to obtain photographs of the area treated, put on an eye pad for 3 to 4 hours, and have the patient take a mydriatic (cyclopentolate 1%) twice a day for 5 days.

FOLLOW-UP STUDY

Before embarking on a course of treatment, one should tell the patient that optimal results can be obtained only if a total committment to frequent follow-up visits and possibly repetitive treatment that may require four or five treatments over a 4 to 6-week period. They are told that the vision for the rest of their lives in that particular eye depends on their degree of commitment. The patients are seen at intervals of 3 to 14 days after the treatment. On the repeat visit, visual acuity, a central field, a color photograph, and a fluorescein angiogram are obtained. With green, yellow, and red light, a fluorescein angiogram is readable within 2 days after photocoagulation because the inner layer of the fovea, which contains the foveal xanthophyll, has not been coagulated and remains transparent. Many cases require four or five episodes of treatment before two consecutive examinations show absence of abnormal subretinal vessels.

For a long-term follow-up study a reexamination of the three basic parameters of visual acuity, central field, and fluorescein angiogram are performed at 6 to 12-month intervals. In the 52 treated cases (follow-up study at 16 months) 42% of treatments were in the first 2 months and 20% in the period between 8 to 12 months. In addition, patients are given a special grid with which they test themselves on a periodic basis. The parallel lines go in the horizontal direction on one side and vertically on the other. With these it is easier to determine if scotomas are enlarging.

In these patients with loss of central vision, the function outside the area of treatment is important. In some instances, there is an abrupt change and the areas immediately outside are functioning quite well. In other instances, there is some deterioration of function in this area immediately about the photocoagulation. This can be determined by the slope of the isopters in the central field. Low vision aids can be very helpful, depending on the size and depth of the central scotoma.[14]

REFERENCES

1. Bird, A.C.: Recent advances in the treatment of senile disciform macular degeneration, Br. J. Ophthalmol. **58**:367-376, 1974.
2. Chandra, S.R., Gragoudas, E.S., Friedman, E., Van Buskirk, E.M., and Klein, M.L.: Natural history of disciform degeneration of the macula, Am. J. Ophthalmol. **78**:579-582, 1974.
3. Gass, J.D.M.: Pathogenesis of disciform detachment of the neuroepithelium, I to V, Am. J. Ophthalmol. **63**:573-688, 1967.
4. Gass, J.D.M.: Drusen and disciform macular detachment and degeneration, Arch. Ophthalmol. **90**:206-217, 1973.
5. Gifford, S.R., and Cushman, B.: Certain retinopathies due to changes in the lamina vitrea, Arch. Ophthalmol. **23**:60-75, 1940.
6. Gregor, Z., Bird, A.C., and Chisholm, I.H.: Senile disciform macular degeneration in the second eye, Br. J. Ophthalmol. **61**:141-147, 1977.
7. Hirose, T., and McMeel, J.W.: Argon laser coagulation in subretinal neovascular membranes in the posterior pole, Jpn. J. Ophthalmol. **30**:65-72, 1976.
8. Hogan, M.J.: Bruch's membrane and disease of macula, Trans. Ophthalmol. Soc. U.K. **87**:113-161, 1967.
9. L'Esperance, F.A.: Argon and ruby laser photocoagulation of disciform macular disease, Trans. Am. Acad. Ophthalmol. Otolaryngol. **75**:609-625, 1971.
10. Nussbaum, J.J., Pruett, R.C., and Delori, F.C.: Macular yellow pigment: the first 200 years, Retina **1**:296-310, Feb. 1982.
11. Pomerantzeff, O., Lee, P.-F., Hamada, S., Donovan, R.H., Mukai, N., and Schepens, C.L.: Clinical importance of wavelengths in photocoagulation, Trans. Am. Acad. Ophthalmol. Otolaryngol. **75**:557-568, 1971.
12. Sarks, S.H.: New vessels formation beneath the retinal pigment epithelium in senile eyes, Br. J. Ophthalmol. **57**:951-965, 1973.
13. Sarks, S.H.: Ageing and degeneration in the macular region: a clinico-pathological study, Br. J. Ophthalmol. **60**:324-341, 1976.
14. Trempe, C.L., Mainster, M.A., Pomerantzeff, O., Avila, M.P., Jalkh, A.E., Weiter, J.J., McMeel, J.W., and Schepens, C.L.: Macular photocoagulation optimal wavelength selection, Ophthalmology **89**:721-728, 1982.

24

Choroidal ischemia

Alan C. Bird

When compared with retinal vascular disease, choroidal ischemia has received little attention in the ophthalmic literature. The records that exist describe two well-defined and distinct manifestations of reduced choroidal blood flow in patients with generalized vascular disease. Large triangular infarcts may be seen in the acute phase as areas of opacification of the retinal pigment epithelium and outer neuroretina[11,16] or later as well-defined regions of scarring.[1,2] These lesions have been ascribed to obstruction of short posterior ciliary arteries and have their counterpart in experimental arterial obstruction in animals.[19] The second form of disease occurs typically in accelerated hypertension in which there is multifocal opacification of the outer retina and serous detachment of the neuroretina. Doubt has been expressed concerning the source of subretinal fluid in such circumstances. Clapp[5] proposed that it was an extension of cerebral edema, Lapco[23] suggested that it was related to generalized edema, whereas Moore[25] and Friedenwald[12] believed that detachment was secondary to retinal vascular disease. However choroidal vascular damage has been shown histopathologically in accelerated hypertension,[22,33] and recent clinical reports of eclampsia imply a choroidal source of the subretinal fluid.[15,24]

During the last decade there has been progressively more support for the concept that choroidal vascular disease may be responsible for retinal pigment epithelial ischemia in the young in the absence of vascular disease elsewhere. Gass[13] described a disease in which there was multifocal opacification of the subretinal structures causing rapid visual loss followed by recovery that was often incomplete and left well-defined scars; he called this condition "acute posterior multifocal placoid pigment epitheliopathy." During fluorescein angiography the pigment epithelial lesions appeared dark during dye transit and later became hyperfluorescent (Fig. 24-1). He considered two possible explanations for this phenomenon: either the choroid did not fill in the areas of swelling or the lesions obscured the background choroidal fluorescence. Soon after the original description of the disease some support was reported for ischemia as the primary pathogenetic mechanism. Van Buskirk et al.[32] illustrated that at some stage during the recovery period the pattern of choroidal filling was abnormally slow (Fig. 24-2 and 24-3); their patient also had erythema nodosum caused by vasculitis. This angiographic sign was illustrated by many authors soon afterwards.[3,4,6,9,18,21] Further evidence of ischemia was recorded when it was shown that major choroidal blood vessels could be identified within the dark lesions showing that obscuration of the choroid could not totally explain the dark appearance

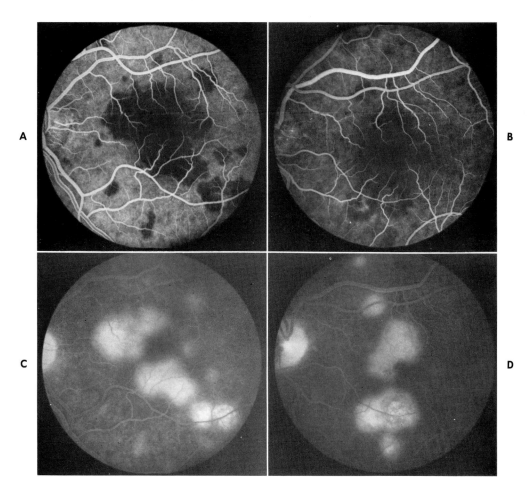

Fig. 24-1. Fluorescein angiography showing dark areas of choroid, **A,** which gradually fade as the study progresses, **B,** and finally by 5 minutes become hyperfluorescent, **C** and **D.**

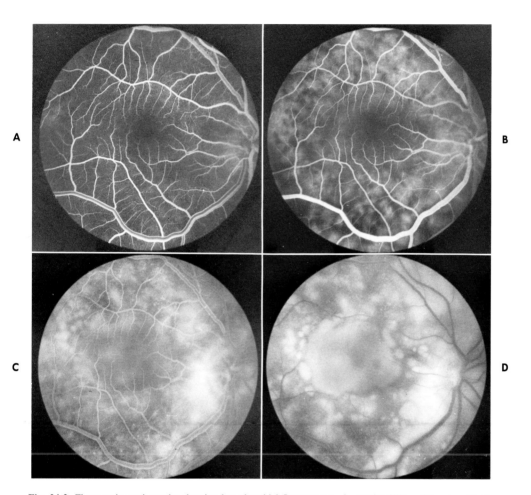

Fig. 24-2. Fluorescein angiography showing late choroidal fluorescence, **A,** patchy filling of the choroid, **B,** and subsequent progressive dye leakage into the subretinal space, **C** and **D.**

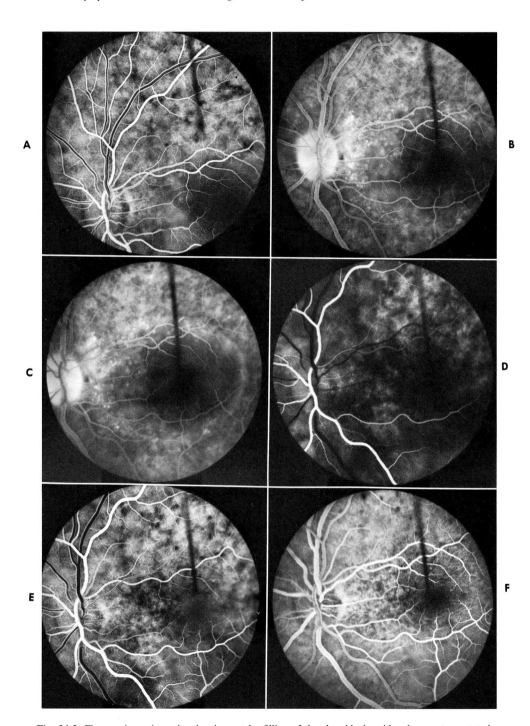

Fig. 24-3. Fluorescein angiography showing patchy filling of the choroid, **A,** with subsequent punctate hyperfluorescence and filling of the subretinal space, **B** and **C.** Within 1 week the retinal detachment subsided, but the fluorescein angiographs still show slow choroidal filling, **D** and **E,** and some irregularity of retinal pigment epithelial pigmentation, **F.**

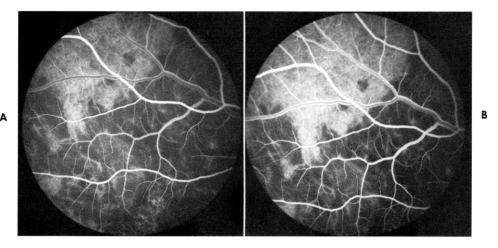

A B

Fig. 24-4. Angiographs during the early stage of acute pigment epithelial swelling show lack of choroidal fluorescence, but large choroidal vessels are seen within the lesion.

of the lesions[6,9,26] (Fig. 24-4). Finally there has been evidence of neurologic functional loss[29,32] and in one case occlusion of cerebral blood vessels was demonstrated.[29]

A few reports have demonstrated that the condition is not as well defined as it originally appeared. Changes similar to those described originally in acute posterior multifocal placoid pigment epitheliopathy[13] have been observed in eyes with limited serous retinal detachment[4] (Fig. 24-2) and in eyes with optic disc swelling.[21] Wright, Bird, and Hamilton[34] described an apparently continuous spectrum of disease from acute posterior multifocal placoid pigment epitheliopathy to Harada's disease and illustrated the difficulties in identifying specific clinical entities within their group of patients on the basis of fundus appearances and the clinical course of the disease. These patients had multifocal retinal pigment epithelial swelling in common and many showed choroidal filling patterns that those authors believed indicated abnormal choroidal perfusion.

Young et al.[36] studied patients with acute pigment epithelial disease in which there was evidence of choroidal ischemia without systemic or retinal vascular disease. From their observations it is possible to define three stages of disease caused by choroidal ischemia. It was identified that significant choroidal perfusion deficit was compatible with a normal fundus appearance and may not give rise to functional deficit. Furthermore abnormal perfusion was demonstrated during the recovery period. More severe ischemia produced two patterns of disease. Some patients had serous detachment accompanying the retinal pigment epithelial disease, which resolved rapidly, and there was rarely scarring or residual deficit (Fig. 24-3). Others had multifocal or single confluent lesions without serous detachment and after resolution of the attack there was well-defined scarring of the pigment epithelium. It is tempting to conclude from this experience that serous detachment without scarring represented the result of less severe circulatory disturbance than in placoid pigment epitheliopathy as described by Gass.[13]

The validity of this interpretation can be tested when one seeks evidence derived from experimental choroidal ischemia and from observations in patients with well-documented systemic vascular disease.

EXPERIMENTAL EVIDENCE

The concept of focal choroidal infarction would have been difficult to defend at a time when anatomic studies implied that the choriocapillaris was a continuous network of capillaries supplied by many arterioles.[27,35] However, Dollery et al.[7] showed that the choriocapillaris in pigs with increased intraocular pressure filled not as a continuous layer, but as a series of dots that later enlarged to become uniform. They concluded that this filling pattern indicated the presence of individual choriocapillaris units. Hayreh[17] demonstrated the lobular pattern of choriocapillaris filling in the posterior pole of normal animals, and other injection studies[8,10,28] have supported the conclusion that lobules of choriocapillaris in the submacular choroid are supplied by short, nonanastomosing precapillary arterioles without functional anastomoses between adjacent capillary units in the normal eye. This lobular arrangement is less well defined in the anterior choroid.

Further information about the choroidal circulation has been derived from experimental occlusion of vessels at different levels.[8,20,30] Hayreh and Baines[20] found that occlusion of the lateral short posterior ciliary arteries in the orbit resulted in nonperfusion of the temporal half of the choroid with a watershed at the optic disc. The disturbance of blood supply was sufficient to produce infarcts of the pigment epithelium and outer retina, which appeared as large oval patches in the posterior fundus or as triangular areas more peripherally; these areas stained with fluorescein late in the study and became atrophic during a period of 2 to 3 weeks.[3] Within 2 weeks of the occlusion, the temporal choroid filled but the filling was delayed; there was still some delay after 3 months. Their work demonstrated the presence of potential anastomotic channels that rapidly became functional after an acute arterial occlusion. Ernest, Stern, and Archer[8] have shown that this may occur more rapidly if the venous drainage of the choroid is also compromised.

Stern and Ernest[30] also identified changes in the retinal pigment epithelium and overlying retina after embolic occlusion of vessels within the choroid. Injection of embolic microspheres into the lateral short posterior ciliary arteries resulted in delayed choroidal filling with spotty leakage through the retinal pigment epithelium. Histologic studies showed focal necrosis of the pigment epithelium and a concentration of microspheres at the posterior pole. Within 4 days, the whole choroid filled rapidly and simultaneously, and by 2 months the only detectable angiographic abnormality was hyperfluorescence through the small atrophic pigment epithelial defects. Retinal detachment accompanied these changes in the acute phase in animals with experimentally induced hypertension. The pattern of pigment epithelial infarction contrasted with that seen after occlusion of the short posterior ciliary arteries in that it was multifocal and was seen only at the macula despite the widespread distribution of microspheres.

Thus experimental evidence demonstrates the polymorphism of lesions induced by choroidal ischemia and that retinal detachment occurred in the mildest experimental model of choroidal vascular compromise.

CLINICAL EVIDENCE

Evidence of choroidal perfusion abnormalities was sought by Gaudric[14] in patients with well-defined generalized vascular disease. It was shown that apparently severe and prolonged choroidal perfusion deficit may not cause funduscopic changes. Choroidal ischemia associated with serous detachment resulted in little permanent functional deficit and little scarring of the pigment epithelium. Infarction of the choroid is often not associated with detachment, and when there is subretinal fluid, the fluid is derived from the edge of the lesion. It was concluded that pronounced perfusion deficits of the choroid need not produce ophthalmoscopic or functional change. The ability of the retina to withstand the effect of choroidal nonperfusion, although of gradual onset, is illustrated by a case of total choroidal replacement by amyloid without causing receptor atrophy.[31] More severe perfusion deficit caused serous detachment of the retina but without permanent scarring. It is possible that ischemia of this degree resulted in ''pump failure'' as a manifestation of ischemic dysfunction of the pigment epithelium without causing cell death. The most severe ischemia caused cell death and consequent scarring but did not result in abnormal fluid movement across the pigment epithelium. These conclusions support concepts derived from observations on young patients with presumed acute choroidal ischemia as described by Young.[36]

These observations imply that choroidal ischemia is much more common than has been appreciated in the past. In some instances the deficit can be detected by fluorescein angiography alone, and in many instances minor pigmentary disturbances are the only long-term consequence of the ischemia. It is clear that if sectorial atrophy alone is used as the index of previous choroidal hypoperfusion many cases will not be detected.

REFERENCES

1. Amalric, P.: Le territoire choriorétinien de l'artère ciliaire longue postérieure: étude clinique, Bull. Soc. Ophtalmol. Fr. **63**:342-351, 1963.
2. Amalric, P.: Acute choroidal ischaemia, Trans. Ophthalmol. Soc. U.K. **91**:306-322, 1971.
3. Annesley, W.H., Tomer, H.L., and Shields, J.A.: Multifocal placoid pigment epitheliopathy, Am. J. Ophthalmol. **76**:511-518, 1973.
4. Bird, A.C., and Hamilton, A.M.: Placoid pigment epitheliopathy: presenting with bilateral serous retinal detachment, Br. J. Ophthalmol. **56**:881-886, 1972.
5. Clapp, C.A.: Detachment of the retina in eclampsia and toxemia of pregnancy, Am. J. Ophthalmol. **2**:743-785, 1919.
6. Deutman, A.F., and Lion, F.: Choriocapillaris nonperfusion in acute multifocal placoid pigment epitheliopathy, Am. J. Ophthalmol. **84**:652-657, 1977.
7. Dollery, C.T., Henkind, P., Kohner, E.M., and Paterson, J.W.: Effect of raised intraocular pressure on the retinal and choroidal circulation, Invest. Ophthalmol. **7**:191-198, 1968.
8. Ernest, J.T., Stern, W.H., and Archer, D.B.: Submacular choroidal circulation, Am. J. Ophthalmol. **81**:574-582, 1976.
9. Fishman, G.A., Rabb, M.F., and Kaplan, J.: Acute posterior placoid pigment epitheliopathy, Arch. Ophthalmol. **92**:173-177, 1974.
10. Forczynski, E., and Ts'o, M.O.M.: The architecture of the choriocapillaris of the posterior pole, Am. J. Ophthalmol. **81**:428-440, 1976.
11. Foulds, W.S., Lee, W.R., and Taylor, W.O.G.: Clinical and pathological aspects of choroidal ischaemia, Trans. Ophthalmol. Soc. U.K. **91**:323-341, 1971.
12. Friedenwald, J.S.: Pathogenesis of albinuric retinitis, Libman Anniv. Vols. **2**:453-458, 1982, International Press, New York.
13. Gass, J.D.M.: Acute posterior multifocal placoid pigment epitheliopathy, Arch. Ophthalmol. **80**:177-185, 1968.
14. Gaudric, A.: Les occlusions vasculaires choroïdiennes aigues: la vascularisation choroïdienne, Bull. Soc. Ophtalmol. Fr., pp. 67-133, Nov. 1981, annual report.
15. Gitter, K.A., Houser, B.P., Sarin, L.K., and Justice, J.: Toxemia of pregnancy: an angiographic interpretation of fundus changes, Arch. Ophthalmol. **80**:449-454, 1968.

16. Goldbaum, M.H., Galinos, S.O., Apple, D., Asdourian, G.K., Nagpal, K., Jampol, L., Woolf, M.B., and Busse, B.: Acute choroidal ischaemia as a complication of photocoagulation, Arch. Ophthalmol. **94:**1025, 1976.
17. Hayreh, S.S.: Recent advances in fluorescein fundus angiography, Br. J. Ophthalmol. **58:**391-412, 1974.
18. Hayreh, S.S., and Baines, J.A.B.: Occlusion of the posterior ciliary artery. II. Chorioretinal lesions, Br. J. Ophthalmol. **56:**736-753, 1972.
19. See reference 18.
20. Hayreh, S.S., and Baines, J.A.B.: Occlusion of the posterior ciliary artery. I. Effects on choroidal circulation, Br. J. Ophthalmol. **56:**719-735, 1972.
21. Kirkham, T.H., ffytche, T.J., and Sanders, M.D.: Placoid pigment epitheliopathy with retinal vasculitis and papillitis, Br. J. Ophthalmol. **56:**875-880, 1972.
22. Klein, B.A.: Ischemic infarcts of the choroid (Elschnig spots), Am. J. Ophthalmol. **66:**1069-1074, 1968.
23. Lapco, L., Weller, J.M., and Greene, J.A., Jr.: Spontaneously reversible retinal detachment occurring during renal insufficiency, Ann. Intern. Med. **63:**760-766, 1965.
24. Mabie, W.C., and Ober, R.R.: Fluorescein angiography in toxaemia of pregnancy, Br. J. Ophthalmol. **64:**666-671, 1980.
25. Moore, F.: Medical ophthalmology, ed. 2, London, 1925, Blakiston Co.
26. McGuiness, R., and Mitchell, P.: A case of acute posterior multi-focal placoid pigment epitheliopathy associated with erythema nodosum, Aust. J. Ophthalmol. **5:**48-51, 1977.
27. Ring, H.G., and Fujino, T.: Observations on the anatomy and pathology of the choroidal vasculature, Arch. Ophthalmol. **78:**431-444, 1967.
28. Shimizu, K.: Segmental nature of angioarchitecture of the choroid. In Shimizu, K., and Oosterhuis, J.A., editors: XXIII Concilium Ophthalmologicum, Kyoto, 1978, vol. 1., p. 251, Amsterdam, 1979, Excerpta Medica Foundation.
29. Sigelman, J., Behrens, M., and Hilal, S.: Acute posterior multifocal placoid pigment epitheliopathy associated with cerebral vasculitis and homonymous hemianopia, Am. J. Ophthalmol. **88:**919-924, 1979.
30. Stern, W.H., and Ernest, J.T.: Microsphere occlusion of the choriocapillaris in rhesus monkeys, Am. J. Ophthalmol. **78:**438-448, 1974.
31. Ts'o, M.O.M., and Bettman, J.W., Jr.: Occlusion of choriocapillaris in primary nonfamilial amyloidosis, Arch. Ophthalmol. **86:**281-286, 1971.
32. Van Buskirk, E.M., Lessell, S., and Friedman, E.: Pigmentary epitheliopathy and erythema nodosum, Arch. Ophthalmol. **85:**369-372, 1971.
33. Verderame, P.H.: Ueber nichtalbuminurische und albuminurische Netzhautablösung und ihre Wiederanlegung bei Schwangeren, Klin. Monatsbl. Augenheilkd. **49:**452-468, 1911.
34. Wright, B.E., Bird, A.C., and Hamilton, A.M.: Placoid pigment epitheliopathy and Harada's disease, Br. J. Ophthalmol. **62:**609-621, 1978.
35. Wybar, K.C.: Vascular anatomy of the choroid in relation to selective localization of ocular diseases, Br. J. Ophthalmol. **38:**513-534, 1954.
36. Young, N.J.A., Bird, A.C., and Sehmi, K.: Pigment epithelial diseases with abnormal choroidal perfusion, Am. J. Ophthalmol. **90:**607-618, 1980.

25

Macular edema: a major complication of diabetic retinopathy

Frederick L. Ferris III*
and Arnall Patz

Diabetic retinopathy is the leading cause of blindness in young adults in the United States.[20] Blindness results either from proliferative diabetic retinopathy and its sequelae or from diabetic macular edema. Severe visual loss, such as vision less than 5/200, is generally the result of proliferative diabetic retinopathy. Although diabetic macular edema rarely causes visual loss to this degree, it is a leading cause of legal blindness (visual acuity ≤ 20/200). Equally important are the very large number of diabetics who have lost some vision but are not legally blind. Thus our statistics that include the number of individuals who are legally blind only demonstrate the tip of the iceberg. We have no good way to estimate the number of individuals who lose their jobs because they can no longer drive an automobile or perform detailed work. With so many persons affected, the public health importance of finding methods of prevention or treatment of diabetic macular edema is obvious.

IDENTIFICATION OF MACULAR EDEMA

Diabetic macular edema is the accumulation of extracellular fluid within the retinal tissue in the macular area. This causes decreased visual acuity by distortion of the retinal anatomy and in the most severe cases actual tissue destruction. Macular edema can be identified by either careful ophthalmoscopic examination or fluorescein angiography. The stereoscopic view of the macula obtained during binocular slitlamp examination through a contact lens provides the best ophthalmoscopic means of identifying this thickened retina. In the most severe cases the noticeable retinal thickening can be appreciated stereoscopically at any magnification. One can best identify less severe cases by narrowing the slitlamp beam and shining it approximately 5 to 10 degrees off axis. Thickening of the retinal tissue produced by edema will be apparent in the cross section of the retina illuminated by the slitlamp beam.

The other major method for identifying macular edema is through the use of fluorescein angiography. Since both the retinal capillaries and the pigment epithelium are

*M.D., Medical Officer, Office of Biometry and Epidemiology, National Eye Institute, National Institutes of Health, Bethesda, Maryland.

normally impervious to fluorescein molecules, there is no fluorescence of normal retinal tissue during fluorescein angiography. However, in diabetics with macular edema, leakage of fluorescein into the retinal tissue is seen. During the angiogram the fluorescein dye can be seen to leak into the retina either from discrete leakage points (Fig. 25-1) or from diffuse sections of the retinal capillary bed (Figs. 25-2 and 25-3). In the later phases of the angiogram the retina will fluoresce in the areas of edema. This can be readily identified in the late stages of the fluorescein angiogram (Fig. 25-1, *D,* 25-2, *D,* and 25-3, *D).*

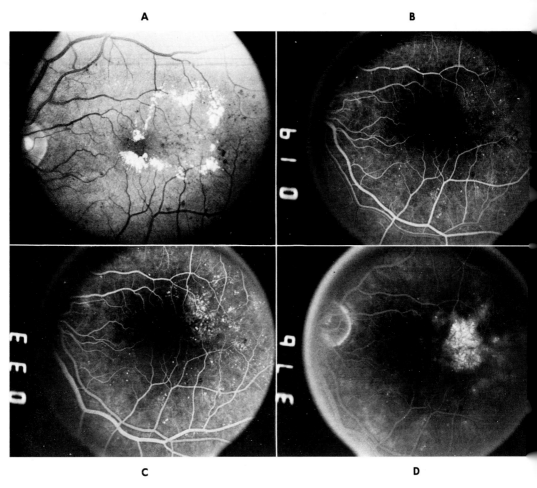

A   **B**

C   **D**

Fig. 25-1. A, Fundus photograph of an eye with focal leakage and a cercinate lipid ring that involves the perifoveal area. **B,** Early phase fluorescein angiogram showing individual microaneurysms. **C,** Capillary-phase angiogram showing fuzzy bordered aneurysms caused by leakage of fluorescein dye from the microaneurysm. **D,** Late-phase angiogram showing pronounced fluorescein accumulation in the area of edema within the cercinate ring. Some cystoid changes are visible.

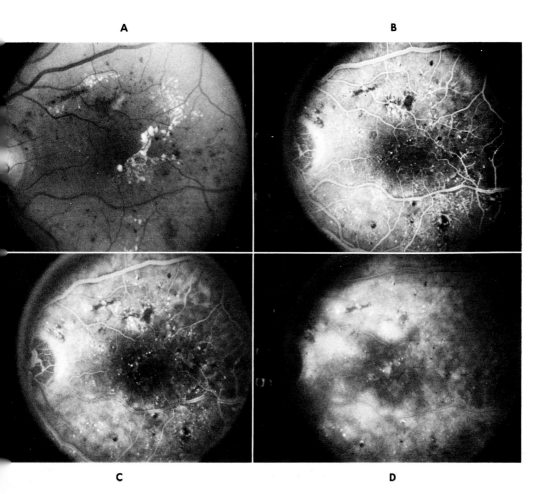

Fig. 25-2. A, Fundus photograph of an eye with multifocal macular edema and confluent rings of cercinate lipid. **B,** Early capillary phase angiogram showing abnormalities of the capillary bed with microaneurysms, areas of nonperfusion, and nipped-off arterial branches. **C,** Midphase angiogram revealing focal leakage from microaneurysms and some diffusely leaking capillaries. **D,** Late-phase angiogram showing diffuse macular edema with cystoid changes.

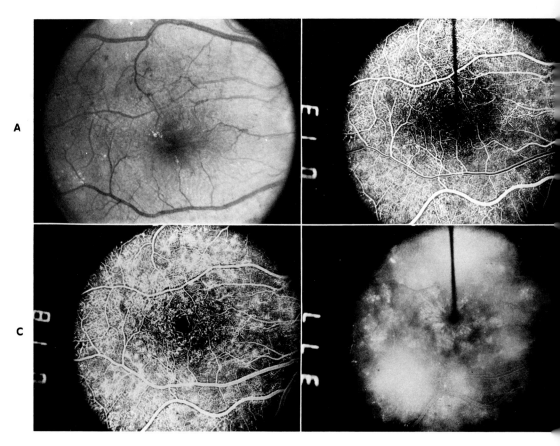

Fig. 25-3. A, Fundus photograph of an eye with macular edema and diffuse capillary abnormalities. **B,** Early capillary phase showing dilated capillary bed. **C,** Diffuse leakage from virtually all the dilated capillary vasculature. **D,** Late-phase angiogram revealing diffuse macular edema and cystoid changes.

PATHOGENESIS

We have discussed the fact that macular edema is associated with the abnormal leakage of fluorescein molecules into the retina. This provides an important clue toward understanding the cause of macular edema. The tight junctions of the endothelial cells of the retinal vasculature prevent macromolecules such as proteins and lipids from passing from the intravascular space into the extravascular retinal tissue. When a breakdown of this barrier occurs, these large molecules can pass from the intravascular to the extravascular space (Fig. 25-4). As large molecules such as lipoproteins gain access to the extravascular space, they cause an oncotic influx of water into the space resulting in retinal edema.

Although most intraretinal edema in diabetics may come from leakage of macromolecules from the vessels, an additional source of edema may result from a breakdown of the tight junctions between retinal pigment epithelial cells[19] (Fig. 25-5).

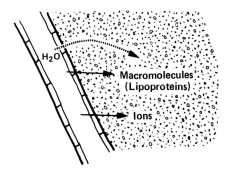

Fig. 25-4. Pathogenesis of macular edema. Defects in retinal capillary endothelium allow passage of substances across the blood-retinal barrier into the sensory retina.

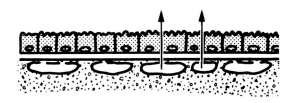

Fig. 25-5. Loss of competence of retinal pigment epithelial barrier between the choroidal circulation and retina allows diffusion of fluid from the choroidal circulation into the retina.

NATURAL HISTORY

Edema of the retina in the macular region caused by diabetic retinopathy can spontaneously resolve, but frequently it is a chronic process resulting from continued multifocal "leakage."[5,13] Classically, this is associated with edema in the immediate area of the "leakage" sites and the deposition of intraretinal lipid exudates peripheral to these sites. In these peripheral areas there is often relatively normal vasculature with an intact blood retinal barrier (Figs. 25-1 and 25-6). The fluid and small ion components of the blood can be reabsorbed in this area leaving behind the lipoproteins, which tend to aggregate as lipid deposits, particularly in the outer plexiform layer.[17] Fluid accumulation is particularly pronounced in the macula, probably because of the larger potential extravascular spaces created by the obliquely running nerve fibers in the Henley fiber layer.

When leakage is limited to a small area of the retina, this area will seem to be edematous, and there is often a circinate pattern of lipid deposition surrounding it (Fig. 25-1). The retina is thickened with accumulated fluid within this circinate ring. Beyond the ring the retina is often not identifiably edematous. In diabetic retinopathy the leakage sites are generally not localized to one area, and lipid deposition may be scattered in the posterior pole or take the form of multiple intersecting rings (Fig. 25-2). Individual leaking sites can spontaneously resolve, with the resultant resolution of edema and eventually the lipid. More frequently, the process is chronic, with new leakage sites replacing the resolved ones, and persistent edema results. This chronic process leads to continued visual loss. In groups of diabetics with macular edema who were untreated, approximately one half lost two or more additional lines of visual acuity in a 2-year period.[1,3,17,18] Perifoveal capillary dropout, which can be identified as loss of the normal retinal capillaries in the foveal area, is often associated with macular edema and has a particularly poor prognosis.[15] Finally, although chronic edema fluid itself may result in some disarray of the outer retinal segments, lipid deposits, though possibly transient, are more destructive. Large placoid lipid deposits generally indicate little hope of restoration of visual function.[10,16,18]

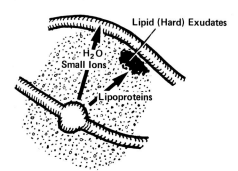

Fig. 25-6. Diffusion of fluid and lipoproteins from defective retinal capillary results in macular edema. The adjacent healthier capillary reabsorbs water and small molecules, but the larger lipoprotein complexes (hard exudates) accumulate about the border of the healthier capillaries.

MEDICAL TREATMENT

Medical treatments for diabetic macular edema can be divided into two different approaches. The first is an attempt to normalize the metabolic abnormalities associated with diabetes mellitus.[12] Although these approaches are theoretically appealing, they have never been carefully tested. This is at least in part because it has become routine to make all reasonable attempts to normalize elevated blood glucose, decrease elevated blood pressure, and improve the cardiac or renal status of any patient who is developing complications of diabetes. Preexisting macular edema does not consistently benefit from these attempts, and without a control group the effects of medical therapy are impossible to interpret. However, improvement of edema concurrent with the improvement in circulatory or renal function does occur, and since this is part of good medical management, it should be a consistent adjunct to any other treatment in the management of macular edema.

A question that remains to be tested is whether further measures aimed at tight control of blood glucose such as multiple daily insulin injections or the use of an insulin infusion pump can reduce the morbidity of diabetic maculopathy. Early results of such studies are promising,[9] and additional research is being planned at a number of centers.

The second major medical approach toward helping patients with macular edema has been the reduction of serum lipids. It was hoped that by reduction of the serum lipids a concomitant decrease in intraretinal lipid accumulation would occur with the eventual prevention of the destructive effects of this lipid. Direct attempts to lower fat intake and reduce circulating cholesterol by substitution of unsaturated for saturated fats in the diet have resulted in some reduction of the total serum lipids.[10] Pharmacologic methods such as the use of clofibrate have also been used to decrease the circulating lipids.[4,6,8,10] Only one published report indicates that lipid lowering may have a beneficial effect on vision[4] though in every study there did seem to be a reduction in the amount of lipid in the retina. Because the pharmacologic approach to lipid lowering has some potentially serious side effects and has not been definitely shown to improve the visual prognosis, it has been virtually abandoned as a specific treatment for diabetic maculopathy except in extreme circumstances.[2] However, attempts to reduce circulating lipid levels by dietary means have become widespread throughout our society. The effect of these dietary modifications on diabetic maculopathy remains unknown and is probably untestable at this point.

PHOTOCOAGULATION TREATMENT

Many investigators have reported a beneficial effect of photocoagulation on diabetic macular edema.[1,3,11,14,15,18] Three randomized clinical trials have been performed to evaluate the effect of photocoagulation on diabetic macular edema.[1,3,14] In each of these trials one of the patient's eyes was randomly assigned to the treatment group, whereas the opposite eye served as an untreated control. For the most part, patients in these studies had bilateral macular edema without proliferative diabetic retinopathy though in the British study some patients had proliferative retinopathy and the definition of maculopathy was not restricted to edema of the macula. Dr. Blankenship and the British collaborative study divided their patients into subgroups according to initial visual acuity and type of leakage. The follow-up period in the three studies is different, but a summary of 2-year follow-up data is possible and is presented in Table 25-1. Since the

Table 25-1. Pooled data from three randomized clinical trials of photocoagulation for diabetic vascular edema

Three randomized studies pooled*	Changes in visual acuity† 2 years after treatment			Total eyes
	Vision improved by 2 or more lines	Vision unchanged ± 1 line	Vision worse by 2 or more lines	
Treated eyes	30 (22%)	83 (61%)	23 (17%)	136
Control eyes	10 (7%)	54 (40%)	71 (53%)	135‡

*From Blankenship, G.W.: Ophthalmology **86**:69-75, 1979; Cheng, H., et al.: Lancet **2**:1110-1113, 1975; Patz, A., Schatz, H., Berkow, J.W., et al.: Trans. Am. Acad. Ophthalmol. Otolaryngol. **77**:34-42, 1973.
†The follow-up period in one study[14] averaged 26 months. Not all patients were seen at 2 years.
‡One initially untreated eye developed proliferative retinopathy and was photocoagulated; it is not included.

results in all three studies are quite similar, it seems appropriate to pool the data from the three studies. Each study demonstrated a statistically significant beneficial treatment effect, and of course the pooled data also demonstrate this. Although some eyes in each study had an improvement in visual acuity after treatment, the main difference between the treated and untreated eyes was the much larger number of untreated eyes that lost two or more lines of visual acuity over the 2-year follow-up period. Attempts to evaluate the subgroups of patients (with very small sample sizes) did suggest that initially poor visual acuity and relatively diffuse leakage as determined on the fluorescein angiogram were poor prognostic factors.[1,18] Other studies, though not randomized, have also emphasized this point. If such subgroups are important, one cannot conclude from the data presented that treatment should be applied in all eyes with macular edema. The beneficial treatment effect that is demonstrated may represent an effect only in certain subgroups of the patients with diabetic maculopathy. This beneficial effect on the subgroup could make it appear that treatment was useful on all diabetics with maculopathy. Many investigators believe that eyes with focal leakage and clearly identifiable circinate rings are the most amenable to treatment.

PHOTOCOAGULATION—CURRENT RESEARCH

The Early Treatment Diabetic Retinopathy Study is currently evaluating the effect of photocoagulation and aspirin therapy in approximately 2500 patients with diabetic macular edema, as well as in diabetics with early proliferative and preproliferative diabetic retinopathy. Specific photographic and clinical criteria are being used to define macular edema, and enough patients will be enrolled in the study to evaluate treatment effect in subgroups. One eye of each patient will be randomized to treatment by argon laser photocoagulation, whereas photocoagulation of the other eye will be deferred. Both panretinal photocoagulation and focal treatment of areas of fluorescein leakage in the posterior pole will be evaluated in eyes with macular edema in this study. Discrete leakage points demonstrated by fluorescein angiography will be photocoagulated directly. Areas of nonperfusion or diffuse leakage within two disc diameters of the fovea will have 200 µm burns scattered throughout the involved area, with a spacing of one burn width between burns. Fluorescein angiograms are repeated at regular intervals throughout this 5-year study, and if macular edema persists, any treatable lesions are photocoagulated.

The specific protocol is available[7] for use by ophthalmologists who are treating while we await the results of this study.

SUMMARY

Diabetic macular edema is a major cause of visual loss in diabetics. The edema occurs because of a breakdown in the endothelial cells of the retinal vasculature or retinal pigment epithelium allowing lipoproteins and fluid to accumulate within the retinal tissue. The natural history of the disease is one of gradual progression, with reduction of visual acuity to 20/200 being a common occurrence.

Medical treatments for macular edema have met with limited success. Attempts to decrease elevated blood pressure and improve cardiac or renal status of any patient who has diabetic macular edema is recommended. Although there is no definite evidence that tight blood glucose control will reduce macular edema, attempts at improving blood glucose control in a diabetic with macular edema are also recommended. Finally, it has been shown that reducing serum lipids in patients with exudative retinopathy does result in reduction of lipid accumulation in the retina. Certainly dietary attempts at lipid reduction should be attempted. Unfortunately, there is little strong evidence to suggest that pharmacologic reduction of serum lipids will result in stabilization or improvement of vision.

Photocoagulation is probably helpful in some patients with diabetic macular edema. Stabilization of visual acuity rather than improvement after it has decreased seems to be the major benefit. Eyes with localized sites of "leakage" seem to be the most amenable to treatment. Whether treatment in the long run will prevent these eyes from going blind and will be beneficial for eyes with more diffuse leakage is uncertain. Answers to these questions must wait until long-term follow-up results of the patients currently being enrolled in the Early Treatment Diabetic Retinopathy Study are available.

REFERENCES

1. Blankenship, G.W.: Diabetic macular edema and laser photocoagulation, Ophthalmology **86**:69-75, 1979.
2. Butera, R.T., and de Venecia, G.B.: Exudative diabetic retinopathy and elevated serum triglyceride levels, Invest. Ophthalmol. Vis. Sci. **16**(4; suppl.):37, 1977 (Abstract 1).
3. Cheng, H., Kohner, E., Keen, H., Blach, R.K., and Hill, D.W.: Photocoagulation in treatment of diabetic maculopathy, Lancet **2**:1110-1113, 1975.
4. Cullen, J.F., Ireland, J.T., and Oliver, M.F.: A controlled trial of Atromid wherapy in exudative diabetic retinopathy, Trans. Soc. Ophthalmol. U.K. **84**:281-295, 1964.
5. David, M.D.: The natural history of diabetic retinopathy, Sight Sav. Rev. **97**:102, Summer 1969.
6. Duncan, L.J., Cullen, J.F., Ireland, J.T., et al.: A three-year trial of Atromid therapy in exudative diabetic retinopathy, Diabetes **17**:458-467, 1968.
7. Early Treatment Diabetic Retinopathy Study (ETDRS): Manual of operations, ETDRS Coordinating Center, Department of Epidemiology and Preventive Medicine, University of Maryland, 600 Wyndhurst Avenue, Baltimore, MD 21210.
8. Harold, M., Marvin, M., and Gough, K.: A double-blind controlled trial of clofibrate in the treatment of diabetic retinopathy, Diabetes **18**:285-291, 1969.
9. Job, D., Eschwage, E., et al.: Effect of multiple daily insulin injections on the course of diabetic retinopathy, Diabetes **25**:463-469, 1976.
10. King, R.C., Dobree, J.H., Kok, D.A., et al.: Exudative diabetic retinopathy, Br. J. Ophthalmol. **47**:666-672, 1963.
11. McMeel, J.W., Trempe, C.L., and Franks, E.B.: Diabetic maculopathy, Trans Am. Acad. Ophthalmol. Otolaryngol. **83**:476-487, 1977.
12. Miki, E., Fukuda, M., Kuzuya, T., et al.: Relation of the course of retinopathy to control of diabetes, age and therapeutic agents in diabetic Japanese patients, Diabetes **18**(11):773-780, 1969.

13. Patz, A., and Berkow, J.W.: Visual and systemic prognosis in diabetic retinopathy, Trans. Am. Acad. Ophthalmol. Otolaryngol. **72:**253-258, 1968.

14. Patz, A., Schatz, H., Berkow, J.W., et al.: Macular edema: an overlooked complication of diabetic retinopathy, Trans. Am. Acad. Ophthalmol. Otolaryngol. **77:**34-42, 1973.

15. Rubinstein, K., and Myska, V.: Treatment of diabetic maculopathy, Br. J. Ophthalmol. **56:**1-5, 1972.

16. Sigurdsson, R., and Begg, I.: Organized macular plaques in exudative diabetic maculopathy, Br. J. Ophthalmol. **68:**392-397, 1980.

17. Toussaint, D., Cogan, D., and Kuwabara, T.: Extramacular lesions of diabetic retinopathy, Arch. Ophthalmol. **61:**42-47, 1962.

18. Townsend, C., Bailey, J., and Kohner, E.M.: Xenon arc photocoagulation in the treatment of diabetic maculopathy, Trans. Ophthalmol. Soc. U.K. **99:**13-16, 1979.

19. Ts'o, M.O., and Shih, C.-Y.: Experimental macular edema after lens extraction, Invest. Ophthalmol. Visual Sci. **16:**381-392, 1977.

20. U.S. Department of Health, Education and Welfare: Statistics on blindness in the model reporting area, 1969-1970, Washington, D.C., 1973, U.S. Government Printing Office.

26

Tears of detached retinal pigment epithelium

Alan C. Bird
Kulwant S. Sehmi*

Tearing around the border of detached retinal pigment epithelium has been described only recently and yet appears to be a common complication of retinal pigment epithelial detachments.[1] At present the pathologic determinants of this response are unknown and there is little doubt that the clinical appearances of the lesion have yet to be fully described.

PATHOGENESIS

It has been recognized that retinal pigment epithelial detachments that are at risk of tearing have a distinctive appearance when compared with those in which this complication does not occur. The variation in appearance and subsequent behavior of the lesions allows some conjecture concerning the structural changes occurring at the site of separation of pigment epithelium from Bruch's membrane.[1]

In some cases of retinal pigment epithelial detachment, drusen can be seen on the undersurface of the detached tissue by biomicroscopy. During fluorescein angiography these lesions become hyperfluorescent during the early phases of the study and the hyperfluorescence is irregular. These lesions have been contrasted with those in which the detached tissues have a homogeneous surface appearance and which exhibit even but late hyperfluorescence during angiography (Figs. 26-1 and 26-2). The former lesions appear to be less highly detached than the latter. These observations call into question the plane of separation when pigment epithelium detaches from Bruch's membrane. In the first case it appears that the pigment epithelium has detached, together with the abnormal material on the inner surface on Bruch's membrane consisting of phagosomal debris and reduplicated pigment epithelial basement membrane.[4,5] In the second case no such features are seen, and it has been suggested that in these lesions the site of cleavage is within the abnormal basement membrane so that the epithelial detaches without an intact basement membrane. In some cases the lesion appears to have two parts, one with abnormal debris on its undersurface and the other with a homogeneous appearance (Fig. 26-3).

---
*Senior Medical Photographer, Retinal Diagnostic Department, Moorfields Eye Hospital, London, U.K.

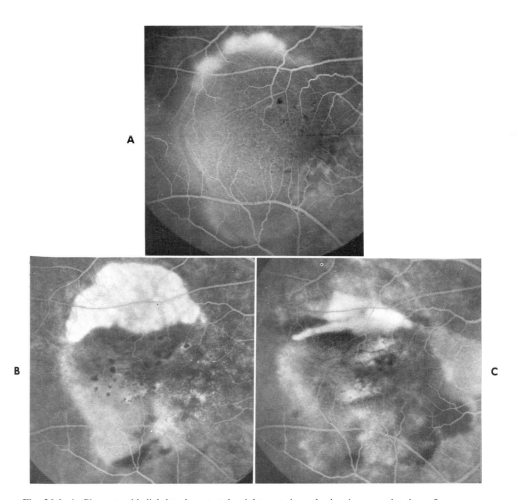

Fig. 26-1. A, Pigment epithelial detachment at the right posterior pole showing even, late hyperfluorescence. **B,** Within 3 weeks there was a pigment epithelial tear along its upper border and angiography showed a well-defined defect corresponding with the exposed Bruch's membrane. **C,** Within 4 months the defect was filled with fibrous tissue and there was invasion of fibrous tissue by new vessels.

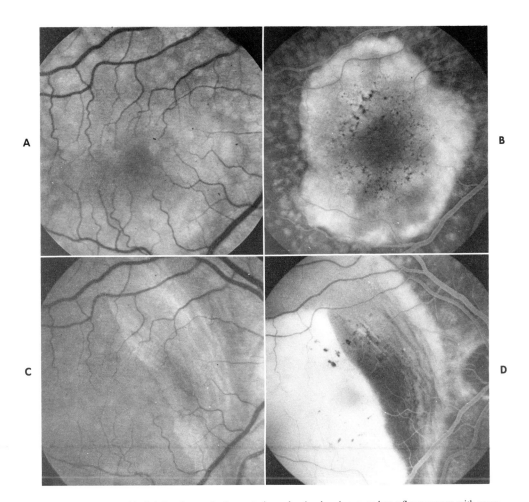

Fig. 26-2. Pigment epithelial detachment in the posterior pole, **A,** showing even hyperfluorescence with some obscuration by pigment centrally, **B.** Within 4 months, **C** and **D,** there was a tear along the temporal border of the lesion exposing Bruch's membrane and the free flap of pigment epithelium, which was thrown into folds.

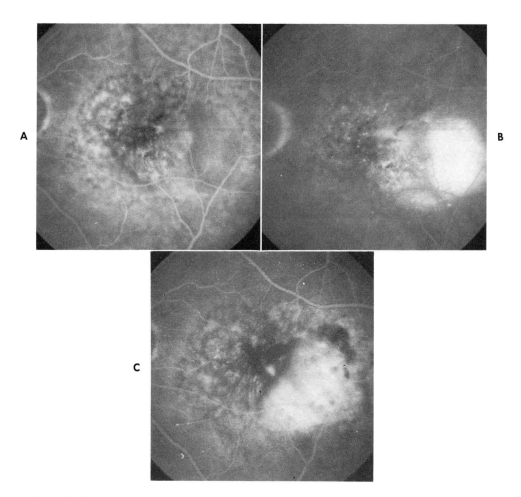

Fig. 26-3. Pigment epithelial detachment in the posterior pole showing two parts. **A** and **B,** The nasal half had early irregular hyperfluorescence, whereas the temporal half showed late, even hyperfluorescence. **C,** Within 8 weeks there was a tear around the temporal border of the lesion.

Predictably the two lesions would have different physical characteristics determined by the presence or absence of tissue on the outer surface of the detached pigment epithelium. This is illustrated by the different height of detachment of the two types of lesion. Most significant is the observation that tears of the pigment epithelium appear to occur almost exclusively in those lesions with high detachment, no deposits of the undersurface of the detached tissues, and even late hyperfluorescence. This observation would certainly be in accord with theoretical predictions of the differential physical behavior characteristics of these lesions. It is also significant that tears have not been seen in pigment epithelial detachments in the young in which basement membrane changes are not believed to exist.

CLINICAL PRESENTATION

Tears of the pigment epithelium cause acute visual loss if they involve the fovea, and in one study it was found that the visual loss was more profound and more acute with this complication than with subretinal neovascularization.[6]

Although those lesions at risk of developing this complication can be identified, there are no changes as yet recognized that signal the likelihood of tearing in the immediate future. In the acute phase after tearing, the area of exposed Bruch's membrane and choroid is well defined and slightly lighter in color than the surrounding fundus and the choroidal blood vessels are well seen. The flap of pigment epithelium may be well seen, with a free edge apparently floating in the subretinal space (Figs. 26-1 and 26-2). Folds are often evident in the pigment epithelium, a finding that suggests retraction of the tissues (Fig. 26-2). On angiography the exposed choroid is immediately hyperfluorescent, and dye may fill the subretinal space rapidly (Figs. 26-1 to 26-4). The pigment epithelium may be very dark, a finding that suggests intense obscuration of the background choroidal fluorescence. In some cases the rip may be accompanied by hemorrhage, which may

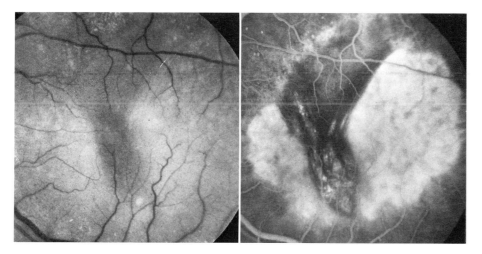

Fig. 26-4. Tearing of pigment epithelium on both sides of a detachment with the residual pigment epithelium forming a bridge centrally.

obscure the true nature of the lesion though even in these lesions the free flap of pigment epithelium may be seen over the surface of the subretinal blood.

During the recovery period, the evolution of the lesion varies from one case to another. In some the pigment epithelium may flatten onto Bruch's membrane leaving a well-defined area of apparent tissue defect, with the pigment epithelium remaining dark and well defined (Fig. 26-5). In others the free edge of pigment epithelium may become reattached to Bruch's membrane at a new site leaving a smaller detachment than before. Finally in a few cases with tearing on two sides of the original detachment, the free edges have been seen to curl toward the sensory retina giving rise to the appearance of an open tube (Fig. 26-6).

The area of apparent tissue deficit may remain unchanged over long periods (Fig. 26-5), or it may become covered by tissue resembling normal retinal pigment epithelium. However, in the majority of cases the defect becomes covered with fibrous tissue, which appears to be derived from the edges of the defect (Figs. 26-7 and 26-8). This process may be accompanied by invasion of the area by new blood vessels, which appear to be derived from the choroid. This neovascularization does not appear to an extension of preexisting subretinal blood vessels but rather a secondary process in response to the tearing.

Fluorescein angiographic changes during the period of repair reflect largely those tissue changes recognizable by ophthalmoscopy, except that soon after the tear and while there is still a tissue deficit leakage of dye into the subretinal ceases so that the hyperfluorescence is limited to the level of Bruch's membrane.

The pattern of healing appears to be analogous to that seen after experimental trauma to the retinal pigment epithelium in animals.[2,3] In small lesions the defect is made good by sliding of cells over the area with limited division of pigment epithelium cells. In larger defects the pigment epithelial cells proliferate and become fibroblastic.

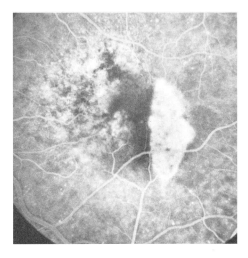

Fig. 26-5. Old tear of the pigment epithelium showing darkening of the pigment epithelium and well-defined atrophy on its temporal side.

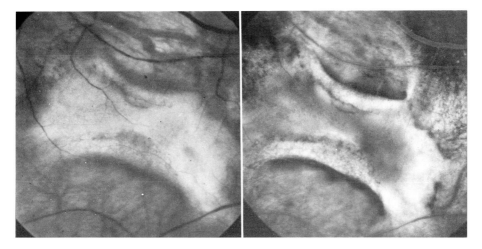

Fig. 26-6. Pigment epithelial detachment that has torn along the superior and inferior borders of the pigment epithelial detachment. The pigment epithelium has curled anteriorly giving rise to an open tube.

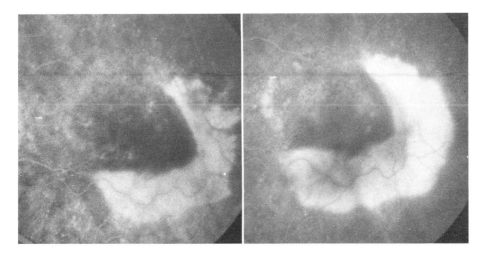

Fig. 26-7. Old pigment epithelial tear showing a dark central area of pigment epithelium with the exposed Bruch's membrane covered in fibrous tissue.

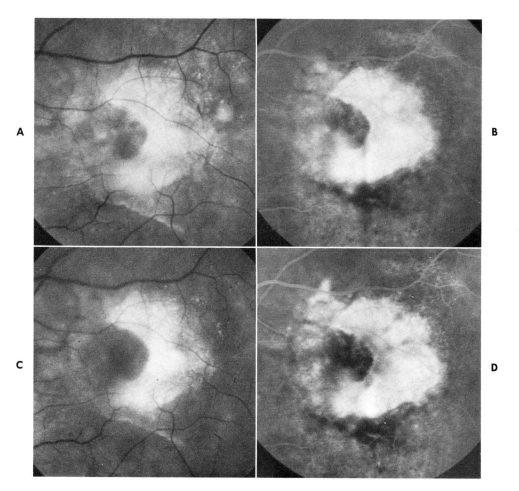

Fig. 26-8. Progressive fibrosis occurring within the lesion at 3 months, **A** and **B,** and 6 months, **C** and **D,** after tearing.

CONCLUSION

Clinical experience suggests that tearing of the retinal pigment epithelium is not rare and causes profound visual loss. The recognition of this complication allows reinterpretation of previous experience and in particular invites reassessment of old case material.

There is little doubt that a fresh tear with hemorrhage around it would have been understood to indicate the presence of subretinal blood vessels in the past and the development of subretinal new vessels and fibrosis would have reinforced this impression. It now appears likely that invasion of the subretinal space by blood vessels from the choroid is not the only precipitating event of a lesion with these familiar characteristics. The presence of marginal hyperfluorescence in lesions occurring before tearing and bleeding immediately after the event suggests the possibility of blood vessels proliferating on the posterior surface of the detached pigment epithelium, but they have not been well defined clinically at this time. Although subretinal neovascularization may yet be shown to be important in the genesis of retinal pigment epithelial tears, there is little evidence to support this proposition at present. Furthermore, the neovascularization seen after the tear is clearly a late event and not an extension of a preexisting new vessel complex. A lesion with well-defined atrophy of the retinal pigment epithelium may have been recognized as geographic atrophy caused by age-related cell loss in the past. It is now evident that the pigment epithelial rips may produce this fundus appearance. In such a case, a history of sudden visual loss, which is incompatible with geographic atrophy, might imply the correct diagnosis.

In both these situations the true nature of the lesion may be indicated by a well-defined area of dark retinal pigment epithelium and well-defined and regular atrophy; each of these regions are often better defined by angiography. It is clear, however, that the progressive invasion of the lesion by fibrovascular tissue may obscure the characteristic clinical features of a tear such that the true origin of the lesions becomes unrecognizable with time.

Although some of the circumstances that lead to tearing of detached pigment epithelium may be signified by the morphology of the lesion at risk, there is little evidence to indicate the events that determine its timing or precipitate its occurrence. It is interesting that the tear is always at the border of the detachment where the physical stresses are likely to be different from those elsewhere in the lesion.

The significance to clinical practice goes beyond the reinterpretation of lesions. It has been shown that a tear may follow photocoagulation of a retinal pigment epithelial detachment and be precipitated by it.[6] One study has implied that photocoagulation with argon laser energy confers no benefit to visual prognosis in such lesions. However, if further studies demonstrate any benefit with a different therapeutic technique, recognition of cases likely to suffer this complication may be important. Furthermore, there is little doubt that cases with recent tears have received photocoagulation under the mistaken impression that the area of hyperfluorescence represented an area of subretinal neovascularization.

REFERENCES

1. Hoskin, A., Bird, A.C., and Sehmi, K. Tears of detached retinal pigment epithelium, Br. J. Ophthalmol. **65**(6):417-422, 1981.
2. Marshall, J., and Mellerio, J.: Disappearance of the retroepithelial scar tissue from ruby laser photocoagulation, Exp. Eye Res. **12**:173-174, 1971.
3. Marshall, J., and Mellerio, J.: Laser irradiation of retinal tissue, Br. Med. Bull. **26**:156-160, 1970.
4. Sarks, S.H.: Ageing and degeneration in the macular region: a clinical-pathological study, Br. J. Ophthalmol. **69**:324-341, 1979.
5. Sarks, S.H.: Drusen and their relationship to senile macular degeneration, Aust. J. Ophthalmol. **8**:117-130, 1980.
6. The Moorfields Macular Study Group: Retinal pigment epithelial detachments in the elderly: a controlled trial of argon laser photocoagulation, Br. J. Ophthalmol. **65**(12):859-865, 1982.

Round table discussions

THE SPECTRUM OF RETINAL TELANGIECTASIA

DR. ROBERT C. WATZKE

Case 1. This was a 25 year old healthy, white male who has noted gradual blurring of central vision in the right eye for approximately 3 years. Vision was 20/40 OD and 20/15 OS with a moderate myopic refraction. In the temporal fundus of the right eye were numerous vascular anomalies (Fig. A-1). These consisted of berry-like dilatations of both arteries and veins. These small terminal vessels were abnormally kinked, tortuous and irregular in caliber. The entire temporal vascular pattern was bizarre with some small, almost capillary sized vessels appearing to arise from the fundus without any connections to larger vessels. There were numerous lipid exudates scattered about these vessels in a circinate fashion. The left fundus was normal.

A work-up consisting of complete blood count, sedimentation rate, protein electrophoresis, chest x-ray exam, antinuclear antibody titer, C reactive protein, rheumatoid factor, serum immunoglobulins, and an FTA [fluorescent treponemal antibody absorption test] were all essentially normal except for a very mild increase of the alpha-2 globulin and gamma globulin fractions and an elevation of IgG and IgA levels.

Fluorescein angiography demonstrated mild leakage of dye from some vascular complexes temporal to the fovea. It also demonstrated widespread enlargement of the entire vascular bed in the temporal midperiphery (Fig. A-2).

No treatment was performed, but the patient was observed 3 months later. At that time there had been no change. The patient was examined 7 months later, and the vision had actually improved to 20/25. There was no change in the abnormal vessels or the exudates. Photocoagulation was deferred.

Case 2. This was a 53-year-old man who had seen his referring ophthalmologist because of blurred vision in both eyes, particularly the left eye, for the past several months. Vision was 20/20 OD and 20/30 OS with a minor correction. The ocular exam was completely normal except for the fundi, both of which showed an unusual vascular pattern. The perifoveal capillaries were dilated, kinked, irregular, and arranged almost in a circumferential pattern. They did not appear to be continuous with the perifoveal vessels but were instead arranged in short segments without any apparent connection to larger vessels. The right fovea had this pattern temporally, whereas for the left fovea there was an anomaly encircling the entire foveal avascular zone (Fig. A-3). The foveal retina appeared mildly edematous, but there was no cystoid degeneration.

On fluorescein angiography the dye collected and stained these abnormal vessels in the transit phase (Fig. A-4). In the late stages there was leakage into the perifoveal retina in both eyes. Leakage was most pronounced in the left eye in the superior fovea though abnormal vessels were present about the entire fovea.

No further work-up was performed.

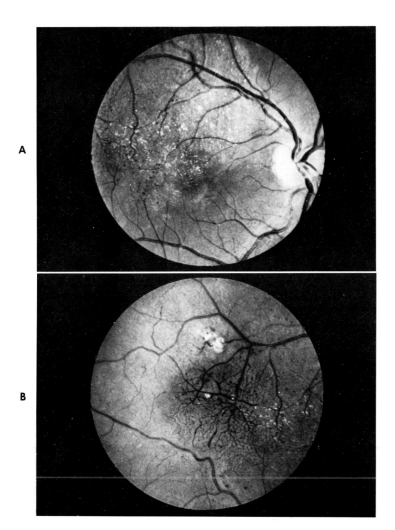

Fig. A-1. A, Case 1: Macula of right eye of 25-year-old man. The temporal retinal vessels are kinked, dilated, tortuous, and sacculated with retinal edema and lipid exudates. **B,** Temporal to the fovea, the retinal vessels are even more abnormal.

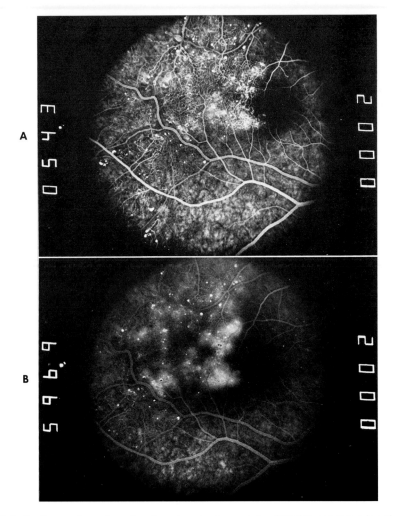

Fig. A-2. On fluorescein angiography, there is extensive vascular dilatation and tortuosity of the retinal vessels, **A,** with late leakage, **B.**

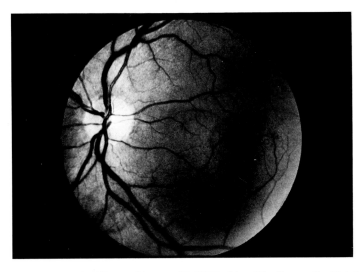

Fig. A-3. Case 2: Left eye of a 53-year-old man with 20/30 vision OS. Abnormally dilated and tortuous perifoveal vessels. The right macula was similar but too subtle to photograph.

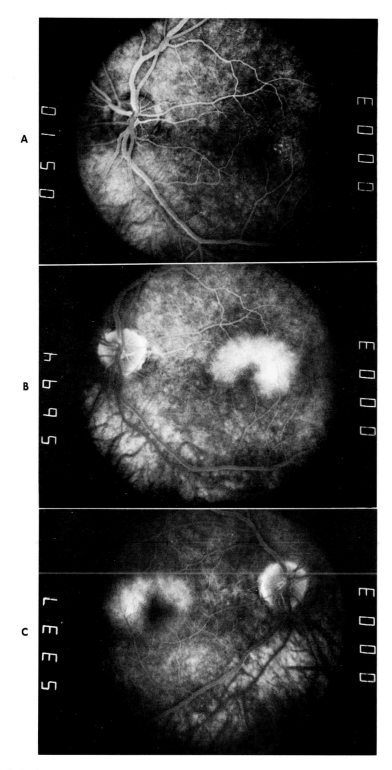

Fig. A-4. On fluorescein angiography, there is early staining of the abnormal vessels, **A,** with late leakage, **B.** The right eye has a similar pattern, **C.**

Discussion

These two cases are chosen to illustrate two varieties of retinal telangiectasia. The first case is an example of Leber's miliary aneurysms. This disease usually affects males and involves usually only one eye. Characteristic vascular changes are found in the equatorial and peripheral retina and are usually restricted to one or two quadrants. The typical vascular pattern is of saccular and fusiform aneurysmal dilatations of the superficial retinal vessels. The capillary network is dilated and leaks fluid. Exudates appear and small intraretinal hemorrhages are common. There is usually persistent cystoid macular edema and often accumulation of lipid material in the fovea.

The second patient's diagnosis is perifoveal telangiectasia. This patient is middle aged and has had normal vision all his life. He was seen 1 year previously by an ophthalmologist who dilated his pupils and performed an ocuar exam. The ophthalmologist cannot certify that small vascular anomalies were not present, but if they were, they would have been very minor in nature. This condition is bilateral, is restricted to the perifoveal area, and consists mainly of dilated irregular and segmental enlargement of the small vessels.

Green, Quigley, De La Cruz, and Cohen have reported an excellent clinicopathologic study of perifoveal retinal telangiectasia.[1] This was a 58-year-old woman with a clinical picture identical to that in case 2. She needed an orbital exenteration for squamous cell carcinoma, and the left eye was removed after photography and fluorescein angiography.

Histologic examination showed the perifoveal retina to have mild edema of the inner and outer plexiform layer with some accumulation of fluid in the ganglion cells. Blood vessels in the area of retinal "telangiectasis" showed narrowing of the lumen of the retinal capillaries with thickening and proliferation of the capillary basement membrane. Retinal trypsin digestion showed thickening of the capillary walls and loss of pericytes.

On electron microscopy the perifoveal capillaries were quite abnormal. They were greatly thickened by a multilaminated basement material with narrowing of the vessel lumen. There was much cellular debris within this basement membrane material and some lamellar material that appeared to be lipid or lipoprotein. The endothelial intracellular junctional complexes were generally normal, but some endothelial cells were degenerative.

In the fundus midperiphery the retinal capillaries were also abnormal with similar but less extensive multilamination of basement membrane material and a lipid deposition, with very little edema. The entire picture resembled the basement membrane degeneration and deposition seen in diabetes. However, there was no history of diabetes in the patient or her family.

Green and co-workers believe that the term "telangiectasia" is inappropriate for this case, though it may represent the mild end of the spectrum of true telangiectasis. They postulated that the fluorescein angiographic picture was one of leakage of the dye through the endothelium into this abnormal basement membrane material.

REFERENCE

1. Green, W.R., Quigley, H.A., De La Cruz, Z., and Cohen, B.: Parafoveal retinal telangiectasis: light and electron microscopy studies, Trans. Ophthalmol. Soc. U.K. **100** (Part 1):162, 1980.

Watzke: Do you think that this is a part of a spectrum of retinal telangiectasis [telangiectasia]? Have you seen cases like this, and do you feel that we are dealing with separate entities, or is it all a congenital Leber's telangiectasis that has simply become manifest in later life? That's quite a tall order. Don, would you comment first of all on the diagnosis and whether you have seen conditions like this? How would you classify and diagnose them?

Gass: Bob, I would like to hear the other members before I show several slides that will summarize what I think of the cases you presented.

Watzke: Okay, let's start with Arnall then.

Patz: Well, I'll agree to calling them "perifoveal telangiectasis." The second case, which had the bilateral, fairly symmetrical perifoveal changes, I would call that "typical perifoveal telangiectasis." The first patient obviously has the lesion more peripheral, and there must be something brewing that I did not catch even though I was sitting in the front row. But I would also put that into the retinal telangiectasis category, the first patient you presented.

Watzke: Arnall, you use the same term "telangiectasia" for both entities. Do you think that they are a single entity with just a variable expression coming on early in life, coming on in just one eye as opposed to a bilateral disease later in life, or do you think that it is all part of this so-called Leber's telangiectasia? Or do you think that they are separate entities?

Patz: I think they are part of a spectrum. I know that Ray Oyakawa, while working with Don, tried to categorize these, and maybe Don's slide will give that classification that he worked up, which I think was under your tutelage. But, I would put them into a variation of a condition of the same basic pathogenesis.

Watzke: Wally?

McMeel: I would agree they are part of a spectrum. The unilaterality of the first example was rather interesting because the other eye was not involved at all.

Watzke: That's right.

McMeel: It appeared as if it was a bit more peripheral and eccentric, a bit farther away from the macular region, plus more edema. Whether this is just a different basic characteristic or whether it is just a little farther along a similar road, I don't think one can tell.

Watzke: Before we ask the next speaker to comment, I would like to emphasize that I don't think that the latter case is a very uncommon condition. I think now we are examining the fovea more critically than we used to, and I have seen seven or eight of these patients just within the last 6 months simply because I am looking for the little abnormally dilated parafoveal vessels. Now, of course, we can see this sort of thing secondary to branch vein occlusions and all sorts of things. You can even see this in patients who have surface wrinkling retinopathy, that is, the cellophane maculopathy seen in so many older patients. You look at the vessels in this slightly distorted, puckered parafoveal area. The retinal capillaries will be sacculated and dilated also, and they will leak. It's hard for me to believe that something that comes on at the age of 50 and is bilateral—in a patient who is completely asymptomatic and has gone through numerous eye examinations without any mention made of this all of his life until the age of 50—that it can be related to Leber's telangiectasia. Dick, what do you think?

O'Connor: I essentially agree with you. I was struck by the fact that they probably represent two different disease mechanisms. When I first saw the pictures that you showed of the young man with the predominantly peripheral disease, I wondered whether it might be an early Coats' disease. I think your later discussions probably ruled that out, but certainly there was evidence of lipoidal exudates in a patient who had prominent telangiectasia. I think that all of these diseases point to a fundamental disorder of basement membranes. And, of course, that's eventually where we are going to get the answer concerning the resolution of the various entities. What is the basic basement membrane anomaly that is causing the problem? I think that we will eventually be able to discern that by chemical means, but we are not at that stage yet, and that's where the answer lies.

Watzke: Steve?

Ryan: I am glad you made those points in regard to the possibility of branch vein occlusion and epiretinal membrane, which may present a similar appearance. In other words, clearly you can have a degenerative or acquired condition that can give a similar appearance to the congenital condition of your first case. On the other hand, in your second case you show bilaterality occurring in a young individual, and that says to me, that there is going to be an inherited disease, or certainly a tendency toward disease. We should keep these points in mind. So I think that really you are going to find two mechanisms, and one of these is acquired by various disease processes that can produce the secondary changes that Dick is talking about rightly and as you showed with your electron microscopy. Thus juxtafoveal telangiectasis can present with multiple different presentations. Until Don gives us the answer, or you from the classification, that would be my opinion—that we are dealing with at least two different types of processes that can lead to similar clinical appearance.

Watzke: She had bilateral disease. I have asked two pathologists whether this basement membrane abnormality could be a part of a spectrum of aging changes. And one doctor, Dr. Green, said that it's conceivable that it could. Dr. Blodi said absolutely not. Morton?

Goldberg: I think it's worth expanding the discussion to include Coats' disease. Does Coats' disease, with the same sort of telangiectatic and aneurysmal blood vessels as shown in your first case but characterized also with massive exudation, represent a disease that is different from your first case? I would say probably not. I think that Coats' disease with massive exudation is the severe manifestation of what has been variously called "Leber's telangiectasis" or "miliary aneurysms," and the latter designation is what I would apply to your first case. In other words, I think there is a spectrum of clinical manifestations of the same basic underlying disease. With regard to the second type of case, so-called perifoveal telangiectasia, it seems clinically to be quite different for all the reasons you stated: it's frequently in older people, is probably acquired, has smaller blood vessels, and is found in a different fundus location. But it's probably a very heterogeneous disease for the reasons you have mentioned. There are lots of other causes, including radiation retinopathy and a form of background diabetic retinopathy. It is sometimes inherited, sometimes not. There is sometimes loss of the foveal capillaries, sometimes not. It is rarely associated with hypogammaglobulinemia, mostly not. So I think it's a diagnostic grab bag and that the causes vary. There is only a limited amount of electron microscopic material available for what has been called "perifoveal telangiectasia," namely, the one case that you have shown us today. As far as I know, there is also only one published report of the electron microscopy of Coats' disease. Now, as different as these two diseases are clinically, the surprising thing, from the limited amount of electron microscopic material available, is that the endothelial cells seem to undergo a very similar sort of degeneration, and they have focal leakage that not only allows fluorescein to stain and leak, but presumably also allows the basement membrane to become thickened by chronic transudation. That's at least one hypothetical pathogenetic sequence of events. That would account for the basement membrane disease that O'Connor has mentioned. If that's the proper sequence of events, then the basement membrane disease is secondary to a primary endothelial abnormality. The reverse sequence of events could also occur I suppose, namely, a primary basement membrane abnormality followed by ectasia of the blood vessel, which is no longer supported by a relatively rigid tubing, and therefore the endothelial degeneration is secondary. I really can't choose between the two hypotheses.

Watzke: Thank you. Alan?

Bird: I would accept that we may be considering the end stages of several disorders and that basement membrane changes may also be a result of different disease states. G. Chaine has just examined 60 such patients. Just over half had bilateral disease, although in one eye the only abnormality may be a reduction in number and elongation of the parafoveal capillaries. One half had peripheral retinal vascular disease. We believe that in some of our patients incompetence of the pigment epithelium may play a part in the pathogenesis of the disorder and in some patients the disease may be initiated by abnormal flow through the pigment epithelium. This would have the effect of altering the contents of the extracellular space. It would not be surprising if such an abnormal environment would induce secondary capillary changes.

Watzke: Greene mentioned in his discussion that these changes that you saw are identical to those seen in diabetes. The patient refused a glucose tolerance test but was not clinically diabetic. Don, what or how would you summarize?

Gass: In regard to your first case, I would agree essentially with what Mort Goldberg had to say. I think that's a case of congenital telangiectasia of the retinal blood vessels including the capillaries, veins, and arteries. This disease may become manifest early in life as a result of massive exudative retinal detachment, or the patient with minimal involvement may have absolutely no symptoms until he is in his sixties, when exudate finally extends into the macular area. Now, regarding the last two patients with juxtafoveolar telangiectasis, I think they are similar but are quite different from your case 1. The following slides illustrate how we subclassify patients with capillary telangiectasis of unknown cause when it is confined to the juxtafoveolar area. They all present with mild visual disturbance usually caused by exudation in the central macular area.

The first subgroup is composed of nine males, mostly young adults, with uniocular involvement. They probably have the same disease as your case number one, except that they had telangiectasis confined to the temporal half of the macular area.

Yellowish circinate exudation occurred in all these patients. Photocoagulation in approximately one half of the patients was successful in stabilizing or improving visual function. The others maintained good visual function without treatment, and some, in fact, had demonstrated considerable improvement of vision with no treatment.

The second group of 12 middle-aged patients, including nine males, had bilateral telangiectasis confined to a small area less than a disc diameter in size involving the temporal half of each foveolar area. Mild edema, but little or no yellowish exudate, occurred in this group.

Group 3 comprising five patients (three females) was similar to Watzke's last two patients in that the telangiectasis involved the entire perifoveolar capillary network in both eyes. Like group 2, these rarely show evidence of yellowish exudation. In groups 2 and 3 the capillary dilatation is more difficult to see biomicroscopically and angiographically. Occasionally patients, however, showed angiographic evidence of unusual dilatation of the deep plexus of the perifoveolar capillaries. This plexus was drained by one or more superfifical retinal venules that centrally appeared blunted where they extended posteriorly into the depth of the retina. Plaques of subretinal pigment epithelial proliferation and occasionally choroidal neovascularization, subretinal hemorrhage and exudation, and chorioretinal vascular anastomosis occurred at the site of the venular drainage of this deep plexus in several patients. Most of these patients, however, show minimal evidence of intraretinal exudation and have a good visual prognosis. They are not good candidates for photocoagulation.

The fourth group of two patients demonstrates capillary changes quite different from those of the other three groups. These two patients showed the following clinical features: both were males, both noted loss of central vision in both eyes during midlife secondary to juxtafoveolar capillary obliteration, capillary telangiectasis, and minimal exudation, and both had optic nerve head pallor and hyperactive deep tendon reflexes. One had other neurologic manifestations and a provisional diagnosis of multiple sclerosis.

We believe that patients in group 1 had a mild form of the congenital retinal anomaly "retinal telangiectasis" or "Leber's miliary aneurysms." Groups 2 and 3 comprised patients who usually were beyond the fifth decade of life when they first became symptomatic. Although the cause of the juxtafoveolar capillary change is unknown, we believe that this is an acquired retinal vascular change that may be related to the retinal vascular pattern peculiar to the macular area, where in nearly every patient the venules draining the macular area cross major retinal arteries before emptying into their parent veins. The two patients in group 4 appear to have a neuroretinal syndrome. It is uncertain as to whether the juxtafoveal capillary changes are congenital or acquired.

It is of interest that in none of the cases of juxtafoveolar and retinal telangiectasis have we been able to identify other family members affected by the same disease.

Watzke: Thank you very much.

DIFFERENTIAL DIAGNOSIS IN TREATMENT OF ACUTE RETINAL PIGMENT EPITHELIOPATHIES

DR. J. DONALD M. GASS

Gass: This will be a brief quiz for the audience, as well as the panelists. I am going to show very rapidly a few photographs of eight specific conditions that either are or may simulate one of the acute pigment epitheliopathies. These will provide a takeoff point for some discussion.

In the first slide this 34-year-old healthy woman woke up one morning with a large scotoma in the central field of her left eye. The right fundus was normal. The left fundus showed this two-disc-diameter-size, round, flat, white lesion centered in the macula (Plate 1, *A*). The angiogram showed a corresponding nonfluorescent zone with a number of other smaller focal nonfluorescent lesions not visible ophthalmoscopically. Her visual acuity was counting-fingers in this eye. The fluorescein angiogram showed no staining except in the later pictures when some staining of the middle of the lesions occurred. Notice that there was no early staining at the edge of these lesions. In the late pictures, all the lesions stain. Two and a half months later, the patient returned with 20/20 vision in both eyes. After a period of 30 months she returned with the same complaints and findings in the right eye. The time for resolution was the same as the left eye and she regained 20/20 vision.

Case 2 is a 35-year-old man who noted blurred vision in both eyes for about 1 week. His past medical history revealed that the man had experienced malaise for the last several weeks, but otherwise was unremarkable. He had numerous white, one-disc-diameter-size lesions scattered throughout the fundus (Plate 1, *B*). These lesions were slightly elevated. Fluorescein angiography early showed some areas of nonfluorescence, corresponding to the lesions. Later, there was irregular staining of these lesions.

Case 3 was a 25-year-old man with a 2-week history of blurred vision, more noticeable in his right eye than his left eye. His visual acuity was 5/200 in the right eye. In the left eye, his visual acuity was normal, but he had a paracentral scotoma. His past medical history was noncontributory. Note the geographic pattern of nonelevated gray lesions at the level of the pigment epithelium extending outward from the optic disc in both eyes (Plate 1, *C*). Notice that the lesions appear more gray along their outer borders. Notice also the multiple flame-shaped hemorrhages scattered widely in both eyes. Fluorescein angiography showed a pattern quite different from that in case 1. These gray lesions are staining along their edges but initially remain hypofluorescent centrally. Later these lesions stained diffusely.

Case 4 is a 22-year-old Latin woman with a past medical history of progressive loss of vision that first started in her left eye and then affected her right eye. She had bilateral patchy areas of serous detachment of the retina and a number of gray or yellowish subretinal patches (Plate 1, *D*). Angiography showed multiple pinpoint leaks underneath the retina. Notice in this eye that she has a discrete area of fluorescence indicative of a serous detachment of the pigment epithelium. Notice that later there is diffuse leakage throughout both eyes.

Case 5 was a 12-year-old girl with rapid loss of central vision in her right eye. Her past medical history again was unremarkable. Notice in the right fundus the scattered multiple, ill-defined, gray lesions (Plate 1, *E*). Angiographically these lesions are partly nonfluorescent. Notice that there was no gray-white lesion present in the center of the macula, and yet this patient's visual acuity was approximately 20/100. One month later, her vision had dropped further to 20/200. The lesions had completely disappeared, and you really see very little alteration in the eye. However, this young girl had a progressive loss of vision down to counting-fingers vision only. Two years later, she has a pale optic disc, narrowing of the major retinal vessels and extensive changes in the retinal pigment epithelium throughout the fundus. The left eye was normal.

Case 6 was a woman 35 to 40 years of age, complaining of floaters in both eyes of several months' duration. Her visual acuity was 20/20 in each eye. On careful questioning, she had mild nyctalopia. Notice this widespread pattern of yellow patches scattered throughout the fundi of both eyes, with relative sparing of the macula (Plate 1, *F*). There were vitreous cells in both eyes. Notice that the angiography was normal. There was no angiographic abnormality corresponding to the yellow choroidal lesions.

Case 7 was a young woman complaining that for about a week she had noticed multiple paracentral scotomas and photopsia in the left eye. Notice the number of little, dark, sort of graylike areas scattered about the left macula (Plate 1, *G*). Her visual acuity in this eye was 20/80. Her history was of significance in that about 1 week before the onset of visual symptoms, she had had an upper respiratory infection. On fluorescein angiography, you really don't see very much at all.

Case 8 was a 40-year-old man with a 1 week history of blurred vision in his right eye. His acuity was normal, but he had these multiple white patches scattered about the fundus (Plate 1, *H*). They appeared to be very slightly elevated, and you will notice that they are nonfluorescent in the early angiogram. During the course of angiography the peripheral portion of these lesions stained. The central portion stained later. There is one important factor in this patient's history. He had lost all sight in his other eye after repair of a corneoscleral laceration 4 months previously followed later by a vitrectomy.

So much for the quiz.

First, let me comment on case 8, because here is the gross photograph of his operated eye that was enucleated the day after the photographs were made in his right eye. Notice the multiple white lesions in the posterior pole. I should mention that this patient was first diagnosed as having acute posterior multifocal placoid pigment epitheliopathy despite the fact that the recent history of a penetrating wound and surgery in the left eye should have immediately suggested the correct diagnosis of sympathetic uveitis. These gray lesions seen in the gross specimen showed multiple focal areas of obliteration of the choriocapillaris by epithelioid cells and surrounding giant cells and lymphocytes. This patient had the posterior form of sympathetic uveitis with multifocal lesions that simulated acute posterior multifocal placoid pigment epitheliopathy [APMPPE].

Now let's return to case 1. In Miami, we made a diagnosis of APMPPE.

Case 2 was proved to have metastatic carcinoma of the lung with lesions simulating those of APMPPE. These multiple lesions, unlike APMPPE, showed less discrete areas of early hyperfluorescence by virtue of the fact that the white lesions

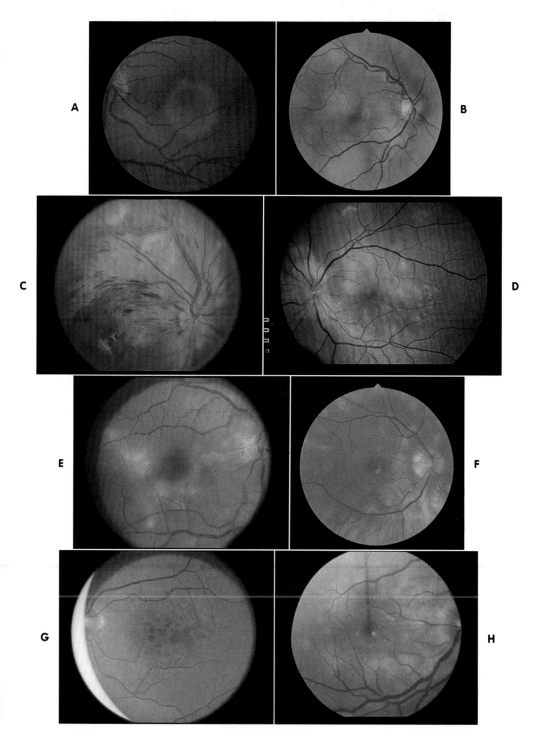

Plate 1. A, Solitary macular lesion in patient with APMPPE (acute posterior multifocal placoid pigment epitheliopathy). **B,** Multifocal areas of metastatic carcinoma of the lung simulating APMPPE. **C,** Multiple branch vein occlusions in a patient with serpiginous choroiditis. **D,** Multiple gray patches and subretinal fluid in a patient with Harada's disease. **E,** Multifocal outer retinal lesions in a child with diffuse unilateral subacute neuroretinitis. **F,** Hypopigmented choroidal patches in a patient with vitiliginous chorioretinitis (birdshot chorioretinitis). **G,** Multifocal lesions associated with acute macular neuroretinopathy. **H,** Multifocal choroiditis in sympathetic uveitis.

were primarily caused by infiltration of the choroid and were not caused by a color change in the retinal pigment epithelium.

Case 3 was a patient with serpiginous choroiditis, sometimes called "geographic choroiditis." An unusual feature was the evidence of multiple-branch retinal venous obstructions. I have now seen three cases of serpiginous choroiditis with evidence of focal retinal phlebitis causing branch vein occlusion. The staining pattern in the active gray lesions at the level of the retinal pigment epithelium is quite different from that in APMPPE because they tend to stain initially along their margins. In APMPPE the acute lesion gradually stains throughout the lesion. The acute gray lesions in both diseases stain diffusely late.

Case 4 was a young woman with the multiple gray patches and the serous fluid and multiple leaks associated with Harada's disease. I put that case in for Dr. Bird particularly, because we have had several of these cases of Harada's disease that do have gray-looking, subretinal lesions that simulate APMPPE. We believe, however, that Harada's disease has nothing to do with APMPPE, but I threw it in because the Moorfields Eye Hospital group has suggested that the two entities are part of a spectrum of the same disease.

Case 5 had deep white lesions caused by a nematode wandering in the subretinal space in a patient who developed all the late features of the unilateral wipe-out syndrome or diffuse unilateral subacute neuroretinitis. This is a disease that is endemic in the southeastern part of the United States and the north midwestern United States. It is caused by at least two different nematodes of uncertain identification. Neither is probably *Toxocara canis*.

Case 6 had vitiliginous choroiditis, better known as "birdshot chorioretinopathy." The multiple yellow spots that did not produce a change in the fluorescein angiogram appears to be caused by loss of melanin from the choroidal melanocytes similar to that seen in vitiligo of the skin. This is a chronic inflammatory disease that probably is an autoimmune disease involving melanin and perhaps retinal tissue.

I don't recall case 7. Steve help me.

Ryan: Neuroretinopathy.

Gass: That's right, that was acute macular neuroretinopathy. The reason I included this disease, which in fact probably does not affect the pigment epithelium, was that the lesions were fairly small and not so large as the ones that were published by Boz and Deutman, and it brings up the question of the entity of acute retinal pigment epithcliitis. I would like to ask the panel, How many of you recognize a disease called "acute retinal pigment epitheliitis" as described by Krill and Deutman, and how many of them do you see in a year's time? Has anyone on the panel seen a case?

Watzke: The retinal fellows keep making that diagnosis. We have seen cases that we labeled as such. Personally, I am not sure that there is such an entity. A presumably healthy person, middle aged or younger, comes in with mild disturbance of vision and a little pigmented spot with a halo of depigmentation around this spot—usually one to three of these things near the fovea. And they just sort of stay there. I don't personally think that this condition is a clinical entity.

Gass: Well, few seem anxious to talk about this disease. We'll skip it for a moment. Dr. Bird, did you want to say something about acute pigment epitheliitis?

Bird: We have diagnosed this several times, and in at least two cases it is now clear that patients had serpiginous choroidopathy. We were observing the first lesion of this disorder.

Gass: Well, I think that the problem is that there is a variety of diseases such as central serous retinopathy that can leave those little rings that they described. The fundus findings are so nonspecific that we just have not been able to nail down the diagnosis. Contrariwise, acute macular neuroretinopathy is a very specific, though rare, disease. I believe that it can be misdiagnosed as acute pigment epitheliitis because the small lesions, which are very hard to see ophthalmoscopically, may cause a distinct scotoma. These patients typically complain of multiple paracentral scotomas and photopsia of a few days' duration. They usually note these soon after experiencing a respiratory or gastrointestinal tract viral syndrome. Well, let me go back to case 1, the case of the lady who had a 30-month delay between involvement of the first and second eye. Although the history was atypical, we made a diagnosis of APMPPE. Does anyone wish to make a different diagnosis? Yes? Mort Goldberg.

Goldberg: Well, I would just like to ask you, Don, why you made that diagnosis. How would you account for the very large, circular, roughly 1½ disc-diameter hypofluorescent zone in the center of the macula of the first eye at the time of presentation?

Gass: Well, we thought that zone was very characteristic of a single lesion in APMPPE. Although the size of the central lesion was considerably larger than the average, she had, in fact, multiple other smaller lesions that we didn't see ophthalmoscopically, but did see angiographically. The course of resolution of the lesions and her visual recovery were typical for APMPPE. The fluorescein angiogram was identical with it. The course was atypical in that there was a 30-month delay in the involvement of the second eye. She is one of two of our patients with APMPPE who have had a significant delay between onset in the two eyes. As far as recurrence of the disease in the same eye is concerned, the longest period that we have observed is 6 months. In most patients no additional lesions occur in either eye after 1 to 2 months from the onset.

Patz: Don, do you think it's rare that the APMPPE lesions will avoid the fovea?

Gass: No, it's not rare. Very often one eye has it in the fovea, and that's what called the patient's attention to it. But by then he's often noticing paracentral scotomas in the other eye. But the fovea has to be involved ophthalmoscopically in our experience in patients with reduced acuity. The patient with DUSN (diffuse unilateral subacute neuroretinitis), the young girl (case 5) that had multiple paracentral gray-white lesions was misdiagnosed initially as unilateral APMPPE. We should have known the diagnosis was incorrect, since she had 20/100 vision, but no lesions in her fovea. First of all, she was 12 years old, which was rather young for APMPPE. Well, one of the reasons I showed case 1 was that she did have atypical features, and another was to raise the question concerning the role of the choriocapillaris occlusion in the pathogenesis of the white lesions seen in APMPPE. Dr. Bird is going to talk later about some of the ischemic fundus diseases, one of which he believes is APMPPE. The clinical and angiographic findings in case 1 demonstrate why I am completely unconvinced that APMPPE has anything to do with closure of the choriocapillaris. Here's a lady who, Alan would suggest, had closure of the choriocapillaris in the entire macular area and counting-fingers vision and yet recovered 20/20 in both eyes. You may want to comment on that now, if you wish.

Bird: There appear to be two features of interest. In the first place the patient appears to have unilateral involvement. We have seen patients with monocular disease in whom angiography shows perfusion deficit in the apparently normal eye. The second point of interest is recurrence. We have seen six patients with recurrent disease, one of whom has had recurrent attacks over 3½ years and yet the disorder simulates placoid pigment epitheliopathy rather than serpiginous choroidopathy. Four of the six patients with recurrent disease were taking antimicrobial drugs recurrently. It seems reasonable that if the disorder could be precipitated by intake of an external agent such as an antimicrobial drug the disease should be recurrent if the precipitating circumstances were repeated.

Gass: Well, that's interesting and we have had no such cases. The only two patients we have seen with a recurrence in the same eye had the recurrence at 6 months and 4 months after onset. About one third of our patients have had a history of some viral infection before the onset of visual symptoms. I might ask, also, in that regard, Have panel members related any systemic disease to serpiginous or geographic choroiditis? We have not. Does anybody want to comment further concerning the role of occlusion of the choriocapillaris in serpiginous choroiditis and APMPPE? Although acute lesions in both diseases look very similar ophthalmoscopically, the angiography does not look similar either during the acute or subsequent stages of the disease. The differences, I believe, have to do with what's occurring in the choroid in the two diseases. But, we will get back to that later. Now, did anybody have questions about case 4 with Harada's disease? We thought that we had the diagnosis of Harada's disease pretty well nailed down, until Peter Hamilton and Alan Bird suggested that it might be related to APMPPE. To date, I have seen no evidence to suggest that these two diseases cannot be clearly distinguished from each other.

Bird: We have seen patients who attended with a fundus appearance typical of Harada's disease and yet who did not behave in a way that we expected in that the detachment resolved within days, leaving multifocal pigment epithelial lesions, and the subsequent behavior was typical of placoid pigment epitheliopathy. It seemed possible that there was a variety of manifestations of choroidal ischemia. That is not to say that the ischemia has the same cause in each patient and that variation in the pattern of disease is determined by a different cause of ischemia. I do not claim that Harada's disease in its typical form, in dark-skinned patients who require steroids for rapid improvement and in whom there is optic neuritis, is caused by ischemia. Nevertheless, when the patient presents to us with a typical appearance of Harada's disease, it is impossible to distinguish at the time of the initial visit between the disorder that will improve spontaneously and the one that requires treatment.

Gass: Was it the history of getting better without treatment that bothered you?

Bird: Yes, of all the patients we have seen with an appearance typical of Harada's disease initially, over half have recovered spontaneously within 7 days. I believe that for Harada's disease this would be most unusual.

Gass: But they can have a very rapid spontaneous resolution in some cases.

Bird: I appreciate that that is correct, but I have difficulty accepting that spontaneous resolution within 7 days is acceptable for Harada's disease.

Gass: Well, at least in Miami that sort of finding is not unique. Have you ever seen a patient with Harada's disease with placoid white lesions and no detachment?

Bird: Yes. We have seen several patients in whom the disorder was typical of Harada's disease on presentation and yet acceptable for placoid pigment epitheliopathy at 7 days.

Gass: Harada's?

Bird: We are talking about a matter of nomenclature. Such patients might be diagnosed as having Harada's disease initially, but the subsequent behavior makes that diagnosis difficult to sustain. Our main argument is one of pathogenesis, and I suggest that such patients with widely differing appearances may all be suffering from choroidal ischemia.

Gass: I see. Does anybody have any questions or comments about vitiliginous or birdshot choroidopathy? No problems with making that diagnosis? I would like to ask the panel concerning the relationship of vitiliginous choroiditis to so-called senile vitritis, which also typically occurs in patients, mostly women 50 years and older, and which is unassociated with vitiliginous patches posteriorly. They may, however, have a more diffuse mottled alteration of the pigment epithelium in the periphery, and some develop a few or scattered, deep, very sharply circumscribed zones of atrophy of the pigment epithelium in the periphery of the fundus. Do you have any feelings about those two groups of patients?

Ryan: Don, I agree with the way you have described and distinguished senile vitritis from the entity listed in your paper as vitiliginous and what other people recognize as birdshot choroidopathy. These cream colored or yellowish lesions of atrophy of the retinal pigment epithelium in the posterior pole, and lots of cells in the vitreous in a group of people 40 to 50 years old, make the basis for this diagnosis. There is support for identifying and grouping cases of a particular disease entity, such as you've made in the past for the DUSN or disease entities before you understand the etiology, as in birdshot choroidopathy. Bob Nusenblatt at the NIH [National Institutes of Health] has taken a series of about eight cases that I have seen in California and at least a similar number from Wilmer and have found them all to have a similar HLA group—A29. This association is statistically significant, you know, beyond a shadow of a doubt. My point is that this is a particular group of patients that does seem predisposed to developing this type of finding, which these patients with birdshot do have.

Gass: These are patients that may not have birdshot choroidopathy. Do they just have the vitritis?

Ryan: No, these patients with birdshot choroidopathy are compared with other examples of intraocular inflammatory disease, including pars-planitis.

Gass: They have included those other cases?

Ryan: I know for sure that they have looked for pars-planitis. Whether they have put in patients with senile vitritis, I can't tell you with certainty.

Gass: All right. One final question. Do the panelists see patients with DUSN or the unilateral wipe-out syndrome? I would particularly like to ask Alan because I know he has been aware of the disease for quite a few years, and yet the last time I had a chance to talk to him he had only uncovered one case at Moorfields. The reason it is of interest is that much of the literature on *Toxocara canis* has come from Great Britain and yet DUSN is apparently very uncommon in Great Britain.

Bird: We have two cases, both from the West Indies; we have not seen one case of unilateral wipe-out syndrome who was born and brought up in England, and yet we are looking at a population where tests have shown a high incidence infection by *Toxocara canis*. It appears that *Toxocara canis* infection in London is not followed by this disorder.

Gass: Okay. Well, I think it's time to call this discussion to a close, and thank you very much.

AVOIDING RUPTURE OF BRUCH'S MEMBRANE IN FUNDUS PHOTOCOAGULATION

DR. MORTON F. GOLDBERG

Goldberg: ...in a generic sense, not just in sickle cell anemia. I think the principles do apply to other proliferative retinopathies such as diabetic retinopathy, branch vein occlusion, and also subretinal neovascular membranes in the posterior pole. In any event, in an attempt to close this fan-shaped neovascular patch, an extremely over-zealous attempt was made. In this case, it happened to be with an argon laser, and there are several areas of ruptures in Bruch's membrane and pigment epithelium. The intent of the therapist was to close the nutrient arterioles and to produce an infarction of the neovascular tissue, after which an attempt was made to close the draining venules. One can see small intense laser lesions, some of which have been complicated by hemorrhagic ruptures from the choroid through the full thickness of the retina into the preretinal space. In addition, even when hemorrhage did not complicate these very intense laser lesions, one can see evidence of ruptures at the level of Bruch's membrane and pigment epithelium in ovoid areas of pigment churning. In fact, the intent of the therapist was achieved acutely, in the sense that the blood supply of the fan-shaped patch of neovascularization was shut off. One can confirm that by the angiographic appearance. There is acute interruption of the nutrient vessels and draining venules, and the preretinal neovascular tissue is completely nonperfused. So, acutely at least, the therapist achieved his goal. Within a period of only 4 months, however, there arose from those rupture sites at the level of Bruch's membrane and pigment epithelium, an enormous fibrovascular stalk of tissue that grew from the choroid through the rupture site and retina into the vitreous. This intravitreal fibrovascular tissue can bleed spontaneously and interfere with visual acuity. Interestingly enough, patients who sustain iatrogenic ruptures of Bruch's membrane and pigment epithelium do not invariably get progressive intravitreal organization and hemorrhage. The abnormal blood vessels may remain tightly confined to the scar tissue in the chorioretinal plane. In monkey experiments we have been able to study Bruch's membrane histologically, and using large diameter burns, we found it difficult to rupture Bruch's membrane. In contrast, Bruch's membrane is more easily ruptured by a highly concentrated, small-diameter laser lesion. In order to show that this problem of rupturing Bruch's membrane, with subsequent growth of neovascular or anastomotic vessels, is not terribly predictable (hence the reason for asking the panelists their opinions on how to avoid it), let me show you an extreme case of a physicist, who in aligning an experimental dye laser, accidentally burned his own foveal pit. There was loss of vision to the count-fingers level and then a rather remarkable good return to 20/100. The acute lesion, within 2 hours of the burn, had blood emanating from the choroid in the center of the foveal pit and coming into the vitreous. This is perhaps somewhat similar, though not precisely identical, of course, to Dr. Ryan's experimental model; that is, it's in the posterior pole, and it's a very intense lesion. To my amazement, nothing happened to the vasculature despite the patient's developing a hole in the macula, with some puckering of an epiretinal membrane. There were no chorioretinal or retinochoroidal anastomoses and no neovascularization. So the problem of vascular growth after intense photocoagulation is a confusing one. The development of these vessels is not predictable, and it would appear, as I pointed out yesterday, that disruption of both the choroid and retina, with defects at the level of pigment epithelium and Bruch's membrane, is necessary but not sufficient for the development of these vessels. There must remain a variety of other factors, about which we have very little information, to explain why neovascular or anastomotic vessels occur or do not occur. Some of these possible stimuli include inflammation, infectious or noninfectious; ischemia at the level of the retina; ischemia at the level of the choroid; possible tumor-induced angiogenesis factors; and, of course, simple fibrovascular organization of a mechanical defect with capillary budding, ultimately with preferential channels of flow developing so that mature or neovascular capillary and arterial connections eventually develop. Fortunately, we have the world's experts here on traditional and innovative photocoagulation methods; so we can find out how to avoid these types of complications. Perhaps I can ask Wally McMeel because he has had the opportunity to photocoagulate for many years with ruby lasers, xenon arc, green lasers, blue lasers, krypton lasers, and so on. Bearing in mind different wavelengths, Wally, how would you avoid rupturing Bruch's membrane and the pigment epithelium?

McMeel: I don't think the wavelength itself is as important as some of the other factors that you have mentioned. I think the duration of the burn and the power density may be much more important. This is a very short burst that you mentioned here. One question that arises relates to the fact that the burn is only 10 nanoseconds; thus an ionizing effect rather than a thermal effect has probably occurred here. And as you see in the photograph, there seems to be a disciform, roundish lesion. Perhaps that is a shock wave from the impact. This may be the effect of that particular burn rather than a thermal effect. I think the power density and the time are the two main considerations. And as your studies have shown, it's the small spot size with high density that produces it.

Goldberg: Thank you, Wally. Alan Bird has reported some of the original work on the use of krypton lasers in disciform degeneration. Reading your paper carefully and trying to read between the lines, Alan, I notice that you do mention that hemorrhage is something that can occur in treating a disciform lesion. Is this liable to be more prevalent with krypton lasers than argon lasers, and, if so, is it caused by bleeding from the neovascular membrane or by rupturing Bruch's membrane with bleeding from underlying normal choroidal blood vessels or both?

Bird: There is a great deal of experimental evidence that suggests that a large proportion of energy from a krypton laser will be absorbed in the choroid rather than in the pigment epithelium when compared with argon. This will result in high-energy absorption by choroidal melanocytes; there appears to be a different wavelength absorption between choroidal melanocytes and pigment epithelial cells. When treating disciform lesions and undertaking peripheral ablations, I notice that hemorrhages do appear to occur, and it is presumed that these are derived from the choroidal capillaries. Histopathologic evidence supports this conclusion. Whether this can be equated to rupture of Bruch's membrane or not is hard to say.

When considering the effects of photocoagulation on Bruch's membrane and in particular the relevance of this to the proliferation of blood vessels beneath the retina, I cannot believe that rupture of Bruch's membrane is the sole factor of importance. There is good evidence that Bruch's membrane represents a barrier to blood-vessel growth, and this is well shown during development. I think we should be considering what changes are necessary in Bruch's membrane to allow blood vessels to transgress this barrier and specifically whether rupture is the correct term to use. In the elderly, Bruch's membrane becomes thinned or altered, and Bruch's membrane is severely disrupted wherever macrophages collect within the sub–pigment epithelial debris. This implies that when treatment is applied to the elderly, Bruch's membrane is already quite abnormal when compared with the young. After photocoagulation there is frequent ingress of macrophages, and this alone may be sufficient to compromise Bruch's membrane further, such that it no longer represents a barrier to blood vessel growth. I think it more sensible to consider the circumstances that alter Bruch's membrane and generate blood vessel growth rather than confining the discussion to physical rupture.

Goldberg: On the issue of the krypton laser, could you tell us what precautions, if any, you take in treating in the posterior pole, to avoid hemorrhage of any sort, particularly in comparison with the more traditional argon-laser modality?

Bird: We tend to be much more careful in increasing the power levels when using the krypton laser than we are with the argon laser. Some certainly believe that quite small increases in power above that necessary to create adequate thermal coagulation may be sufficient to precipitate visually damaging hemorrhage.

Goldberg: And what is your visual stopping point in treating a disciform lesion with a krypton laser?

Bird: Our stopping point is definite opacification of the outer retina and pigment epithelium, but we do not attempt to obtain the dense white opacification that others believe is the correct end point. Arnall Patz may wish to comment on this later.

Goldberg: Could you just give us a sample set of physical parameters with which you begin treating a disciform lesion with a krypton laser: time, power, spot size, and so on?

Bird: We always use 200 μm at 0.2 second initially, but we may increase this to 0.5 second and the initial power setting would be about 300 mW with krypton, increasing this slowly up to 600 or 700 mW. It is rare that we have to go above 700 mW.

Goldberg: Thank you very much. Arnall, what is your approach to using a krypton laser in a disciform lesion, and how do you avoid hemorrhagic complications?

Patz: The parameters that Alan just mentioned are essentially what we were using. We have deliberately gone to a whiter, more intense lesion than what Dr. Bird has used and some other investigators have published. The reason for that has been that in patients who had a recurrence—or at least where we've not completely eradicated the neovascularization around the edge of the lesion—it seems that those were areas that were of less intensity as we look back over the pictures, and it is for that reason that we have gone to a whiter burn. We don't aim for that four-plus white reaction that you try to achieve with the argon laser treating neovascularization, but I think it would be one degree (in other words in terms of one, two, three, four-plus) more intense white than what Dr. Bird has used.

Goldberg: Do you think you are more likely to get hemorrhages with a krypton laser used in the posterior pole than with an argon laser?

Patz: I would say, yes. I have not seen a hemorrhage treated with the argon laser in recent years. I have had approximately 10% of the krypton-treated cases with a very small hemorrhage at the time of treatment that caused no problem.

Goldberg: Thank you, Arnall. Bob Watzke, do you have any comment on avoiding these kinds of complications with any form of photocoagulation?

Watzke: I always tell anybody who is doing this that you don't throw a dart at a balloon and you don't use a small spot size, particularly when treating disciform lesions, never anything less—that is, for treatment not outlining—and I know we are supposed to outline it, and we do on the Macular Photocoagulation Study, though I really don't quite see the need for that in some cases; but I never use less than a 200 μm spot size. If you start out with 500 μm and you are treating close to the foveal avascular zone, you will get such a spread that you almost can't stop treating soon enough. If you get too ambitious and go up to 500, or 400 with 200 μm spot size, you very frequently will get a hemorrhage. And never less than 0.2 second. If the patient has a good retrobulbar block, I like to use 0.5 second because I can control the size and intensity of the lesion. After you make that first exposure, you know what you have to do. You can increase it a bit, or you have got it just right, or you. can decrease it a bit.

Goldberg: Thank you, Bob. Steve Ryan, first, do you have any advice for avoiding these kinds of complications, and, second, do you have any explanation for the clinical course followed by that physicist who burned his foveal pit? Would that be analogous to your experiments, or is it quite different?

Ryan: In terms of specific aspects of treatment, I would basically endorse what the other panelists have said, and I also will use it only to outline a smaller spot size, but for therapy never use less than 200 μm spot size. I use 0.2 second exposure and, with the patient's cooperation, 0.5 second, and I start at a low energy and increase to the energy that's required. In terms of that particular physicist, Mort, I have heard Wally's explanation, and I wonder again, when you've got such a tremendous energy pulse going in there, whether that is in fact similar to what we really attribute to a thermal effect. There is another area, though, as Wally had pointed out, and I would be interested in what you other members of the panel thought when you saw that whitish area that was so extensive. It suggested to me interference with the choroidal circulation possibly at that area, and this energy might, in fact, just have been so intense that it burned back through and destroyed some of the larger feeding vessels as well. In other words, it's a question of just how much is available there for response. You can always argue that eventually you are going to get to the edge of that burn, and something might be able to grow back in, but my point is that you would have had such extensive destruction and there would have been so many macrophages moving in that area that they might not have called out the vascular response. This does bring me to one other aspect, though, in relation to your and my discussion yesterday with Alan Bird. I think that when we are talking about factors that are important to induce subretinal neovascularization after photocoagulation, I very much agree with you that a break or rupture or alteration in Bruch's membrane alone is certainly not enough. And we have enough clinical evidence to support this concept. I think there is a very key role for extracellular factors that are calling out this response. And there is something fundamentally different about blood vessels in the retinal space versus blood vessels in the choroidal space. If you stop and analyze where you find the fenestrations in the normal choriocapillaris in its normal state, it is on the retinal side, whereas you don't see those fenestrations on the scleral side. This observation suggests that there is some extracellular control in the eye telling those vessels that this is the retinal side to open and teleologically to provide the nutrition getting across to the retina. So I think there is very definitely a real role for extracellular control of whether these vessels are open and fenestrated or not. Is the presence of fenestrations just a factor of maturation and growth of these vessels over time, or is it really that different spaces in different extracellular environments produce a very different effect on blood vessels?

Goldberg: Thank you, Steve. Jack Coleman, do you have any advice for avoiding these kinds of complications?

Coleman: I am not totally convinced that the rupture of the tunica ruyschiana or the Bruch's membrane is all that destructive. I think the main concept concerns the edge of the lesion. Should treatment be excessive whether with xenon arc or laser, an additional margin of lighter treatment is afforded to constrict neighboring vessels so that the chances of vessel bleeding is far less. I think the complications in the patient you showed may in part be patterning that was followed. Certain areas of Bruch's membrane were ruptured with sharp margins. My own treatment in this disease is relatively heavy, but I deliberately defocus the beam I am using so that the edges of the lesion are less sharp. I do not recall the complication of neovascularization of the type that you have shown.

Goldberg: Thank you, Jack. Don Gass, aside from not treating at all, how do we avoid these problems?

Gass: I have one comment. I do use 50 and 100 μm under certain circumstances. In the presence of nuclear sclerosis it may be difficult to get the desired intense burn with larger spot sizes. Also, a 50 μm aperture may in fact produce a 500 μm–sized burn because of light scatter. I would like to make one additional comment—it's related to one already made. I don't think breaks in Bruch's membrane are required for blood vessels to go through Bruch's membrane. When you realize that diseases such as Best's disease and rubella retinopathy are complicated by choroidal neovascularization, there is reason to suspect that, under appropriate stimulation, possibly capillary tufts arising from the choriocapillaris may invade and perforate Bruch's membrane. This may also occur in response to photocoagulation damage to the choriocapillaris–Bruch's membrane complex. It has been estimated that as high as 5% of people with idiopathic central serous retinopathy treated with low-intensity laser burns will develop choroidal neovascularization. Although there is always the possibility in some that new vessels were hidden from view before treatment, this observation suggests that even a minimal amount of laser may call forth blood vessels into the subretinal space.

Goldberg: Thank you.

EALES' SYNDROME

DR. ALAN C. BIRD

Bird: I would like to show three cases that I believe fall into the category of Eales' syndrome, though members of the panel may wish to dispute the use of this term in connection with these patients. The first patient has edema of the posterior retina, leakage from retinal capillaries and from major vessels in the posterior pole, and peripheral retinal leakage and in the far periphery retinal vessel closure. The second patient has a similar complex of fundus changes except that the peripheral closure is more pronounced and there are forward vessels on the optic disc. This patient was treated with corticosteroids, and on this regime the forward vessels resolved, implying that inflammation as well as closure is important in causing vessel growth in this patient. The final patient shows an extreme example of the end stage of Eales' syndrome. This is a 26-year-old woman who had suffered repeated vitreous hemorrhages from 18 to 20 years of age and thereafter had been free of further attacks. The fundus shows major distortion of the vessels of the posterior retina, confluent peripheral closure to within 20 degrees of the fovea, and a peripheral part of the perfused retina with a very simplified capillary system. Photographs of the other eye show identical changes.

These patients illustrate the difficulties of defining Eales' syndrome. It is difficult to use Eales' original concept of the disorder, which he characterized as including recurrent vitreous hemorrhages and epistaxis in nervous, constipated young men of southern England. If one is to identify patients in current practice likely to represent the modern eqivalent of this disorder, it would consist of patients whose fundi show peripheral vessel closure and forward vessel growth for which no cause is found. The question arises as to whether intraocular inflammation is part of the disorder and what ocular changes would be acceptable. Inflammation may be reflected as retinal vasculitis only, such as major leakage around retinal veins. All such patients are likely to have retinal capillary leakage also. Under these circumstances it is most unlikely that the vitreous will be normal, particularly if there have been vitreous hemorrhages. It seems unlikely, therefore, that one can insist on a normal vitreous for such a patient to fall in the definition of Eales' syndrome.

The major threats to vision appear to be macular edema, vitreous hemorrhage, and traction detachment.

I would like members of the panel to consider three aspects of the disorder, namely, definition of the disorder, cause of the disorder, and management of the disorder. First, Mort, do you have any strong ideas as to the definition of Eales' syndrome, except that it is not sickle cell disease?

Goldberg: It's definitely not sickle cell retinopathy, but in many cases the angiographic appearance is identical. I don't mean virtually identical I mean absolutely identical. The best evidence for that comes from the work of Manfred Spitzas, who has studied a large population of patients with Eales' disease in Germany. I would return to your point about this being a heterogeneous group of diseases. I think you have shown us several different diseases in this slide presentation, Alan. I do not think they are necessarily the same underlying disease. Actually, I always enjoy citing Henry Eales' original paper, as you did, because Eales' original description, as you pointed out, includes epistaxis and constipation associated with vitreoretinal hemorrhage in young men. Now, if you are a purist, that's Eales' disease. Historically, however, it then became associated with true tuberculous periphlebitis, and there is ample histopathologic evidence in the older literature, including some nice reproductions in the Duke-Elder *System of Ophthalmology,* of true tuberculous periphlebitis associated with recurrent vitreous hemorrhage. Subsequently, in the evolution of the use of the name "Eales' disease," it became associated with any form of retinal periphlebitis. Many of those cases, in retrospect, probably had sarcoid or other diseases about whose cause we know very little. And most recently of all, the term has been used variously by different people to mean either peripheral idiopathic vascular closure with secondary arteriovenous connections, as Spitzas has used the term, or, as is widely used in this country, any form of vitreous hemorrhage associated with idiopathic preretinal neovascularization. Now, whether that's the proper use of the term is anybody's guess. It is a widespread definition, however, in this country. In practical terms, when we see patients with preretinal neovascularization, we put patients through a fairly extensive systemic evaluation, looking for evidence of diabetes, sickle cell disease, systemic hypertension with branch vein occlusion, sarcoid, emboli from talc, atrial myxomas, floppy mitral valves, or rheumatic fever, and rare diseases such as incontinentia pigmenti and dominantly inherited exudative vitreoretinopathy. After we have done all that and go through a list of 15 to 18 entities, we are left with a grab bag where we cannot make a specific diagnosis. That's what we're calling "Eales' disease."

Bird: Can I ask you how many patients are left without a diagnosis when you have undertaken full testing? Are you left with 98% of your total or have you eliminated a large proportion of your patients?

Goldberg: We eliminate most. I'd say we eliminate approximately 90%. This fundus abnormality may represent different diseases around the world. I have had the same experience that you have had in India. For example at the Sitapur Eye Hospital, which is a 1300-bed eye hospital, there is a permanent sign on a door to a large ward that says "Eales' disease", and there are roughly 40 people lying there at any given time who have Eales' disease. That is more than I have seen in my entire lifetime of ophthalmic experience in North America.

Bird: Our experience is not similar to yours. Of our patients with chronic intraocular inflammation, vasculitis, and closure, the majority do not appear to have sarcoid or any other recognizable basic disorder. Would other members of the panel care to consider this problem, and, specifically, is Eales' syndrome a useful term?

Patz: I find it useful as a "wastebasket" term when you can't put a handle on it, as Mort just mentioned. I would add, in terms of your history, that you ought to check the birth weight of the patient. I would like to ask Dr. Bird, or anyone, how many times he has had the occasion to test the vestibular auditory apparatus because, I think you know, Alan, on the survey that we did with Bob Murphy on all or our patients with Eales' disease almost 50% of them had some vestibular abnormality, and I just wondered if you have had an opportunity to examine your patients or if you are aware of that particular associated finding?

Bird: We have not undertaken vestibular testing in our patients. Have others undertaken such a survey?

O'Connor: No.

Bird: I remember during my year in Miami it was considered that Eales' syndrome did not exist. Is this other people's impression?

O'Connor: We encounter it very rarely in our clinic. But there are certain subgroups in our West-Coast population that may have it. One group is an American Indian group; another is a group of aboriginal people from Alaska for surveys. Now, both of these groups, for what it's worth, generally have genetically determined immunodeficient responses to the tubercle bacillus, and both of these groups still have a considerable amount of phlyctenulosis, which we believe may represent a special kind of hypersensitivity to tuberculoprotein. That element of the disease cannot be totally neglected. Now, as you pointed out, some of the patients appear to have associated inflammatory disease in the more anterior parts of the eye, including the vitreous, whereas others do not. I have seen several patients with so-called Eales' disease that have iridocyclitis as well. So I believe that there is an inflammatory component to the disease, and this is a contradiction to the material that Ashton and Eva Kohner have described. They are not calling it an occlusive vasculopathy to differentiate it from a true inflammation. I think their study is open to some question because much of the autopsy material that they have reviewed represents burned-out cases where there was nothing left but organized thrombus in the vessels. They did not in fact see inflammatory disease, but they may have examined the tissue at a late date when it was impossible to detect inflammatory change.

Bird: I would agree that inflammation must be acceptable within the context of Eales' syndrome. Steve, do you have anything to add?

Ryan: I think the question of definition of terms and the role of intraocular inflammation is of fundamental importance. "Eales' disease" is a very broad term with different meanings for different individuals. Mort has clearly recounted the history nicely in terms of Eales' disease or syndrome and its gradually splitting off entities. As an argument ad absurdum, if you were to describe intraocular inflammation in its broadest sense given the extent of retinitis and ischemia, BARN syndrome, as Don described it this morning, would probably qualify as Eales', depending on how extreme you want to be. I guess the place that I've found the term "Eales' disease" to be useful is the alternate term, that is, it's the "I-don't-know" retinal vasculitis or the "I-don't-know" retinal vascular disease, and that's not acceptable to the referring ophthalmologist or to the patient. And so, we nod our heads and wisely say "Eales' disease." Is your name the "wastebasket Eales' disease," or is it the "I-don't-know disease"?

McMeel: We've had two cases that fell into this general category that had really nothing wrong except a very highly positive tuberculin skin test, and they were treated and responded very, very nicely. So I think that's something that should be emphasized.

Bird: The possible presence of tuberculosis cannot be ignored in such patients. Tuberculosis was relatively uncommon in the United Kingdom 15 years ago but is now becoming more common again, particularly in immigrant communities. I would like to consider etiology before we discuss treatment. There are certain factors that cannot be ignored. Eales' syndrome is extremely common in India and becomes progressively less common as one travels west. In India it is frequently found that such patients have tuberculosis, but this is an attribute common to the population from which those patients are drawn. I would reiterate that in the vast majority of patients seen in England with Eales' syndrome, no systemic abnormalities are found. I would ask what investigations might be useful at this stage or in future what investigations are likely to help us in identifying the etiology of Eales' syndrome.

O'Connor: Well, it's only a guess, of course, but Eales' disease has certain parallels with Behçet's disease, which I am going to describe tomorrow in some detail. In both diseases there is abnormal leakage from veins before the time of occlusion, which seems to indicate some kind of an endothelial damage resulting possibly from inflammation. Now, I think that the evidence that Behçet's disease is an immune complex–mediated disease is now very strong, and maybe the same kind of information will eventually come out of Eales' disease. In other words, the disease probably represents a blend of environmental and immunogenetic stimuli that leads patients to express vascular disease in a certain way. Whatever the immunogenetics of the groups that get Eales' disease, it may be their exposure to tuberculosis or to the pathogens of other infectious diseases or it may be the trigger that sparks the deposition of immune complexes in their vessels and ultimately the occlusion of those vessels. So one of the leads that might be pursued is a longitudinal study of the immune complex levels in the circulating blood of patients with Eales' disease. It might not turn up anything, but if I were to push one lead, that's one thing I might suggest. I might also suggest HLA typing, particularly for B and D types. Those are the two HLA's that seem to influence the pattern of immunologic expression.

Bird: We should now consider management. What treatment should be given to a patient with peripheral vessel closure and forward new vessels but no history of vitreous hemorrhage? Management will depend to some extent on the risk of vitreous hemorrhage or, if there has been minor hemorrhage, the risk of further major hemorrhage.

Goldberg: It's almost a matter of definition, isn't it? If the diagnosis of Eales' disease requires vitreous hemorrhage, they all have it. To discuss therapy really requires that we focus in on the minimal essential criteria for making the diagnosis. For the moment, let's think of the type of case you're referring to: preretinal neovascularization surrounded by vascular closure—let's say also, there may be some sheathing of adjacent venules. In that situation, the chance of spontaneous bleeding is rather high, and I'm in the habit of recommending intervention. I recognize that the burden of proof is always on the person who recommends prophylactic therapy, and I have no proof that this is effective in this group of patients because their number in this country, at least defined as the way I have defined them, is rather small. But we treat them as we treat sickle cell retinopathy. If the neovascularization is extensive and highly elevated and has had a large white fibroglial component, then we will use a feeder vessel technique of argon laser photocoagulation. If the lesions are small and relatively flat and don't have too much in the way of a white fibrous component, we'll do a limited panretinal photocoagulation around them to reduce the complications of the feeder-vessel technique. I have also had the same experience you mentioned, in which neovascularization occurred in the posterior pole in association with active panvasculitis, and that responded dramatically to steroid administration. In my experience that's a very unusual circumstance.

Bird: If you believe there is a major inflammatory component, it would be worth trying corticosteroids initially.

Goldberg: I wouldn't have called it "Eales' disease," but I would have treated that unknown disorder with steroids first, yes.

Bird: Okay. Wallace?

McMeel: After getting a PPD [purified protein derivative], I would trust?

Goldberg: Yes, of course.

Bird: Would it make any difference if forward vessels were identified with little closure as opposed to major peripheral vessel closure?

Goldberg: I wouldn't call it Eales' disease. I don't know whether I am correct in being quite so narrow in my definition, but I wouldn't call it "Eales' disease." I have seen preretinal neovascularization in the posterior pole associated with diffuse panvasculitis. I think it was similar to one of the patients you have shown, where virtually every capillary could be seen on the angiogram to be dilated and leaking profusely. There the new vessels arise not in association with local, adjacent zones of ischemia, and I think the pathogenesis of the neovascularization there has nothing to do with hypoxic retina but is related more to local products of inflammation or inflammatory cells, macrophages, or chronic leakage, as Hayreh has recently hypothesized. In that situation, focal obliteration of the neovascular tissue, at least in my hands, has been successful and has not been dangerous. Steroids may also be used.

Bird: Jackson?

Coleman: Those that I have treated with only low-grade inflammation by photocoagulation and even cryopexy, depending on how far in the periphery they were, have done well. Those that have had moderate-to-severe inflammatory change we have been very loath to treat. Recently I did a vitrectomy in one eye because of the hemorrhage and a tractional detachment with a good result.

Bird: Steve?

Ryan: If I can say that again, I admire your courage, Alan, in asking us to discuss Eales' when you hear how we are defining it. And you might be getting very different answers because of how people are using the term up here on the panel. But, to me, I think Mort's point is well taken in terms of how much inflammation determines whether or not you even try steroids. Before doing laser photocoagulation, I insist on hemorrhage at least once, before going ahead and treating them. I haven't treated them on a strictly prophylactic basis, but if they have hemorrhaged once and then clear sufficiently, I go ahead and then do an ablative type of therapy in those particular cases.

Bird: Arnall?

Patz: I'd like to qualify Steve's comment; that is, I would not treat the neovascularization just because it was there, unless there are new vessels in the disc and I see it *increasing* in size probably a little bigger than a standard 10-A DRS photograph, that is, larger than a third of a disc diameter. I would then do treatment of the nonperfused area coming all the way to the disc in that patient, with active proliferation of the disc vessels.

Bird: I would have severe reservations about prophylactic treatment of forward new vessels under these circumstances, since many patients may develop local traction and detachment and this may be precipitated or aggravated by photocoagulation. We have several young patients with traction detachment of retina after photocoagulation of peripheral new vessels. There is no good indication as to the risk of such patients developing vitreous hemorrhage, and I think it is reasonable to wait for hemorrhage before considering treatment. In general, the initial hemorrhage is often quite small and does not necessarily preclude photocoagulation. I would also consider that if there are significant signs of inflammation corticosteroids should be tried initially. I certainly accept that vitrectomies can be undertaken when there is traction detachment, but this may not always be easy and may not be particularly well tolerated by the eye.

O'Connor: I would just like to comment for a minute about steroid therapy. Again, I have no large experience with this disease, but if it's anything at all like Behçet's disease, the patients may appear to show a beneficial response to corticosteroids early in the course of the disease. But later, after there has been considerable occlusion of vessels, they seem to show almost no response. It almost seems as though steroid therapy might be deleterious at this time. In other words, it is as though corticosteroids were occlusogenic in the same way that systemic corticosteroid therapy may lead to peripheral vein thrombosis in the legs. So I question the value of steroid therapy late in the course of the disease.

Bird: It is interesting that once the disorder has progressed beyond a certain point the risk of vitreous hemorrhage may become progressively less. In a situation where peripheral closure is extreme and there is total vitreous detachment, the risk of new vessel growth is small. The situation is reached where vitreoretinal contact is limited to nonperfused retina, such that there is no posterior hyaloid scaffolding upon which forward new vessels can grow.

In summary, Eales' disease is hard to define clinically, and it is made much more difficult by the lack of concrete information concerning its etiology. There is no doubt that such patients are uncommon in England, but the lack of effective therapy renders this disorder a significant clinical problem in specialized practice. Our difficulties do not compare with those in India where this disorder is extremely common, and there is little doubt that any major advance in therapy would have a major impact on clinical practice in that country. I would like to thank the panel for an interesting and informative discussion.

VITRECTOMY IN DIABETES

DR. STEPHEN J. RYAN

Ryan: I would like to show you an interesting case of diabetes that remains the leading indication for vitrectomy. What I would like to ask the panel, and maybe bring out for those of you here in the audience, is to review our current indications for vitrectomy in proliferative diabetic retinopathy and specifically some of the complications, notably neovascularization of the iris and secondary glaucoma and how we might propose managing those. Understandably, not everyone on the panel might be involved with vitrectomy in diabetes, but if you do have views of your own or those of your centers, it certainly will help to keep the rest of us honest. Vitrectomy is ideal to clear the opacity in the media, and our most common indication today is to relieve traction on the retina and resultant tractional detachments. And it has been argued from the series of Ron Michels and Tom Rice as well as George Blankenship that basically a good result at 6 months tends to be a good result at 5 years. I think that we can utilize some of Ron's slides and very nice diagrams that he has put together at Wilmer and just comment briefly on pathogenesis as background information for this discussion. Clearly there is a question initially with proliferative diabetic retinopathy and then with the process going on to vitreous hemorrhage and traction developing, and the fundamental importance of posterior vitreous separation at that time in the process, which then go on to repeated hemorrhage, that proliferation of vessels and tractional detachment is a vicious cycle. But the surgical objectives we realize are to clear the media, to release traction, to divide bridging membranes, and to dissect epiretinal membranes. So, in other words, we start off by trying to cut the anteroposterior traction, relieving the bridging membranes, and then dissecting the epiretinal membranes. As Ron and Gary Leeds and Tom Hengst have shown, there are aspects of relief of the anteroposterior tractions that help relieve the other tractions. Again, this is our concept in terms of relieving traction, and we certainly can do far more than we could a few years ago.

As an illustration there is the case of a young teacher that I had occasion to see some 3 years ago, and I followed him until his macula detached. We then intervened at that time and were able to get a successful result in his left eye. His right eye, however, as you can see, was again a sitting duck in terms of going on to develop similar problems. He was not someone who responded to laser photocoagulation by his ophthalmologist, and again this is to show the progression and what goes on with him. The point is that the left eye had done satisfactorily. This patient had done satisfactorily in both eyes and achieved and maintained 20/30 vision by waiting for his macula to detach. So I think the key question that we'll be asking the panel initially to discuss, if we have a patient like this that may not respond to laser photocoagulation—and I know that Jack Coleman and others have certainly commented and written on this topic—is, What is the role for vitrectomy in management of such cases of active profuse proliferation of new blood vessels as an indication for vitrectomy?

Here's another case where you can have extensive hemorrhage. You can see that there is disc proliferation, and again Mort might want to comment in terms of krypton laser photocoagulation, as he mentioned yesterday, or Arnall or other members of the panel. I have given it away (this is a case that was in the DRVS [Diabetic Retinopathy Vitrectomy Study]) as to how we approach this. But the first series of questions for the panel will relate to the indications for vitrectomy. Now it wouldn't be fair if we didn't point out that obviously we have significant complications. So how do we manage neovascularization of the iris and secondary glaucoma? And I think we will agree that if there is retinal detachment, the first order of business is to reattach the retina. But what do we do with neovascularization of the iris, and how do we manage this problem? Thus we have a fairly complicated series of questions for the panel. We must first address ourselves to the question of the role of vitrectomy and proliferative diabetic retinopathy.

Specifically, first, what are the indications for when you would consider vitrectomy in vitreous hemorrhage? Second, how do you approach traction detachments of the macula? If the macula is detached, how long after it is detached would you operate? And also would you consider surgery for a "macular threatening detachment"? A third group of potential surgical candidates is that group where we showed extensive neovascularization, and a fourth group would be any others that you would care to comment on in terms of the role of vitrectomy as an indication, or what indications there are in proliferative diabetic retinopathy. As I said, perhaps we can start—if you yourself are not doing these, or if you have opinions from your center you would care to relay—that would be perfectly agreeable with the rest of us. Wally, would you start that series of questions?

McMeel: First of all, I think your initial slide with the four different categories is a very convenient way of looking at the overall problem in that there is an escalating degree of capability and risk in each of those four, with the hemorrhage, your anteroposterior traction, then the membrane, and then ultimately the preretinal peeling. I think that most people in the audience know that there is the DRVS going on, and one aspect of it relates to vitreous hemorrhage and the other relates to the second and third, the more advanced stages of change that we have to deal with. The hemorrhage group of the DRVS has been divided into the early and late vitrectomy groups. I don't think that there is anyone at this point who argues that vitrectomy is indicated for the group of patients with severe hemorrhage. It's a matter of timing. We were trying to find out which one is the preferable one. The present consensus is that vitreous hemorrhage is a prime indication for vitrectomy. On AP traction, my own feeling is that if there has been no vitreal hemorrhage and the macula is still on, I would not operate on them. If the macula is being elevated, the vision is down to about 20/100 or 20/200, and there is a documentation of progression, one can go ahead. Also there are cases where one is having repetitive hemorrhage, and the buildup of the fibrotic aspects of the proliferation can be seen, and there may not be the traction at the macula as yet—it's still flat—but the vision is down to the level of 20/100, 20/200, not bad enough to be included in the hemorrhagic group for the DRVS, but it's a deteriorating eye and in those instances I think that vitrectomy is indicated. I would also like to interject here that in these eyes that are really very florid, as one of this group was, we still have to keep in mind the pituitary ablation, which still has a limited place. It need not be used alone. Right now we are using it with cases that also have photocoagulation and vitrectomy, and maybe then they reduce this late complication of iris neovascularization in an eye that has had pituitary ablation.

Ryan: Wally, would you give the rest of us some perspective, roughly, how many times per year would you guess from your group, or the group that you work with there, that pituitary ablation is performed?

McMeel: Maybe three or four. It's really very infrequently. But it is something that shouldn't be totally written off.

Ryan: Could the rest of the panel maybe comment on that before we go on to ask Don his views and perspective on where vitrectomy belongs in the midst of this? Alan, do you want to make a comment on what you think pituitary ablation is useful for?

Bird: Pituitary ablation is rarely if ever undertaken now in London for diabetic retinopathy, though it was firmly believed at one stage that it was helpful under certain limited circumstances. It appeared that pituitary ablation was the only treatment that could truly cause the disease to become reversed, though it did not appear to affect the longevity of the patient; there were certain sudden unexplained deaths in patients who had pituitary ablation. It seemed that life was not extended but the quality of life was better since sight was maintained. We have not come to the position yet where we believe that this treatment is indefensible, but experience suggests that the indications must be extremely limited.

Goldberg: I think the role of pituitary ablation is still an important one for limited indications, as Wally McMeel has said. It's still tough to communicate with people as to precisely what forms of diabetic retinopathy might be best served by utilizing a pituitary ablation approach. I find the term "rubeosis retinae," rubeosis of the retina, helpful in that respect. I would have used it with one of your cases, Steve, where the virtual sheet of naked neovascular tissue was proliferating over the posterior pole. Particularly if those vessels involve the papillomacular bundle and macula itself, an indirect approach to therapy, such as that with the pituitary, seems to be useful. I would agree also with Wally that the number of times one recommends it is very limited. In my own experience, it is only about once every 18 months or so, but for those with exceptional cases it does appear to be a useful last-ditch measure.

Ryan: Jack, before you went to Cornell, New York Hospital was a center where a lot of pituitary ablation was done. What is your opinion?

Coleman: I don't use it at all. My own view in dealing with retinopathy cases that don't respond to laser is to consider a vitrectomy, at least in the first involved eye. I did, as you mentioned, a series of 15 eyes with disease of this type. There were seeing eyes, that is, 20/20 to 20/40 eyes, without any serious complications, at least attributible to surgery. One of them did bleed later and went on to 20/200 with disc and macular changes, but by removing the posterior membrane of the vitreous, the scaffold for these disc vessels is gone. They do not recur. The bleeding complication I had was one that bled anteriorly, perhaps from the scleral wounds or iris. One other complication I had was that we missed a strand of vitreous that remained attached to one of the blood vessels. The traction was ominous, but it has not been a problem yet.

Ryan: Arnall?

Patz: We have not used pituitary ablation at Hopkins in the last 8 years, and I have one case that I would like to briefly refer to. It's a patient of Dr. Thad Prout. He is a nationally recognized diabetologist, who had a patient undergo pituitary ablation.

According to his appraisal on the endocrinology result, this patient had very effective pituitary ablation. The patient's retinopathy was very definitely asymmetric; that is, there were very large disc vessels with vitreous hemorrhage in the right eye, and the left eye had only mild proliferative retinopathy with no disc vessels; within 2 years after the pituitary ablation, the left disc proliferation looked very much like the picture that you showed of the very severe proliferation. So this is a patient who, at least metabolically, had all the signs of good pituitary ablation and who progressed and was documented to show this severe progression of the proliferation at the disc after pituitary surgery. Of course, one case obviously doesn't prove that the procedure is ineffective, but we have not subscribed to it, at least during the last 7 years.

Ryan: So, now that we can demonstrate to everyone our unanimity of opinion and how we can make it more easy for all of you to understand how we approach things, maybe back to the question of vitrectomy and vitreous hemorrhages.

Don, Bascom Palmer and Robert Machemer have certainly got us all going in this area. Do you have any perspectives as you've watched George Blankenship and co-workers go on through diabetes and vitrectomy?

Gass: Steve, I don't think I could really add much to what Wally said. I really don't know the specific indications at this moment in regard to what stage the diabetic with vitreous hemorrhage gets a vitrectomy. I think that most of the patients coming to the [Bascom Palmer] Eye Institute that will fit into those studies that are now ongoing are put into those studies. I know there is still a reluctance to operate on patients with tractional detachments that still have good central vision, and I know that there is still a general feeling that the patients you showed with massive proliferation of blood vessels on the disc and out around beyond the disc have a fairly bad prognosis no matter what you do.

Ryan: Dick, any comments?

O'Connor: Our university is part of the DRVS, and we've generally followed the tenets laid down for that study group. There is, of course, a waiting period after vitreous hemorrhage before anything is done, and that generally is somewhere between 6 and 9 months. I am quite convinced that the procedure of vitrectomy does remove the scaffolding for the proliferation of retinal vessels, and I think that I have seen quite a few people helped. But the final analysis of the study is the proof of the pudding.

Ryan: Bob?

Watzke: Well, our approach, since we are not members of the DRVS, is a very practical one. We have excellent echography, and we don't operate on fresh vitreous hemorrhage. We follow these patients very closely. As long as there is no traction detachment developing, we tend to wait at least 6 months, sometimes longer, particularly if there is vision in the second eye and if there is no developing rubeosis. If there is a tractional detachment, it is watched carefully, and when it seems to be progressive, we don't wait for the macula to detach. That pushes us into an early vitrectomy.

Ryan: Jack, would you care to address all of those issues and specifically, in addition to the time of the hemorrhage, the aspect of ''macula-threatening detachments'' and then the so-called rubeosis retinae type of appearance and anything else you would care to comment on?

Coleman: A vitrectomy procedure is a serious operation to consider. In the best of hands the chances of a complication are at least 10%, including retinal detachment, hemorrhage from the incision site, lens change, infection, or some other problem. I always tell a patient that there is a considerable risk. Clearly the risks escalate, as Steve's slide has shown. If a patient presents with a fresh hemorrhage and sees well with the other eye, I see no reason to recommend surgery. There is every reason to think that a fresh hemorrhage will clear, and it may also produce a retraction or synchysis of the vitreous so that there may be less likelihood that a worse problem may arise. On the other hand, if it's the patient's only eye and he isn't able to function or work, then the time before considering vitreous surgery is shortened, and I would recommend surgery in as little as 2 or 3 months, particularly if it is a very dense hemorrhage that does not indicate any clearing in that time. Once the macula is threatened with the appearance of a progressive traction change developing, I recommend surgery. Concerning the proglem with disc neovascularization, I really believe that this is a matter for the surgeon with his experience to decide. Even dense vascular changes can be photocoagulated inside the eye with endocautery, endophotocoagulation, and endocryopexy. These techniques combined with a gas tamponade reduce much of our concern. I think a major factor has to be the patient and the progression of the disease, particularly in regard to the status of the other eye; for example, loss of macular function in a second eye may merit more radical procedure—as long as the patient understands the risk factor you are describing to him.

Ryan: Mort?

Goldberg: In contemplating vitrectomy for a diabetic patient, I think one has to consider not only the overall success rate, which is not dramatically high—it's of the order of magnitude of 50%, perhaps 65% in very good hands—but one also has to consider the complication rates if one is going to do a clear-vitreous vitrectomy before the macula is actually involved in a tractional detachment. What are the potential complications that could occur from prophylactic surgery? They are really quite substantial, including rubeosis iridis, which again, in the best of hands, has been reported in up to 25% or 33% of cases—cataracts, glaucoma, and so on. If membrane stripping, along with all the other techniques of vitrectomy, is carried out, there is a high incidence of iatrogenic intraoperative holes in the perimacular distribution. This certainly interferes with anatomic and visual rehabilitation. I would come back to the issue of rubeosis and point out that it is probably the least well understood and the least well treated disease in modern ophthalmology, and yet it is a very common complication of vitrectomy in diabetic patients. The incidence of postoperative rubeosis increases when any of the following has already been present: first, *preoperative* rubeosis; second, extensive neovascularization of the retina; and third, detachment of the retina. So we adopt a very conservative point of view, bearing these considerations in mind; namely, a success rate that is not overwhelmingly high and a complication rate that is not insignificantly low. In practical terms, we would therefore generally wait 6 months with a vitreous hemorrhage of 20/200 acuity or worse and not operate on a tractional detachment until the macula actually became involved.

Ryan: Thank you. I think maybe to just briefly try to summarize. Clearly we have some disagreements in certain areas, but as a rule of thumb, those of us in the DRVS clearly will randomize patients with early vitreous hemorrhage, but for those of you who don't have that option or don't consider that option, clearly I think the critical point was made as to what the visual needs of that patient are and what the status of the other eye is. This aspect of visual needs and the risk/benefit ratio will determine when to carry out vitrectomy in such an eye. Again we can say 12 months, 6 months; we argue about those things but won't know that until the results of this study are available in some 3 years, and until then I really think it's the visual needs and the status of the fellow eye that are really the key points in managing vitreous hemorrhage. In terms of traction detachment, at least we have been persuaded by the studies of Wally McMeel and Steve Charles in terms of following tractional detachments until in fact the macula itself is detached. In other words, we will not operate for a so-called macula-threatening detachment. But if and when that macula detaches, we treat that with the same sense of urgency that you manage rhegmatogenous retinal detachment. That patient is acquainted with the symptoms; that patient is advised to come in immediately; and that's someone you don't wait and say "Well, keep your regular follow-up appointment." You have got to see them right away if you are going to approach them that way. Similarly, if you are going to carry out photocoagulation on some of these patients with macula-threatening detachment with significant fibrovascular proliferation—that is, the chance of the macula coming off—again you have really got to follow that patient closely and be prepared to intervene immediately. In regard to the question of neovascularization again, I think that's been handled well in the panel discussion. We tend to follow those patients outside the study. In the DRVS, we will operate on a prospective randomized basis. Other indications that might be considered include those patients who go on to rubeosis with opaque media, where you just can't see to do laser or to do cryotherapy, but I think that it sort of leads in; and maybe very briefly we might discuss with the panel and then the management of—as Mort has pointed out—one of the most difficult and poorly understood areas of ophthalmology, neovascularization of the iris and secondary glaucoma. The panel can address itself to the postvitrectomy stage and that issue too. Arnall, do you have a few comments on how you approach or manage neovascularization of the iris and secondary glaucoma?

Patz: Well, after vitrectomy, if the media are clear, now we go for full panretinal treatment, and I mean treatment with 3000, 4000, or up to 5000 burns to cover as far forward as we can get, and tight burns overlapping, and I will show illustrations of what I mean by really heavy treatment. The other thing is that we have treated by using the Boston technique of focal treatment to the vessels in the angle. But we've found that we have had better results when we can get a more extensive panretinal, very extensive treatment in those cases.

Ryan: Mort?

Goldberg: During vitrectomy surgery, if the media are clear enough and the technology is available, an intraoperative panretinal photocoagulation is desirable. Using an endolaser is technically the easiest way to create many hundreds of burns, sometimes over a thousand burns, because there is no waiting time between applications, and the eye can be filled with air or gas, and the probe tip doesn't have to be very close to the surface of the fundus. Equipment reliability is somewhat of a problem, and widespread commercial availability of this hardware is still somewhat of a problem, but those are problems that can be solved with time. Endophotocoagulation with a xenon arc is also technically feasible, but it's laborious and time consuming. As far as postoperative treatment is concerned, I would agree with Arnall's approach. If the media are not clear, however, then one sometimes has to decide whether or not blind cryotherapy will be performed. Some of you in the audience have told me, and I have heard this from others in the past, that equatorial cryotherapy does have a favorable effect in iris neovascularization. I have not been able to make that observation myself in substantial numbers of patients, and I look forward to a systematic study of that particular issue.

Ryan: Jack?

Coleman: You've covered most of the points. The only thing I would say in addition is that the presence of a lens makes a great deal of difference to the development of anterior neovascularization and glaucoma. If the lens is present, in our series the incidence of neovascularization is not so high as has been reported here. It's really less than 8%, and it's far more easily controlled. When the lens is absent, I agree, the problem is greater. Certainly, I agree with the use of intraoperative endophotocoagulation. I do not do an extensive one. I limit the treatment primarily to the disc region and posterior to the equator, hoping to be able to do the rest of the treatment later with cryopexy or with external photocoagulation.

One modality that we are working on, on an experimental basis, is the use of therapeutic ultrasound to create filtering blebs in treatment of some of these eyes with neovascular glaucoma. This technique can lower the pressure and help control that part of the problem. It does not affect the neovascularization itself.

Ryan: Don, any comments?

Gass: No, not concerning how they manage rubeosis before, during, or after surgery. In regard to the recent comments expressing very little enthusiasm for photocoagulation of rubeosis, I would like to say that there is considerable enthusiasm at the Bascom Palmer Eye Institute for its possible use in glaucoma.

Ryan: For direct goniophotocoagulation, but will they do ablation of the retina?

Gass: Oh, yes. Then they do cryopexy. And in some cases, I believe, cryotherapy has been used when they couldn't visualize the fundus adequately on photocoagulation.

Ryan: Wally.

McMeel: We've been working with Dr. Richard Simmons and his group, who actively use both iris and angle photocoagulation. They usually do the work-up and treat the anterior segment. In all of these, we also treat the fundus if the media are sufficiently clear. If we cannot get through with the laser, we have been using the cryoprobe sometimes just going into the fornix. Occasionally we do a peritomy and go far back posteriorly. In that instance, however, treating where you cannot see well can be very dangerous. When I treat rather far back, I can usually get a glimpse of the indentation before I make the cryoprobe application. If one gets too far back, particularly on the temporal side, the macula can be destroyed and any hope for useful vision is lost. I have seen one lady recently who developed a small tear at the edge of one of the cryoprobe applications and developed a rhegmatogenous detachment. Thus it is not without hazard.

Ryan: Alan, would you want to comment on this—are you still doing Molteno tubes, or filtering procedures—or can you tell us that aspect of things for neovascularization of the iris: How would you approach these problems?

Bird: There is an alternative management, namely, the use of drainage tubes as described by Molteno, not only for postoperative rubeosis but also for neovascular glaucoma in general. If an eye has useful vision and the drainage angle is totally closed, one might consider the use of a Molteno tube in the first instance. As the media clear, it may be possible to undertake photocoagulation. We have several eyes in which the pressure has been well controlled over long periods with drainage tubes. In the majority of cases clinical circumstances mitigate against a good acuity, but one eye has normal vision now, an implication that the use of drainage tubes does not necessarily cause irreparable damage to the anterior segment. I believe this management is better than blind cryotherapy.

Ryan: I would like to ask Alan to comment further. Our own limited experience has been with a glaucoma surgeon who has used Krupin valve tubes for advanced rubeotic glaucoma, and to my amazement many of those iris vessels do involute dramatically within days or a week or two after the successful placement of a shunt. That suggests some theoretical grounds that one is rather quickly liberating an angiogenic factor to the outside of the eye. Whether or not the theoretical explanation is correct, I have no idea, and Dr. Patz can comment on that better than I can. But the observation is a fascinating one, and may times these vessels will go away. What have you seen with the Molteno tubes?

Bird: It is certainly true that within 24 hours of inserting a Molteno tube the new vessels on the surface of the iris cannot be seen by biomicroscopy and iris angiography shows a dramatic change in their perfusion. These observations would support the concept that drainage is causing a washing-out of a diffusible agent that has an influence on blood vessels.

Ryan: So, in summary then, I think we've heard that it's certainly a difficult problem to manage. We must individualize each case as to the state of the media:—Is the retina attached or detached? Is the angle open or closed? What can you do? It's going to influence matters tremendously, and there is this possibility of filtering surgery that some have reported on recently.

I thank the panel very much for the fine discussion.

DRAINAGE OF SUBRETINAL FLUID DURING SCLERAL BUCKLE OPERATION

DR. J. WALLACE McMEEL

McMeel: This section is to elicit under what conditions the retinal surgeon will or will not drain subretinal fluid and then, as regards drainage itself, what thoughts you might have with regard to its location, the meridian, whether you go in the bed or out of the scleral bed or underneath your area where you make your buckle, what preparations you do for making your perforation, any particular thoughts on perforation itself, any caveats and any other things that might be of interest to us. This may be an oversimplification, but probably everyone has an area in which he shifts from where he does not drain subretinal fluid to where he does. In this slide we have the severity of the detachment situation on the x axis. To the left we have no drainage, and to the right, toward drainage. Most would probably agree that a flat hole that is traction-free and has no fluid would probably not be drained. At the other end of the spectrum, you have MPP, MVR or MPR [massive preretinal proliferation, massive vitreous retraction, massive preretinal retraction]. Somewhere, we all shift from nondrainage to drainage. The three things that may be important are the extent of the detachment, how much traction there is, and the degree of elevation. So this is a two-dimensional, philosophical chart. What is a sufficient amount of subretinal fluid for drainage? That probably is different for each person as well. How close should the break be to the buckling indentations? Some people like this closer than others. Some people can live with this a little farther apart and be happy and either not drain or stop drainage. In the preparation I think one thing we try to do is to avoid choroidal bleeding at the sclerotomy site, and I would just like to mention a couple of things here with regard to the location of the vessels, transillumination, and the diathermizing of your exposed choroid. Now, my own prejudices are showing through here; so just bear with me. In the fundus the area that has the least amount of choroidal vasculature seems to be the meridian just above and below the long ciliaries and at the 6 and 12 o'clock meridians. Those areas, if perforation is performed, would be less likely to have bleeding. Also the choroidal vascular network is less dense as one goes more anteriorly, and, of course, the regions around the vortex veins have an increased risk to them. The long ciliary structures, the arteries and nerves, are at the 9 and 3 o'clock meridians. Sometimes one can see them while making a dissection. Transillumination can often accentuate this. It can also tell you if you are over a vortex when you're attempting to perforate either in the bed or outside the scleral bed. In a transilluminated eye the light goes in through the pupil while the observer views the sclera. Diathermizing of the choroidal knuckle is another way to decrease hemorrhage at the time of perforation. This electrode is insulated except at the tip, greatly reducing shrinkage of the sclera. You have your exposure of your choroidal knuckle. Some people like to get a knuckle, some people make a small tangential perforation, and others may go perpendicularly. Some like a very small aperture; some produce a little wiggle as they go in or come out to make it a bit larger. Some prefer to go within the bed, others preferentially perforate outside the bed, and many make no bed at all. Perforation outside the bed may be preferable in a detachment that is extensive and elevated and in which one anticipates implant manipulation during surgery. In this instance, one may be more comfortable not having to drain and then reopen the bed because one can tighten sutures across the implant and still continue to drain. Another situation in which having the perforation site out of the bed would be preferable is when readjustment of the implant may be necessary with plans to reinflate the contents of the globe with a gas or fluid. Dr. Watzke, would you just give us a run-through of these various facets, if you would, as to what you do and what the group at Iowa does? How do you approach the perforation and how do you plan? What are your indications for perforating a rhegmatogenous detachment?

Watzke: First of all, at Iowa there are four of us doing these detachments now, and there are four different, or somewhat different, points of view. First, I think we should all realize that there is a point at which those who drain, like myself, tend to drain more than they need to. I am sure that many detachments where I drain could be equally well managed without drainage, and for those who say I never drain, or very seldom drain, will have to go back and have some cases where they will take the patient back into the operating room and drain because it turns out that in the next few days the retina will not have gone on. So you can't be very dogmatic about this. The second point is that with experience all of us develop a technique that works most of the time, and when you try to change that technique, say "Well, I think I'm not going to drain so much," you have to go through a certain learning experience, and those who do not drain and then decide to drain will have some learning problems, and vice versa. George Hilton completed a beautifully randomized control study in which he found that by assigning patients before the surgery into drainage or nondrainage patients and then following through on the surgery there really was no significant difference in the operative result between drainage and no drainage. So, I think none of us can be too dogmatic about which method is best; it's mainly which is best in our hands. But be that as it may, my first assessment is on considering the severity of the detachment and particularly the height of the detachment and the mobility of the retina. I like to get the retina on in the operating room, and if a retina is very mobile and preoperatively shifts and moves with the position of the patient, I tend to use that as an indication for drainage because I want to get that retina back in place. I am afraid that otherwise, with motion of the patient postoperatively, something that looks as if it will go on by the next morning, instead that night the patient moves about a bit, and I look at it the next morning, and the fluid is still there, and we are in for a reoperation. The second is the assessment of the tear—both the number of tears and whether there is a certain amount of preretinal fibrosis around the tear. Is it a tear that's liable to fishmouth? Is it one that you are going to have to drain close to the tear and end up with a fold that, if that's the case, I tend to try not to drain? I tend to try to put a buckle under there in the operating room and assess that maybe I can get by without draining. These are just clues that you sometimes have to use. Another is your assessment of where you are going to drain. There are six places where one is safest in draining subretinal fluid, 6 o'clock, 12 o'clock, and then along the margins of the horizontal recti. And if the detachment is such that these safe places put you very close to the tear, obviously, you'll start out with a game plan of probably not draining, and also if I am going to drain, I don't like to drain temporal to the fovea. That is in, under, or near the lateral rectus because hemorrhage from your drain site there can dribble right down into the fovea and practically never will the patient get 20/20 vision after that happens, assuming that the patient's macula is detached. So if I have to drain in that area—I tend to try not to drain—I try to choose the case so that I will not drain. Finally, no matter what your game plan is, when you mark the tear or tears, you have to be able to change your mind and change your game plan. If, for example, when you are marking the tear, you can approximate the cryoprobe to the retina and you get up very close to it, make an indentation on the detachment, and then put a buckle under it and see if it looks as if it's in good position. You may have started out saying you are going to drain and then say, "No, I don't think we are going to need to." So these are in a rather sketchy fashion I am afraid, the ways I assess the patient.

McMeel: I think that is a very good rundown. I think also there are two or three very excellent specific points that were brought out. Steve? Would you like to continue— regarding how things are done at USC [University of Southern California]?

Ryan: As Bob [Watzke] has pointed out, everybody is going to have to have his own variation in how he does it, and certainly if you take some people like those on our full-time faculty or on our voluntary faculty in town, you will find very different and widely divergent approaches to this. I think when you start off saying, "Are you going to drain in the bed or outside the bed?" there are some for whom you must answer the historical "What is a bed?" since we all use explants. But, seriously, we do have some people that you have exported from Boston or Philadelphia so that we get to see the results of diathermy and scleral beds. I think that does make a real difference, though, and certainly, the question that you brought up concerns the sclerotomy site itself and whether you are going to support this with the buckle or not. In general, I like to support the sclerotomy on the buckle. I think we would all agree that the major and important aspect is that our goal is to close the hole, in addition to the points that Bob made, virtually all of which I would subscribe to. My philosophy is that I'm not quite as far along as Harvey Linkoff, but I am toward his end of the spectrum. I will be worried if I do see preretinal membranes, if there is an inferior tear, if there is shifting fluid—those sorts of things are all going to add up and make me much more anxious to get the retina flat right there at the table. Certainly, if we are dealing out of the extreme, as what you pointed out in your talk yesterday about MVR or MPP, in those cases I think it's absolutely essential that the retina be flat at the completion of the operation. Thus I will drain all those cases. And again, although we do a fair number of vitrectomies, I would emphasize that again, in keeping with your philosophy of yesterday, it's less than 10% of the time in those cases that there has not been a previous buckle done in those cases, either by ourselves or someone else. So we are going to try with a buckle first whenever it's feasible, no matter how bad a lot of those membranes look. In terms of the aspect of the site and the location, we must drain where there is the most fluid that is the safest to drain. The advantage of different sites in relation to decreased complication has been discussed. But I am sure Wally and Bob drain where the fluid is greatest. After cryotherapy, there may be choroidal engorgement in that area. The importance of maintaining intraocular pressure and avoiding hypotony during the course of drainage is a key one. We find ourselves using air and gas on occasion, and certainly with vitrectomy and MPP or MVR, we find ourselves doing so-called internal drainage through a hole within the retina posteriorly, where there are no epiretinal membranes in that area, just to get the retina flat in that area. So again we will individualize every case, and I will subscribe to most of the points Bob has made.

McMeel: What do we hear from the London post?

Bird: I believe in London we drain subretinal fluid less frequently than what is common in the United States. In a London series reported by Peter Lever, the average time for resorption of subretinal fluid was over 7 days, which implies that the presence of subretinal fluid on the first or second day after surgery does not imply a bad final outcome. Furthermore, if the eye has not been opened, it is absolutely safe and we are happy to discharge patients from the hospital with residual subretinal fluid.

I am particularly happy that in a teaching institute such as Moorfields draining only a small percentage of patients is the habit. Residents at Moorfields usually undertake 50 or 60 detachment operations during their residency period. Detachment surgery undertaken without drainage becomes a perfectly safe procedure, since the most dangerous part of the operation has been avoided and there is no reason to believe that this technique is unsuitable for the vast majority of patients with retinal detachment.

I agree with most of the points made concerning drainage, but there is one additional precaution that may be taken. In London most surgery is undertaken under general anesthesia, and whenever draining subretinal fluid is contemplated patients are overventilated to reduce blood Pco_2. This causes closure of the choroidal blood vessels, reducing considerably the risks of hemorrhage. Ventilation is guided by an expired Pco_2 monitor. Wallace Foulds has shown that with hyperventilation the choroid can be cut with Vannas scissors and it does not bleed.

McMeel: That's a very interesting point. Dr. Goldberg?

Goldberg: This is another example of Sutton's law. You all know about the famous bank robber, Willie Sutton who, when asked why he robbed banks, said ''That's where the money is.'' In this case, one should try to drain where most of the fluid is, so that one avoids perforating the retina. Having said that, I would agree that the safest places are alongside of the long posterior ciliary vessels and in the vertical meridians. I would also agree with the idea that, in general, it is desirable to drain nasally rather than temporally, not only avoiding hemorrhage into the macula, but also avoiding a retinal pucker involving the macula if there is herniation of retina or loss of vitreous through a drainage site. In addition, I try, whenever possible, to drain under the buckle, either in the bed of a scleral dissection or under an exoplant, giving up some of the versatility that you mentioned for some added safety, that is, having a potential iatrogenic retinal break already localized to the middle of the buckling site. As far as technique is concerned, I like to have the choroid fully exposed without any residual scleral fibers. Because I tend to drain where I have previously put cryotherapy (and that is somewhat hazardous because of engorged uveal vessels), I then use a diathermy pin to heavily diathermize the exposed choroid where perforation will actually occur. Then I take that one step further and perforate with a hot diathermy pin. Sometimes that doesn't work, and then I use different instruments, if necessary, to get fluid, including a sharp spatula needle. Some of our surgeons use a Wilder probe, which is a variant of a punctum dilator. I personally prefer a sharp diathermy pin or suture needle. One final point: if one is draining very posteriorly in association with MPP or MVR, there is a tendency to pull the eye away from the surgeon so that he can see what he is doing when he is inserting a perforating pin or needle. That will, on occasion, tend to roll fluid away from the site of perforation and bring the retina closer to the site, so that if the needle is inserted too perpendicularly there is a very definite hazard of perforating the retina. In that circumstance, it's important to remember not to push or pull the eye too far away from the surgeon who is doing the perforating (if he's looking externally at the site of the perforation). It's important to emphasize in that situation, as in most, that there is value to a tangential entry rather than a perpendicular entry.

McMeel: Dr. Colemen, have you been more of a settler since you have gone over and rubbed elbows with Harvey Linkoff?

Coleman: That's a major point. I grew up with draining and feel very comfortable with it. I would agree with all the concerns that have already been raised and would like to add one more. Just before draining, I make sure the assistant does not put any pressure on the globe, releasing all traction, letting the eye become completely still. This is less likely to produce a sudden gush of fluid that can cause an incarceration.

Harvey Lincoff is a strong advocate of nondrainage. I must say I have been very impressed with his results that we have seen on rounds. He makes a great deal of effort to localize prior to surgery. He uses bed rest I think more than many of the rest of us would. He uses the balloon and his sponge explants and drains very rarely. The use of bed-rest settling and precise localization, I think, can reduce the amount of drainage that is required. I do agree completely with Alan that if you don't drain, it's one less major complication that you are likely to have from bleeding, incarceration or inflammation. The tunica ruyschiana has to be punctured to release subretinal fluid, and this does reduce the nosologic barrier for infection as well. Nevertheless, with the proper techniques already amply described, I think drainage is relatively safe and often necessary to get the hold on the band. If I can't obtain that with variations in the position or height of the buckle or with gas, then I do drain.

McMeel: Don, would you like to wind up the panel?

Gass: I'll comment on the Gass way of skinning the cat. I do not drain when it's comfortable not to drain and by that I mean when there is only one hole to close. In general, multiple holes, inferior holes, uncertainty of where all the holes are, and evidence of traction are all reasons for drainage.

McMeel: We'll be looking for the answer to that one at the next panel in 6 years. I think we have had a very broad range of very good advice. Thank you.

MANAGEMENT OF PATIENTS WITH SEVERE DISC NEOVASCULARIZATION IN DIABETIC RETINOPATHY

DR. ARNALL PATZ

Patz: I would like to discuss management of advanced disc neovascularization in the diabetic patient and to remind you that the cooperative Diabetic Retinopathy Study, which was completed in the mid-1970s, showed a very striking difference in terms of treated versus control eyes, particularly in terms of the response of disc neovascularization. But there are some problems in management of patients who have severe new vessels at the disc. I would like to present a challenging case. This is a patient, 26 years of age, who came with this condition 3 months pregnant and, having had previous miscarriages, was very anxious to go through a complete pregnancy. This is January 1980, at 3 months of pregnancy. She went on to develop disc vessels, and we started treatment. This is her left eye, and I think one can see the large caliber of these new vessels. This is following standard PRP [panretinal photocoagulation], and without taking you through all the sequences of her treatment, I picked this stage, which is approximately 2 months after what you saw initially. She went through the development of disc vessels and panretinal treatment, and she still has these vessels, which are continuing to proliferate in each eye. And here we see this patient again 1 month later. Additional peripheral panretinal treatment was extended anteriorly past the equator, yet significant disc vessels presented, and in her right eye the disc vessels had bled. She had extensive PRP, but the vessels persisted with extensive hemorrhage occurring. Well, we persisted with a panretinal treatment, and here she is when she was 8 months pregnant, and indeed we re-treated. We treated almost between every single burn and went out almost to the ora 360 degrees, with approximately 5000 burns in each eye. At this particular time, at 8 months, she still has a little residual hemorrhage, but no residual new vessels. And here's that eye about 1 month after delivery. The hemorrhage has cleared. She was able to complete her pregnancy successfully, and we were able to control the severe proliferative diabetic retinopathy. One reason I wanted to show this case is to show her Goldman fields. So, this patient has a significant visual-field impairment, which is bilateral. Yesterday hypophysectomy was discussed; certainly, in this young pregnant patient, that cannot be considered, and she is very happy that she has central vision and some useful visual field. She cannot drive her car, but she is able to function fairly well.

I would like to show the next picture of severe disc vessels and ask the panel for their comments on this patient. Dr. Ryan yesterday showed a type of neovascularization quite similar to this—what he described as "rubeosis retinae." I would like to ask the panelists and start with Dr. Bird. In terms of your management of this patient, would you attempt PRP or would you wait for a hemorrhage, or would you automatically consider hypophysectomy? This patient has severe disc vessels in both eyes.

Bird: Is this patient pregnant?

Patz: This is a male patient who is 31 years of age, diabetic since age 14, not pregnant and not considering it.

Bird: Most of the patients with diabetic retinopathy in Moorfields are managed by Peter

Hamilton, Ralph Blach, and Eva Kohner. It is certainly considered that the primary treatment of such a patient would be panretinal photocoagulation, and it would be undertaken in very much the way that you have shown. There would also be a thorough assessment of the patient's diabetic control and, if poor, the patient would be admitted to obtain the best possible control of blood glucose levels, including the use of an insulin pump, if this is necessary.

In such case we may discuss the indication for hypophysectomy, but I do not know of one case that had had a hypophysectomy for a very long time. Nevertheless, there is no consensus yet that hypophysectomy is never indicated although the practice suggests that the indications for this must be very rare.

Patz: Bob?

Watzke: Well, we've dealt with these patients. In fact, I had a patient who was really almost identical to the pregnant lady that you described. There was a difference between these two patients, I think. The first patient, who had not only florid neovascularization, but also cytoid bodies, macular edema, lots of superficial hemorrhages, a very wet-looking, leaking retina in addition to these long, stringy, florid vessels, I think has a much poorer prognosis. Obviously, we'll do a panretinal photocoagulation, but in the patient who has a lot of leaks and a very florid, wet, hemorrhagic-looking retinopathy in addition to these vessels, I think we will do a staged PRP; that is, we'll do about half a retina, and then within 2 weeks to a month we will do the second half, which is not our practice in the usual panretinal photocoagulation. Now, in the patient whom you have just showed, who has mainly a lot of florid vessels but not a lot of the other attributes, we'll do an immediate panretinal photocoagulation, and I think the prognosis is not good, but I think if it's present in both eyes, it's not invariably bad. I think frequently one eye will end up with at least 20/200 vision or such, and I really don't know what else you can do because by the time you consider whether you should do more photocoagulation, you have waited a month to 8 weeks to see what the result of the first is, and by that time, if the eye is going to go down the tube, it's probably already started to bleed. So that's basically our approach to both of those.

Patz: Dick? Would you comment?

O'Connor: I think we would do a PRP on the second patient that you showed. We have studied a large series of hypophysectomy patients at our institution. It was begun long ago in the Donner Laboratory in Berkeley. A moratorium was called on hypophysectomy a few years ago in order to give us the chance to stand back and analyze the results of the cases. We have not proceeded with hypophysectomies since that time, not because of the difficulty in controlling the hormonal imbalance of those patients, but because we were not convinced of the basic worth of the procedure. Considering the level to which this second patient's disease had already progressed, we would not do hypophysectomy but would perform PRP alone.

Patz: Wally?

McMeel: I think that one of the points that Bob Watzke made is an important one here, and in a sense separating the background retinopathy from the neovascular appearance at the disc is important, and the more edema and cytoid bodies and blot hemorrhages that one has, the less likely you are to have a good response from the panretinal photocoagulation. With regard to the pregnant lady, I think a point should be made that if a young married woman is diabetic, counsel should be made to have her children as early as possible so that she doesn't get to this later stage where you have to make these difficult decisions. May I at this time show a couple of photographs, Arnall, of pituitaries before and after treatment? I have them on the slide here.

Patz: Put them on.

McMeel: This is one that we did a number of years ago. This is the pretreatment pituitary appearance, and some people would probably do a panretinal photocoagulation at this point. At the time we did this—and I myself might well at this juncture also. This is the posttreatment appearance, and there was a definite drying out, and this woman has maintained a 20/20 vision in this eye. Now, these next two—this is a very florid one with a segmentation, and the posttreatment shows how this has dried up, and she also has a good vision at 20/40 or 20/50. As you see, there's an ectopia of the macula, and that has been drawn. The pituitary ablation is holding the vision in approximately 70% to 75% of the patients that are in this category, and it is something that should continue to be considered. One of the points that Dr. Watzke made is that you're losing time by doing a PRP and waiting a month or two. There is a time window that is quite vital in a pituitary ablation, and that is before much fibrotic tissue develops around these florid vessels. By doing panretinal photocoagulation and waiting, an opportunity for an optimal result may be lost. In the massive disc vessels, you can treat directly on the vessels at a later date if PRP is not effective.

Patz: Thank you, Wally. In reference to that first patient, the pregnant patient with extensive field damage, obviously, we treated so many areas that the photoreceptors were destroyed in a very large area. But do you think that the green laser, inasmuch as you would have less damage in the sensory retina, might theoretically preserve some field in this type of patient?

McMeel: I think with burns of the intensity that were done here, no matter what wavelength you used, you would probably destroy everything. We did two patients in whom we did a panretinal photocoagulation of approximately 1200 burns of identical size and energy and milliwattage. In both patients we did the PRP, one eye with the blue-green, the other with the green. With the 1200 spots in each eye, we were unable to determine the difference in dark-adaptation field, peripheral fields, or flicker fields, in either eye.

Patz All right. Jack, in that patient with the very florid disc vessels, the second, the male patient, would you go right to PRP or would you consider other treatment?

Coleman: Several years ago, I did vitrectomies on a series of 15 patients with disc neovascularization almost identical to the picture you showed. In my series the complication rate was extremely low. Only one patient had a complication, a hemorrhage 4 months after surgery. Technically, these are easy to do. The membrane can be peeled away near the optic nerve. There is a risk of bleeding at that point, but it was not a problem in my limited series. I have not continued that series because the Diabetic Vitrectomy Study is going to be answering this question. For the past 4 years, I have been initially treating these patients with photocoagulation. I do treat a little differently. I don't treat as extensively peripherally. I treat in close to the optic nerve head in a C-shaped, fairly heavy fashion adjacent to the nerve out to about the region of the equator. I have had about a 60% success in doing that but have had to proceed with vitrectomy in several patients. I treat just as heavily in the peripapillary region as you did. I think you had a good result.

Patz: Mort, how would you manage the second patient?

Goldberg: I would also use a PRP as the mainstay of intial treatment. Having said that and agreeing that the proper diagnosis is rubeosis retinae, if the first eye doesn't do well, I would talk about pituitary ablation with the patient and would tend to encourage it. If there is a only a partial response after a PRP, there are still other things one can consider. If one does a very early phase fluorescein angiogram, one can sometimes find the feeder vessels, the nutrient arterioles supplying patches of either epipapillary of peripapillary neovascularization, and there is a role for focal feeder vessel treatment in this situation. There is another clinical situation that arises, where the epipapillary vessels are supplied by posterior ciliary vessels as shown by angiography. In that situation, my experience is somewhat similar to Dr. Coleman's in that intense peripapillary photocoagulation, very close to the nasal border of the disc and the superior and inferior borders of the disc, can sometimes result in closure of those posterior ciliary vessels with involution of intravitreal vessels. Most of the time, however, the new vessels aren't supplied by those more posteriorly located ciliary vessels, but one can still occasionally see a feeder vessel and focally obliterate it. The risks, of course, are that you induce thermal optic neuropathy if the disc is directly treated. This can irreversibly drop acuity to the 20/400 level or worse. This form of treatment involves a calculated risk. It requires retrobulbar injection, very early phase magnified fluorescein angiograms, and an understanding patient, but I think there is a role for that approach in some cases.

Patz: I think, in reference to what Dr. Goldberg just mentioned, we come tightly to the disc and come into the arcade in this type of patient.

Steve, the second patient with the very florid retinopathy—would you consider PRP as your first approach.

Ryan: I would consider PRP as the first approach. If I could make just one or two comments in relation to diabetes and pregnancy and recognizing that Larry Singerman is in the audience, and perhaps he or Sandy Brucker certainly have far more informaton in terms of the role of pregnancy and its effect with diabetes in the management of these patients, I wish to tell you about two cases that I have been involved with in the past year. Both of these cases, after going through all the moral and medical decisions, elected to go on with their pregnancies, and in one of these we put 7000 laser burns in one eye and 8000 laser burns in the other eye and it looked very much fried, just like your cases, and yet we still did not get the involution of the vessels. Fortunately, she completed the pregnancy and has maintained those small central islands after clearing of relatively minimal hemorrhages, but I just want to point out that, at least to me, there are those times that you can go and treat and re-treat and still not get the involution of the vessels.

Another young woman is one that did in fact go into the study, and it is of note that in one eye, the eye that underwent vitrectomy, has been her only eye that she has maintained. This is after laser photocoagulation therapy failed to induce regression of those vessels, and the eye that underwent vitrectomy is her only seeing eye. I wish that I could tell you that everything went smoothly on her. However, she did develop neovascularization of the iris and secondary glaucoma, which we have had a difficult time controlling, but currently are controlled. The lens had to be removed in that case. Again we, like you, Jack, and everyone, want to leave the lens in place, but there are those patients with cataracts in which to do the operation it's essential that the lens be removed. The point that I'd say is that certainly in both these cases we just flat out would not recommend hypophysectomy. I think the points that Jack made are quite true. Ron Michels, Bob Machemer, Steve Charles, and others have emphasized that as horrible as those vessels look the point is that they're on a plane and they're on the posterior surface of the vitreous, and when you gain access to that plane, you'll find that whole area to lift up; and again it comes down to a matter of cauterizing and segmenting and removing that particular membrane. So I have no question, but that technically those eyes can be successfully operated on. The critical question is the one that Mort raised yesterday about the risk/benefit ratio to these patients, and again obviously these operations are fraught with tremendous hazard and complication later on as well. So I think that that is— as Jack pointed out today and yesterday—what this DRVS is all about, it's to try to answer the question of what the role of vitrectomy in those patients is. No one can honestly tell you in the absence of a trial and its results. Today what my approach would be is to try to get involution with PRP as the first therapy. If that is not successful, go on and enroll the patient in the study.

Patz: Don, in reference to management at Miami, that second patient. . .

Gass: Well, I'm pretty sure that George Blankenship would probably do a PRP in the second case. I would like to make a comment about your first patient. Since there is still some question about the intensity of photocoagulation required to get the desired effect, and realizing that Dr. Aiello apparently got the effect from using ruby laser, which did almost no damage to the eye, I think in a patient with bilateral and symmetrical proliferative retinopathy it would be prudent to use the standard recommended treatment in one eye and to use less intense treatment in the second eye in the hope that that eye will retain some additional visual field. I think it is important to try to determine if the British are correct in using much less intense photocoagulation than that used in the Diabetic Retinopathy Study. The reported results of ruby-laser treatment by Aiello and the experimental work of John Weiter and Maurice Landers suggest that laser damage to the pigment epithelium and outer retina allowing more diffusion of the oxygen into the inner retina may be one of the most important effects of laser in causing resolution of proliferative retinopathy. It is important that we not accept the DRS recommended treatment as the last word in management, and we use patients with bilaterally symmetrical disease as an opportunity to learn.

Patz: I think your point is well taken, but I would like to disagree on the laser treatment by Dr. Aiello in a small way, Don. The patients that he treated, for the most part, did not have significant disc vessels, and indeed early in the argon-laser period Lloyd sent me patients who developed disc vessels and had had his scatter ruby-laser treatment, and I was impressed with the fact that when they had disc vessels they did not completely regress and they would develop disc vessels after his "full scatter with a ruby." I think your point is well taken. Maybe in hindsight we might have taken one eye and stopped at 2500 burns. But with her bleeding in both eyes we felt pressed. The fact is that I have other patients who don't have quite that tight a PRP who get away with a fairly useful field, although constricted, of course, but here again I think I would do just as you have suggested.

Patz: Despite the fact that the Diabetic Retinopathy Study was published, and several publications have come out of it going back 5 or 6 years, there is still a role for the ophthalmic community, not only to educate the internists and diabetologists, but also to be sure that our colleagues are aware of the results of the Diabetic Retinopathy Study and patients who have proliferative retinopathy should be under close surveillance and treated promptly when indicated.

Thank you.

TRAUMA: TIMING OF REPAIR

DR. D. JACKSON COLEMAN

Coleman: I began this discussion the other day by questioning the timing of surgery in ocular trauma. Clearly there are differences of opinion on this issue. This is not surprising because of the large constellation of problems that relates to evaluation of the severity of injury, the techniques of surgery, and the emotional and sociological implications that relate to trauma. We all understand the patient's grave concern after an injury, with the attendant effect on their lives, for example, their subsequent choice of occupations. There are also great social implications that relate to the cost of treating this type of injury and its relation to the extent of surgery that might be contemplated. There are certainly legal implications. Whereas our patients don't blame us for their misfortune, they do blame fate and feel the need for redress. Thus most of these cases involve litigation, involving third-party insurers, drivers of other cars in automobile accidents, manufacturers of possibly defective items, employers, or whomever the patient and their attorney chooses. Careful documentation is thus important to verify the patient's pre- and postoperative clinical status and to substantiate valid claims. We also have to include the adequacy of facilities for handling complex trauma for both diagnostic evaluation and the full scope of surgical intervention.

We all recognize the need not to perform unnecessary surgery. Clearly there are many cases of trauma that do not require extensive surgery, or referral beyond the initial evaluation and treatment; for example, mild vitreous hemorrhage after non-penetrating trauma would generally fall in this category. Yet we all pretty much agree on the need for extensive surgery in certain situations. These would include cases where there has been penetrating injury of the eye with vitreous involvement and secondary problems, for example, lens rupture mixed with hemorrhage, ciliary body laceration with massive hemorrhage and posterior perforation or retained intraocular foreign body, which is usually associated with hemorrhage, and the inability to examine the retina for occult tears, and finally retinal detachment with vitreous hemorrhage.

We should define the concept of posterior perforation. We often use the term "double perforation" in this situation, although some of the wordsmiths among us would take the point of view that the globe is a unit, and therefore "double perforation" is redundant. Most of us use this term "double perforation" to indicate a penetrating entrance wound and a posterior exit wound.

Although the panel may not accept all of these indications, once the decision for surgery is made, we then have to determine when we are going to operate. There are clearly major differences of opinion here. I've used the term "windows" and showed you a diagram that relates to the timing of surgery. We have long recommended that patients with these clinical indications have vitrectomy as part of the initial repair, or at least early after the initial procedure. There have been others who have also recommended this approach. Faulborn et al.* reported on 77 cases in the *British Journal of Ophthalmology.* He did note the fact that one of the major com-

---

*Faulborn, J., Atkinson, A., and Olivier, D.: Primary vitrectomy as a preventive surgical procedure in the treatment of severely injured eyes, Br. J. Ophthalmol. **61:**202, 1977.

plications is recurrent hemorrhage. Muga and Maul* did a prospective series of early surgery that related primarily to lens rupture. This was reported in the *British Journal of Ophthalmology* of 1978. This series contrasted alternate cases of lens rupture where the eye was closed and observed, to those in which lensectomy and vitrectomy made up the initial procedure. The results were so strongly in favor of early lensectomy as part of the primary repair that they limited the series to 27 cases.

Other very competent surgeons have recommended a delay after injury before performing vitrectomy. This is certainly reasonable for the reasons that they have given. But, as I see it, part of the problem relates to the fact that many of these series are self-engendering. If vitrectomy surgeons recommend waiting several days, they will not have patients referred within the initial 1- to 3-day period to properly compare the results of those referred and treated in a 7- to 14-day interval. In my view, the initial period before inflammatory changes have developed is an ideal window. If we are able to accurately choose the cases that both (1) need surgery and (2) are not likely to bleed, we have an excellent chance of maximizing our visual results. By way of laboratory support for this concept, I would like to bring to your attention a paper by Burke and Smith†, which appeared in *Investigative Ophthalmology,* describing tritiated thymidine injections of blood in rabbit eyes. These investigators determined that there was a great increase in cell production of small leukocytes in the inner nuclear layers and the nerve fiber layers that started at the second or third day. Their calculated response curve of inflammation corresponds well to the diagram that I created on clinical grounds some years ago‡.

With this introduction, I would like to invite the panel, on the basis of Bertram Russell's theory that "truth is that which is stated to be believed by all competent observers," and on recognition of the fact that our limited panel does not include all competent observers, albeit some very respectable ones, to see if we can arrive at some consensus on two basic questions: (1) should all trauma surgery be delayed or is there some indication that some categories of trauma should be operated on early, and (2) if some cases should be operated on early, how do we select those specifically, and how do we deal with problems that relate to bleeding? I have discussed this issue many times with Steve Ryan and know that he will have a ready response. Steve, why don't you start the discussion.

Ryan: In the interest of our lively discussion, we have different windows from the ones Jack uses in New York. Although every case of trauma must be individualized, I will discuss our general principles. When there are cases for immediate intervention such as endophthalmitis or fulminant chalcosis or a rhegmatogenous retinal detachment that we can repair more quickly and efficiently by getting in earlier, sure, we'll go in earlier. But the other cases, we're going to go in 5 to 14 days. For young

*Muga, R., and Maul, E.: The management of lens damage in perforating corneal lacerations, Br. J. Ophthalmol. **62:**784, 1978.

†Burke, J.M., and Smith, J.M.: Retinal proliferation in response to vitreous hemoglobin or iron, Invest. Ophthalmol. Vis. Sci. **20:**582-592, 1981.

‡Coleman, D.J.: The role of vitrectomy in traumatic vitreopathy, Trans. Am. Acad. Ophthalmol. Otolaryngol. **81:**406-413, 1976.

children we tend to move up the time for vitrectomy by some 2 days. I, for one, briefly tried Jack's good advice for early intervention. I went to Los Angeles anxious to make something out of vitrectomy, in terms of its role and indications in trauma. We went through a series of cases and were operating on these cases in the middle of the night. There is no disaster for a vitreous surgeon quite like uncontrolled bleeding, which we encountered in a few early cases. We support the philosophy of Professor Neubauer and Heimann in Germany. There are temendous advantages if you are going to consider vitrectomy in having the nursing team and anesthesiology on a scheduled basis. Experienced surgeons must be involved. So I certainly agree that there are some cases with indications for earlier, more rapid intervention. In general, the injuries characterized by predominantly sharp penetration have less uveal engorgement and inflammation and can have earlier intervention. Those injuries with a major blunt component do better with vitrectomy at the latter portion of the 5- to 14-day interval after injury that we continue to recommend.

McMeel: Our people would be more likely to go in a few days later.

Coleman: Mort?

Goldberg: Let me describe two clinical situations: first, perforation of the cornea where the lens is also lacerated and has relatively clear vitreous coming through it. In that situation, if we are assured that the retina is attached, we teach our residents to perform wound closure initially followed *immediately* by pars plana lensectomy, vitrectomy, and anterior segment reconstruction. The second and more serious situation, where the vitreous is completely filled with red blood, is a very dangerous situation for vitrectomy in the acute phase. It is like operating in tomato soup. The surgeon has difficulty knowing where the surface of the fundus is relative to the tips of his vitrectomy instruments. There is often fresh red bleeding that obscures one's view. The media are too cloudy to allow endophotocoagulation or underwater diathermy. Simple elevation of the infusion bottle is often insufficient to stop the bleeding.

Coleman: What blood pressures do your patients have?

Goldberg: Lower than mine under those circumstances. I prefer to wait for thrombosis and decongestion of the traumatized retinal and choroidal vessels and detachment of the posterior hyaloid face.

Coleman: Bob?

Watzke: If echography shows hemorrhagic choroidal detachment, there is a significant advantage in waiting at least 2 weeks for vitrectomy.

Coleman: Steve?

Ryan: Ron Michels and I have a very similar philosophy.

Coleman: Alan?

Bird: At Moorfields Eye Hospital we usually wait until the end of the surgical window.

Colman: The second window?

Bird: Yes.

Coleman: The question of sympathetic ophthalmia is something that does enter significantly in forming our opinions at around the fourteenth day. In this country at least, we tend to believe that this is the time we need to make a decision regarding enucleation in some of these injured eyes. Does sympathetic ophthalmia seem to be as much a problem for you in England as it is here?

Bird: I believe most people when faced with an eye without visual potential, which would be cosmetically poor and is inflamed, would consider enucleation to be correct before the fourteenth day. There would also be a consensus that an eye with reasonable visual potential would not be enucleated. The only disparity of opinions would come with an eye with little or no visual potential and yet an eye that would remain cosmetically good. Some would elect to try and retain the eye, whereas others would elect to undertake enucleation. Opinion is often governed by the previous experience, and anyone who has seen visual loss from sympathetic ophthalmitis may behave differently from one who has not. I would be inclined to try and retain an eye where I belive the cosmetic result would be good even though visual potential of the eye is strictly limited.

Coleman: Perhaps we could answer Don's question, which has to do with the management of an eye that has an anterior penetrating injury, relatively clear media, and a steel foreign body at the back of the eye. The question is, Do we need vitrectomy in this situation? Mort, do you want to start it off?

Goldberg: We have undertaken the care of a fair number of patients who have a foreign body that's known to be iron-containing, but the visual acuity is excellent. The foreign body is often imbedded in the wall of the eye. At one time I thought the external magnetic approach to the back of the eye would be desirable, but this can lead to macular puckering if the exit site is near the posterior pole. Now, I prefer the pars plana approach with a foreign-body forceps. Nevertheless, we don't operate on those foreign bodies automatically but wait for documented reduction of ERG [electroretinogram] voltage. If we document early siderosis, we then subject the patient to surgery. On the other hand, we are talking about an eye that has 20/20 visual acuity; so there is every reason to avoid surgery when we can. When one begins to see ERG changes, however, one has to bite the bullet and take the foreign body out before the retina is destroyed.

Coleman: Steve, any difference of opinion?

Ryan: Just to underscore and agree with Mort's points that we do not have to do vitreous surgery but rather can remove the foreign body with a magnet. Or as you pointed out in your talk the other day, Jack, where there's injury and a foreign body located in the vitreous, in those cases we take those foreign bodies out through the pars plana. On the other extreme, when it's in the sclera and has produced early changes and siderosis, those would be our indications for prompt removal. Otherwise, just as Mort pointed out, we basically use a vitrectomy approach. In other words, I basically agree with the approach outlined by Mort.

Coleman: I would disagree again, even in this issue, with you. I think that if it's definitely a metallic foreign body with iron content, and a large piece that you can visualize, there is little question that the patient will develop siderosis with changes that may be irreversible. I recently saw a patient from Iran with a small foreign body in the eye just above the macula. He had relatively good vision for a long period of time, but gradually developed siderosis, and the vision was essentially lost. He then unfortunately lost the other eye in an accident. I do agree that surgery may not be necessary with small metallic fragments. They can be relatively quiet and encapsulated, and certainly one must weigh the risk of surgery against the removal. On the other hand, I don't think there is any question that if you can see a large fragment, the eye is going to develop siderosis, and to wait to document this process is unnecessary. Basically, I think that a fragment that is visible and exceeds 1 mm in any dimension is a large fragment. I think that with some smaller ones, slivers, or those that do not demonstrate magnetic response, I would follow your advice. There is a risk in any surgical intervention. I believe that any iron fragment over a millimeter in size will eventually develop siderosis over an extended period of time.

Goldberg: Is anything lost by waiting and doing ERG's every 4 to 6 weeks?

Coleman: I think that there are a couple of things that can be lost: First, I think that there is a risk that the loss of time and cost to the patient as you continue to observe the eye may cause him to be lost to follow-up study until after an opportune time for rehabilitation. Second, after a period of time the fragments do become more heavily fibrosed so that not only is surgery more difficult, but also, as I described, certain changes may become irreversible. I would like to draw a clear distinction between severe injuries with blood and large reactive fragments that I think will require surgery and those with clear media and normal vision that may not require surgery. If the need is questionable, a delay is amply justified. I think that if the eye sees well it certainly is reasonable to wait more than the immediate postinjury period or even to defer surgery altogether. Blood in the eye is a severe irritant, and if it can be removed early, there is less chance of complication, not only in terms of fibrosis, but also of iris adhesion, iris and lens adhesions, and neovascularization of secondary membranes. In the series of my own patients with severe injuries of the type I have specified, I have found a better recovery of visual acuity in those groups operated on early. This relates to macular changes that develop with blood or inflammatory changes in the eye for periods of time, since the chronic effects of inflammation are profound. Simply stated, if surgery is to be done, consider doing it early. If it may not need to be done, delay until the indications are clear.

Judgment in this area of surgery obviously reflects differences in personal experience that will take additional review until we can reach a more complete agreement. Ultimately, we may obtain answers from eye trauma centers. Ron Michels and Len Parver in the Washington-Baltimore area have instituted an emergency trauma service that expedites the referral of patients. The opportunity to evaluate these patients earlier may confirm the effectiveness of earlier repair and better define those patients who will benefit most.

Gass: The reason I brought the subject up was that in our area there is a great fear on the part of some physicians that it's imperative to remove an intraocular steel foreign body within a few days or he may be medicolegally liable. I think that there's a good reason to believe that not all intraocular metallic foreign bodies, and particularly those buried in the depth of the wall of the eye, cause siderosis. And I would just like to say that I think it's a perfectly reasonable approach, particularly if they are seeing well at the time, to follow what Mort Goldberg has suggested and observe them. Some of these patients may go through life with 20/20 vision and avoid the risks of operation.

Ryan: I would just like to thank you for the background remarks that you keep providing whenever another alternative point of view comes up!

Coleman: Alan, a last comment?

Bird: In defense of Mort Goldberg's view, it is quite possible to salvage an eye with good vision even if there is early siderosis by removing the foreign body and possibly adding desferrioxamine. For this reason, I think it quite defensible if there is a small metallic foreign body in an eye with excellent vision to await events rather than undertake early surgery, and to review the eye at regular intervals for signs of siderosis.

Coleman: I don't disagree with that point about eyes that are clear and may not require surgery. My point is that if they *are* going to require surgery, then the surgery performed earlier in the presence of less inflammation is more rational.

Thank you, panel.

THE USE OF IMMUNOSUPPRESSIVE AGENTS IN DISEASES OF THE EYE

DR. G. RICHARD O'CONNOR

O'Connor: I should like to present a few slides concerning my basic philosophy about immunosuppressive agents in the treatment of intractable inflammatory diseases of the eye. I would then like to question the other members of the panel on some issues having to do with this subject. When you get down to the end of a long list of potential treatments for various forms of uveitis, you come to a group of patients that form a residue of relatively resistant cases. These include, but are not limited to, Behçet's disease, sympathetic uveitis, and rheumatoid sclerouveitis. In patients of this type, there is an indication that they may be relieved or considerably improved by the use of corticosteroids, but in some cases the disease progresses beyond the point where they can be helped by corticosteroids. They can be helped, but they have such serious secondary complications that they no longer can continue to take these medications. My indications for immunosuppressive therapy are as follows: I would use immunosuppressive agents for an intractable, potentially blinding uveitis, one that appears to be steroid resistant or relatively so; I would use them for a condition where steroids are contraindicated for some particular physical or mental reason (I will give you some examples of that in just a few minutes) I would use these agents for a condition in which loss of vision has already occurred in one eye and the second eye seems seriously threatened.

The next series of slides shows an example of what I am talking about. This is a 62-year-old woman with rheumatoid sclerouveitis. She had both anterior and posterior scleritis. She also had severe secondary glaucoma requiring her to take Diamox [acetazolamide] and potassium supplements as well as local epinephrine drops. She had received so much systemic corticosteroid treatment for her rheumatoid arthritis that she was wheelchair ridden because of multiple pathologic fractures. She was hypertensive. She had bled three times from peptic ulcers. She had had two admissions to a mental hospital for steroid-induced mental changes. She had extensive acne and hirsutism. She suffered from obesity, and in short she was a serious problem for herself, her family, and her doctor. I think you will agree we had to do something else for this woman besides more steroid therapy.

Now, this was the picture of her right eye, and this was the picture of her left eye, which had similar involvement. She already had a dense cataract in one eye, but she had 20/25 vision in the remaining eye. We elected to treat this woman with chlorambucil, an agent with which our local rheumatologist had had a great deal of experience. Within about 5 weeks we were able to note considerable improvement in her condition, such that she was able to be taken off her steroids altogether. She showed a very pronounced improvement of her sclerouveitis. Her secondary glaucoma improved to the point that she required no Diamox or epinephrine. Her inflammatory disease is now controlled on a single drop of diluted corticosteroids per day. She is out of her wheelchair. She is totally rehabilitated. Her mental status is enormously improved. She has had no more gastrointestinal hemorrhages. This is the appearance of her other eye, now much improved. This woman has been in a state of remission for the last 9 years. I think it's reasonable to assume that a patient like this has profited from immunosuppressive therapy and its use was justified.

Behçet's disease is another disease that, as you know, I consider one of almost uniformly bad prognosis. If we elect to treat Behçet's disease with immunosuppressive agents, we must do so before there are irreversible changes. And one of the potentially useful handles on the progress of this disease is the reversal of ERG changes. Initially we may see retinal vasculitis that appears to respond to corticosteroid therapy, but later, as more massive occlusion takes place and more retinal atrophy develops, we will notice not only grave morphologic changes, but physiologic changes as well, indicating a steady deterioration. Certainly, patients must be treated before this state of affairs takes place.

Once again, the potential advantages of immunosuppressive therapy are (1) to preserve visually important structures that are at risk, (2) to induce, if possible, a permanent remission of inflammatory disease, and (3) where this is not possible, to reduce the dependence that the patient may have on corticosteroid or other anti-inflammatory drugs. Against this background, we must point out some of the disadvantages of this form of therapy. There is the possibility of inducing permanent hematopoietic changes and of inducing the formation of neoplasms, particularly those of the hematopoietic system. Here I am referring particularly to leukemia. We realize that we may be reducing the defenses of the patients against opportunistic pathogens such as *Herpesvirus, Candida,* or other organisms with which we normally live in concord, but which may proliferate wildly when the normal immunologic defense mechanisms are interefered with. We may possibly cause the induction of sterility, and this is particularly true of the agent chlorambucil. Then there are other local effects such as skin rashes, gastrointestinal disturbances, and hemorrhagic cystitis, which is a particular problem with Cytoxan [cyclophosphamide].

I believe that there are certain specific contraindications to immunosuppressive therapy, and I would like to poll the panel on this issue also. I will not give immunosuppressive therapy in the face of chronic infectious disease. I will not give it to a patient who has had a previous history of neoplasm, where the long-term status of that patient is unclear. I will not give it to a pregnant patient because of possible teratogenic effects, or to a patient in whom there is poor compliance. With regard to the latter, if we start treating a patient and then we can't get him back for his appropriate blood counts, or we can't get him back for the monitoring of his condition, we must stop his immunosuppressive therapy. This is the patient who has to be told "either you take the drug under our instructions or we can't handle you." One must pause in the administration of immunosuppressives in cases where the ability to give informed consent can be questioned. California has some strange regulations about this sort of thing, and recently when we had occasion to give a child some immunosuppressive therapy, the issue was raised: "How can you or the parents decide whether it's more important for this child to see than to procreate when he gets to be age 21? How can you make that decision for the child?" This is an area where the ability to give informed consent might be questioned.

The following slides show just an example or two of what I mean. Here's chronic herpetic keratouveitis, and sometimes these cases are indeed severe and intractable. These patients are sometimes sent to me regarding the question of immunosuppressive therapy. I wouldn't touch that patient with immunosuppressive therapy because we know that in a condition like this, or in toxoplasmosis, the infection itself may go wild under conditions of immunosuppression. If we do elect to treat with cytotoxic immunosuppressive agents, we have quite a few to choose from, including some new ones that I will just mention briefly. They fall into three broad categories: the alkylating agents, and we learned something about these as the result of experience with war gases, such as the nitrogen mustards. Among these agents, which interfere with the cross-linking of DNA, we have two powerful drugs, cyclophosphamide and chlorambucil. Chlorambucil has been the one that most ophthalmologists have been giving for chronic, intractable, inflammatory diseases because it's relatively easy to give on an outpatient basis and has relatively few unpleasant side effects. In this sense it is unlike cyclophosphamide, which may cause a very serious hemorrhagic cystitis and other undesirable side effects. There's methotrexate and there's pyrimethamine, our old friend, as folic acid antagonists. Finally we have the purine antagonists such as 6-MP and azathioprine (Imuran). In addition to these, one new agent has come upon the horizon very recently that seems to hold great promise. This is cyclosporin A, which is an agent that has had absolutely fantastic results in the retardation of organ transplants. It seems to have a specific effect on T lymphocytes, and therefore it has certain advantages, particularly in autoimmune diseases such as those that have been induced by retinal autoantigens. Robert Nussenblatt at the NIH now has some indication that this agent is particularly effective in the treatment of ocular autoimmune conditions. However, like the other cytotoxic immunosuppressants, it too can do serious damage to the body, and this is particularly true as far as the renal system is concerned.

I would like now to poll some of the panel members about what they believe are some of the ophthalmic diseases that might well be treated with immunosuppressive agents. Alan, may I start with you?

Bird: There are certain specific disorders where immunosuppressive agents are used routinely, specifically Behçet's disease. Any of our patients who have proved Behçet's disease are routinely given immunosuppressive agents, usually chlorambucil. Azathioprine is often used in patients in whom steroids are contraindicated because of such diseases as diabetes or systemic hypertension. Immunosuppressive agents may also be used with corticosteroids when a patient's vision is very poor and the effect of steroids is insufficient to cause visual recovery compatible with good function. Most such patients will have chronic low-grade intraocular inflammation with macular edema. Finally, some consider it advisable to use immunosuppressive agents in children who have not yet completed their growth period, since steroids may cause major growth retardation.

O'Connor: Let me just make a comment before we go on. I personally feel that if a child of my own were to have sympathetic ophthalmia that was difficult to treat with corticosteroids and required a high constant dosage of corticosteroids, I would rather see that child take chlorambucil and run the risk of sterility than go through the grotesque changes of secondary steroid effects, the stunting of growth, the cushingism, the rejection by school classmates, and so on. Now, that's a personal choice, but I think I would rather see that patient treated with chlorambucil than with long-term systemic corticosteroids. Mort, may I ask your opinion about this?

Goldberg: I subscribe to your list of indications and contraindications and would add one disease to the list: Wegener's granulomatosis. We've had a very good response using cytoxan.

O'Connor: Did your patients develop hemorrhagic cystitis by the way?

Goldberg: We have not had that complication from cytoxan. The usual dose has been between 50 to 150 mg a day.

O'Connor: Let me ask the panel this: Has anyone seen in his practice, or in his department, a death from cytotoxic immunosuppressive agents?

Gass: No, but they have been reported.

O'Connor: Has anyone seen an irreversible hematopoietic complication from the use of these agents? Well, I believe that from that experience there's something to be learned. We now have considerable experience with these agents. Even with possibly life-threatening situations, we have in fact seen no emergence of lethal complications from the use of these agents. I know of one patient in our series who was treated with chlorambucil for a pars planitis–like syndrome. She achieved a permanent remission, but some years later she died of a *Listeria* brain abscess. Now, that's an unusual organism. Except in obstetrical situations, *Listeria* is ordinarily regarded as an opportunistic pathogen. The brain is an odd place for it to wind up. So I don't know, in fact, whether that death might have been related to immunosuppressive therapy. However, it's the only serious complication that I know of in our series, which now includes several hundred patients. So I would offer this form of therapy to the audience as a possible way out of an intractable situation. I would urge you again to exercise great caution in any case in which you believe there is an infectious background for the disease. There I am referring particularly to diseases such as herpes and toxoplasmosis and perhaps the new BARN [bilateral acute retinal necrosis] syndrome or ARN [acute retinal necrosis] syndrome. I would advise you to work in close collaboration with an internist, preferably a hematologist or an oncologist, who has some experience with these agents. You should not feel that you are running the show all alone, without an effective backup in case there are problems.

Thank you.

New Orleans Academy of Ophthalmology

Officers

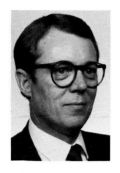

MOSS L. ANTONY, M.D.
President

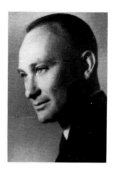

ROBERT A. SCHIMEK, M.D.
President-Elect

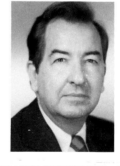

H. FRANK BOSWELL, M.D.
Vice-President

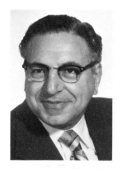

GEORGE S. ELLIS, M.D.
Secretary

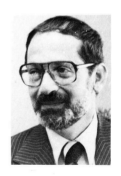

MILES H. FRIEDLANDER, M.D.
Treasurer

EXECUTIVE COMMITTEE

Walter D. Cockerham, M.D.
J. William Reddoch, Jr., M.D.
Robert J. Cangelosi, M.D.

PROGRAM CHAIRMAN

James McComiskey, M.D.

EXECUTIVE SECRETARY

Bud Robinson

ACTIVE MEMBERS
1982

NEW ORLEANS ACADEMY OF OPHTHALMOLOGY

ABERNATHY, Edward A.
ADAIR, Bonnie
ADLER, Hartwig
ALLEN, James H.
ANTONY, Moss L.
AREND, Laurence
AZAR, Robert F.
BALDONE, Joseph A.
BAXTER, Robert S.
BLAKENEY, C.C.
BOLES, William McDonald
BOSWELL, H. Frank
BOTERO, Alfredo
BRECHNER, Ross J.
BRINT, Stephen F.
BROCK, Joseph R.
CALDWELL, Delmar R.
CANGELOSI, Robert J.
CAPLAN, Dan
CAPLAN, Harry B.
CARROLL, Denis
CLARK, Charles E.
COCKERHAM, Walter D.
COHEN, Gerald
COHEN, Sam C.
DABEZIES, Oliver H., Jr.
DIAMOND, James G.
DIAZ, Walter P.
DIMITRI, George J.
DOZIER, Horace B.
ELLIS, George S.

FINKELSTEIN, Wilfred
FRANKLIN, Rudolph
FRIEDLANDER, Miles H.
GAINES, Shelly R.
GITTER, Kurt A.
GORDON, Robert A.
GRAETZ, Roger T.
GUARNIERI, Joseph
HABEEB, Albert F.W.
HAIK, George, Jr.
HAIK, George, Sr.
HAIK, Hilliard M.
HAIK, Kenneth
HANLEY, Jeanne R.
HART, N. Leon
HESSE, Richard
HOLLAND, Monte G.
KALIL, Rodney F.
KAUFMAN, Herbert E.
LANDRY, Ronald
LEA, Martha Ellis
LEADER, Barry
LECKERT, Edmund L., Jr.
LONG, Robert A.
McCOMISKEY, James
McKENNA, Warren P.
McNEILL, David L.
MEDLEY, Jerome T.
MORGAN, Keith S.
NAUGLE, Thomas C., Jr.
NAUGLE, Thomas C., Sr.

NELSON, Earl L.
NEWSOM, Samuel R.
NIX, Ralph R.
O'BYRNE, Alvaro
OCHSNER, Rise
PAILET, Sanford L.
POLLARD, Joel B.
PURYEAR, G. Porter
RACHAL, William F.
REDDOCH, J. William, Jr.
REITMAN, Howard S.
ROSENTHAL, J. William
ROSSNER, Charles W.
RUBIN, Richard L.
RUMAGE, Joseph R.
SAFIR, Aron
SAMSON, C. L. M.
SANDERS, C. Drew
SCHIMEK, Robert A.
SCHOEL, Robert E.
SCHOENBERGER, Martin
SIBLEY, Riley C.
SONNIER, Earl J.
STAHEL, Edward
STANBERY, Marie
STRAUSS, Howard B.
TUMAN, Walter C.
TURKISH, Lance
VAN DYK, H. J. L.
WOOD, Betty Jean
ZIMMERMAN, Thom. J.

ASSOCIATE MEMBERS

NEW ORLEANS ACADEMY OF OPHTHALMOLOGY

AFEMAN, Charles E.,
ARCHER, Dewey Dale
AZAR, Paul J., Jr.
BLOCKER, Donald R.
BOHN, Barry A.
CAFFAREL, Randal C.
CASANOVA, Thomas
COOKSEY, John
EMERSON, Samuel M.
FALGOUST, Quentin D.
FARGASON, Crayton A.
GREGORY, Conrad
GUPTA, Satyarthi
HEMARD, Bryan
JOFFRION, Van Cleave
JONES, George H.
KALIL, Harvey H.
LACOSTE, Alan D.
LaFLEUR, Kenneth C.

LANDRY, Robert J.
LeVINE, Jerome E.
LONG, Daniel
MAXWELL, Ralph III
MIXON, William A.
MURTAGH, James J.
PERRY, Priscilla
PHILLIPS, Donald C.
PLANCHARD, Thomas
SINGH, Harcharan
STEIGNER, John B.
SYLVESTER, Roland J.
TEXADA, Donald
VIDACOVICH, Richard P.
WELCH, James W., Jr.
WHEAT, Margaret Taylor
WHEAT, Reginald David
WYBLE, Merrick J.

Index